Primary Biliary Cholangitis

Editor

BINU V. JOHN

CLINICS IN
LIVER DISEASE

www.liver.theclinics.com

Consulting Editor
NORMAN GITLIN

November 2022 • Volume 26 • Number 4

ELSEVIER

1600 John F. Kennedy Boulevard ● Suite 1800 ● Philadelphia, Pennsylvania, 19103-2899

http://www.theclinics.com

CLINICS IN LIVER DISEASE Volume 26, Number 4
November 2022 ISSN 1089-3261, ISBN-13: 978-0-323-97294-9

Editor: Kerry Holland
Developmental Editor: Ann Gielou M. Posedio

Clinics in Liver Disease (ISSN 1089-3261) is published quarterly by Elsevier Inc., 360 Park Avenue South, New York, NY 10010-1710. Months of issue are February, May, August, and November. Business and Editorial Offices: 1600 John F. Kennedy Blvd., Ste. 1800, Philadelphia, PA 19103-2899. Customer Service Office: 3251 Riverport Lane, Maryland Heights, MO 63043. Periodicals postage paid at New York, NY and additional mailing offices. Subscription prices are $329.00 per year (U.S. individuals), $100.00 per year (U.S. student/resident), $782.00 per year (U.S. institutions), $421.00 per year (international individuals), $200.00 per year (international student/resident), $813.00 per year (international instituitions), $382.00 per year (Canadian individuals), $100.00 per year (Canadian student/resident), and $813.00 per year (Canadian institutions). Foreign air speed delivery is included in all *Clinics* subscription prices. All prices are subject to change without notice. **POSTMASTER:** Send address changes to *Clinics in Liver Disease*, Elsevier Health Sciences Division, Subscription Customer Service, 3251 Riverport Lane, Maryland Heights, MO 63043. **Customer Service: Telephone: 1-800-654-2452 (U.S. and Canada); 314-447-8871 (outside U.S. and Canada). Fax: 314-447-8029. E-mail: journalscustomer service-usa@elsevier.com (for print support); journalsonlinesupport-usa@elsevier.com (for online support).**

Reprints. For copies of 100 or more of articles in this publication, please contact the Commercial Reprints Department, Elsevier Inc., 360 Park Avenue South, New York, NY 10010-1710. Tel.: 212-633-3874; Fax: 212-633-3820; E-mail: reprints@elsevier.com.

Clinics in Liver Disease is covered in *MEDLINE/PubMed (Index Medicus)*, Science Citation Index Expanded, Journal Citation Reports/Science Edition, and Current Contents/Clinical Medicine.

Contributors

CONSULTING EDITOR

NORMAN GITLIN, MD, FRCP (LONDON), FRCPE (EDINBURGH), FAASLD, FACP, FACG
Head of Hepatology, Southern California Liver Centers, San Clemente, California, USA

EDITOR

BINU V. JOHN, MD, MPH, FACG, FAASLD
Associate Professor, Division of Hepatology, Miami VA Medical System, Department of Medicine, University of Miami Miller School of Medicine, Miami, Florida, USA

AUTHORS

ROSANNA ASSELTA, PhD
Department of Biomedical Sciences, Humanitas University, Pieve Emanuele, Italy; Humanitas Clinical and Research Center, IRCCS, Rozzano, Italy

ARIANNA BERTAZZONI, MD
Department of Biomedical Sciences, Humanitas University, Division of Internal Medicine and Hepatology, Department of Gastroenterology, Humanitas Research Hospital IRCCS, Milan, Italy

CHRISTOPHER L. BOWLUS, MD
Lena Valente Professor and Chief, Division of Gastroenterology and Hepatology, University of California, Davis School of Medicine, Sacramento, California, USA

KERI-ANN BUCHANAN-PEART, MD
Division of Digestive Health and Liver Diseases, Department of Internal Medicine, Jackson Memorial Hospital, University of Miami Miller School of Medicine, Miami, Florida, USA

MARCO CARBONE, MD, PhD
Division of Gastroenterology and Hepatology, Department of Medicine and Surgery, University of Milano-Bicocca, Milan, Italy

RUILING CHEN, PhD
Division of Gastroenterology and Hepatology, Key Laboratory of Gastroenterology and Hepatology, Ministry of Health, State Key Laboratory for Oncogenes and Related Genes, Renji Hospital, School of Medicine, Shanghai JiaoTong University, Shanghai Institute of Digestive Disease, Shanghai, China

FRANCESCA COLAPIETRO, MD
Department of Biomedical Sciences, Humanitas University, Division of Internal Medicine and Hepatology, Department of Gastroenterology, Humanitas Research Hospital IRCCS, Milan, Italy

CHRISTOPHE CORPECHOT, MD
Reference Center for Inflammatory Biliary Diseases and Autoimmune Hepatitis,
Saint-Antoine Hospital, Assistance Publique–Hôpitaux de Paris, Inserm UMR_S938,
Saint-Antoine Research Center (CRSA), Sorbonne University, Paris, France

MIRIAM M. DÜLL, MD
Department of Medicine 1, Gastroenterology, Hepatology, Pneumology, Endocrinology,
University Hospital Erlangen, Friedrich-Alexander-University of Erlangen-Nürnberg,
Erlangen, Germany

RAPHAELLA D. FERREIRA, MD
Division of Hepatology, Miami VA Medical System, Miami, Florida, USA

M. ERIC GERSHWIN, MD
Division of Rheumatology-Allergy and Clinical Immunology, University of California at
Davis, Davis, California, USA

ALESSIO GERUSSI, MD, PhD
Division of Gastroenterology, Department of Medicine and Surgery, Center for
Autoimmune Liver Diseases, University of Milano-Bicocca, Monza, Province of Monza
and Brianza, Italy; European Reference Network on Hepatological Diseases
(ERN RARE-LIVER), San Gerardo Hospital, Monza, Italy

GIDEON M. HIRSCHFIELD, MB BChir, FRCP (UK), PhD
Professor of Medicine, Staff Hepatologist, Department of Medicine, Division of
Gastroenterology and Hepatology, University Health Network, University of Toronto,
Toronto, Ontario, Canada

NASIR HUSSAIN, BSc, MBBS, MRCP
National Institute for Health Research Birmingham Biomedical Research Centre, Centre
for Liver and Gastroenterology Research, University of Birmingham, United Kingdom;
Liver Unit, University Hospitals Birmingham Queen Elizabeth, Birmingham, United
Kingdom

PIETRO INVERNIZZI, MD, PhD
Division of Gastroenterology, Department of Medicine and Surgery, Center for
Autoimmune Liver Diseases, University of Milano-Bicocca, Monza, Province of Monza
and Brianza, Italy; European Reference Network on Hepatological Diseases (ERN RARE-
LIVER), San Gerardo Hospital, Monza, Italy

BINU V. JOHN, MD, MPH, FACG, FAASLD
Associate Professor, Division of Hepatology, Miami VA Medical System, Department of
Medicine, University of Miami Miller School of Medicine, Miami, Florida, USA

ANDREAS E. KREMER, MD, PhD, MHBA
Department of Medicine 1, Gastroenterology, Hepatology, Pneumology, Endocrinology,
University Hospital Erlangen and Friedrich-Alexander-University Erlangen-Nürnberg,
Erlangen, Germany; Department of Gastroenterology and Hepatology, University Hospital
Zürich, Switzerland

KRISTEL K. LEUNG, MD, FRCPC, BSc (Hons)
Autoimmune Liver Diseases Research and Clinical Fellow, Department of Medicine,
Division of Gastroenterology and Hepatology, University Health Network, University of
Toronto, Toronto, Ontario, Canada

CYNTHIA LEVY, MD, AGAF, FAASLD
Professor of Clinical Medicine, Arthur Hertz Chair in Liver Diseases, Division of Digestive Health and Liver Diseases, Associate Director, Schiff Center for Liver Diseases, University of Miami Miller School of Medicine, Miami, Florida, USA

CHUNG-HENG LIU, BS
Drexel University College of Medicine, Philadelphia, Pennsylvania, USA

ANA LLEO, MD, PhD
Professor of Internal Medicine, Department of Biomedical Sciences, Humanitas University, Division of Internal Medicine and Hepatology, Department of Gastroenterology, Humanitas Research Hospital IRCCS, Milan, Italy

XIONG MA, MD
Division of Gastroenterology and Hepatology, Key Laboratory of Gastroenterology and Hepatology, Ministry of Health, State Key Laboratory for Oncogenes and Related Genes, Renji Hospital, School of Medicine, Shanghai JiaoTong University, Shanghai Institute of Digestive Disease, Shanghai, China

NATALIE MANSOUR, MD
Assistant Professor of Medicine and Liver Diseases, Herbert Wertheim College of Medicine, Florida International University, Miami, Florida, USA

ERIC F. MARTIN, MD
Assistant Professor of Clinical Medicine, Program Director, Transplant Hepatology Fellowship, Medical Director, Living Donor Liver Transplant University of Miami Miller School of Medicine, Miami Transplant Institute, Miami, Florida, USA

MIKI SCARAVAGLIO, MD
Division of Gastroenterology and Hepatology, Department of Medicine and Surgery, University of Milano-Bicocca, Milan, Italy

MINA SHAKER, MD, MSc
Division of Hepatology, Miami VA Medical System, Department of Medicine, Miami, Florida, USA

ALEXANDER M. SY, MD
Department of Medicine, University of Miami Miller School of Medicine, Division of Hepatology, Miami VA Medical System, Department of Translational Medicine, Clinical Associate Professor, Florida International University, Herbert Wertheim College of Medicine, Miami, Florida, USA

RUQI TANG, PhD
Division of Gastroenterology and Hepatology, Key Laboratory of Gastroenterology and Hepatology, Ministry of Health, State Key Laboratory for Oncogenes and Related Genes, Renji Hospital, School of Medicine, Shanghai JiaoTong University, Shanghai Institute of Digestive Disease, Shanghai, China

PALAK J. TRIVEDI, BSc (hons), MBBS, MRCP, PhD
National Institute for Health Research Birmingham Biomedical Research Centre, Centre for Liver and Gastroenterology Research, University of Birmingham, United Kingdom; Liver Unit, University Hospitals Birmingham Queen Elizabeth, Birmingham, United Kingdom; Institute of Immunology and Immunotherapy, University of Birmingham, Institute of Applied Health Research, University of Birmingham, United Kingdom

Contents

Primary biliary cholangitis (PBC) is a cholestatic liver disease with potential evolution to liver cirrhosis when left untreated. Despite being rare, PBC has a substantial impact on the quality of life and survival of affected patients. Women are the most diagnosed worldwide; however, male subjects seem to have more aggressive disease and worse prognosis. Changing epidemiologic trends are emerging in PBC, with increasing global prevalence and slight smoothing of sex differences. In this review we present available data on incidence rates and prevalence of PBC worldwide, highlighting geographic differences and factors impacting clinical outcomes.

Primary biliary cholangitis (PBC) is a rare disease of the liver characterized by an autoimmune attack on the small bile ducts. PBC is a complex trait, meaning that a large list of genetic factors interacts with environmental agents to determine its onset. Genome-wide association studies have had a huge impact in fostering research in PBC, but many steps need still to be done compared with other autoimmune diseases of similar prevalence. This review presents the state-of-the-art regarding the genetic architecture of PBC and provides some thoughtful reflections about possible future lines of research, which can be helpful to fill the missing heritability gap in PBC.

Primary biliary cholangitis (PBC) is an autoimmune liver disease with a female predisposition and selective destruction of intrahepatic small bile ducts leading to nonsuppurative destructive cholangitis. It is characterized by seropositivity of antimitochondrial antibodies or PBC-specific antinuclear antibodies, progressive cholestasis, and typical liver histologic manifestations. Destruction of the protective bicarbonate-rich umbrella is attributed to the decreased expression of membrane transporters in biliary epithelial cells (BECs), leading to the accumulation of hydrophobic bile acids and sensitizing BECs to apoptosis. A recent X-wide association study reveals a novel risk locus on the X chromosome, which reiterates the importance of Treg cells.

Primary biliary cholangitis (PBC) is a chronic immune-mediated liver disease characterized by a lymphocytic cholangitis, with subsequent cholestasis, progressive liver fibrosis, and ultimately complications arising from end-stage liver disease. Testing for autoantibodies is important in the diagnosis of PBC, as well as stratifying prognosis. This review focuses on the role of autoantibodies in the diagnosis of PBC, as well as the relationship between autoantibodies with pathophysiology and prognostication, along with a discussion regarding novel and other related disease autoantibodies.

Primary biliary cholangitis (PBC) is a complex, chronic disease with a heterogeneous presentation, disease progression, and response to therapy. Several prognostic models based on disease stage and/or treatment response enhance risk stratification and therapeutic management. Recent work on disease modeling proposed early prediction of outcomes at PBC onset, yet this has not been implemented in clinical practice. Although early stratification of patients based on their individual risk of developing end-stage liver disease may prove cost-effective and actually become matter of medical deontology to timely offer the best therapeutic option, given the forthcoming availability of novel, disease-modifying drugs. This review outlines established and novel prognostic systems in PBC and provides some perspectives on the potential role of omics-derived biomarkers in developing reliable risk prediction models and promoting the implementation of personalized medicine in PBC.

Primary biliary cholangitis (PBC) is an immune-mediated chronic liver disease characterized by progressive cholestasis, bile duct destruction, biliary fibrosis, and cirrhosis. Patients who respond to ursodeoxycholic acid have an expected survival similar to the general population. Although PBC primarily affects females, the prevalence in males is higher than was previously believed, with contemporary studies suggesting a female-to-male ratio of 4–6:1. A diagnosis of PBC is often delayed among males because of the myth that PBC is rare in males.

The term 'PBC/AIH-overlap' has been applied when features of autoimmune hepatitis (AIH), be they biochemical, serological or histological, coexist with primary biliary cholangitis (PBC), either at first presentation or sequentially during disease course. Several treatment paradigms have been proposed, extrapolated from those of the primary conditions.

However, there are no randomised studies showing improved survival with combination therapy compared to bile acid monotherapy. In the absence of high-quality evidence, multidisciplinary patient-specific approaches must be used to individualise treatment pathways, with appreciation that disease phenotypes are not always static, differ in treatment responses, and have the potential to evolve over time.

Efficient therapy consists of topical treatment combined with systemic options such as anion exchangers, rifampicin, bezafibrate, μ-opioid receptor antagonists, selective-serotonin receptor uptake inhibitors, and gabapentinoids. Future therapeutic approaches may contain the selective blockade of the enterohepatic cycle by inhibiting the ileal bile acid transporter, the agonism at κ-opioid receptors, and antagonism of the mas-related G protein–coupled receptor X4. As nondrug treatment, ultraviolet B therapy, albumin dialysis, and biliary drainage are available at specialized centers.

Primary biliary cholangitis is a chronic autoimmune disease characterized by inflammation and the progressive destruction of small intrahepatic bile ducts. Current first-line treatment includes ursodeoxycholic acid; however, a significant number of patients have an inadequate response to therapy. These patients are at risk of liver failure requiring liver transplantation and experience a poor quality of life due to refractory symptoms. This manuscript aims to shed light on the current and prospective treatment options that may slow disease progression and improve these patients' symptoms.

Despite a significant increase in the total number of liver transplants (LTs) performed over the last 3 decades, primary biliary cholangitis (PBC) has become an uncommon indication for LT, which likely reflects the benefits of earlier diagnosis and available treatment, such as ursodeoxycholic acid (UDCA). Nonetheless, LT remains the only cure for patients with progressive PBC despite medical therapy with survival rates that are among the highest of all indications for LT. Post-LT PBC patients, however, are at increased risk of rejection and disease recurrence.

CLINICS IN LIVER DISEASE

SERIES OF RELATED INTEREST

Gastroenterology Clinics of North America
https://www.gastro.theclinics.com

THE CLINICS ARE AVAILABLE ONLINE!
Access your subscription at:
www.theclinics.com

Preface

The Evolving Landscape of Primary Biliary Cholangitis

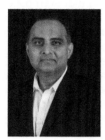

Binu V. John, MD, MPH, FACG, FAASLD
Editor

Primary biliary cholangitis (PBC) is an autoimmune liver disease characterized by the destruction of intrahepatic bile ductules, resulting in chronic cholestasis, that can progress to advanced fibrosis, cirrhosis, portal hypertension, and hepatocellular carcinoma (HCC), and if untreated, requires liver transplantation. Ursodeoxycholic acid (UDCA) has been an effective first-line agent for this condition for approximately three decades; however, approximately one-third of patients are not complete responders to UDCA. The second-line treatment agent obeticholic acid is associated with significant side effects, including worsening pruritus and hyperlipidemia, and is contraindicated in patients with portal hypertension and/or hepatic decompensation. Over the past 5 years, there has been a rapid evolution in our understanding of the epidemiology, genetics, and pathophysiology, and an increase in the number of potential agents and therapeutic targets for PBC. This issue of *Clinics in Liver Disease* addresses the evolving landscape of PBC.

One of the most interesting aspects of PBC is the sex predisposition among women. Although contemporary epidemiologic studies indicate that PBC is more common among men than previously thought, we now have a better understanding of the progression of PBC among men. Recent studies have shown that men are more likely to present at a more advanced stage of disease, but even among patients presenting with compensated cirrhosis, male sex is associated with higher overall and liver-related death, compared with women.

Genome-wide association studies (GWAS) have identified a number of HLA and non-HLA loci showing strong association with PBC. Approximately 20 novel risk loci have been identified in a recent international meta-analysis, pointing to a total of 22 genes. Although due to its female preponderance, genetic loci located on the X chromosome may be an obvious target in genetic studies, X chromosome is often less studied in many existing GWAS analyses. Recent studies have linked loci located on

Clin Liver Dis 26 (2022) xiii–xv
https://doi.org/10.1016/j.cld.2022.06.006
1089-3261/22/© 2022 Published by Elsevier Inc.

the X chromosome to PBC, and it is hoped, these data will improve our understanding of the female predisposition to this disease. Genetic studies have suggested that IL-12 and IFN-γ are two key drivers of immune-mediated cholangitis, as observed in both human and animal models of PBC.

Another area of development in PBC has been in risk-stratification scores. While many of the commonly used scores in the past, including the Toronto and Paris classifications, dichotomized patients with PBC into UDCA responders and nonresponders, there has been an evolution in our understanding that even patients who do not normalize their alkaline phosphatase derive some benefit with treatment and are now referred to as partial responders. Instead of dichotomous variables, we now also have continuous scores, including the GLOBE score and UK-PBC scores, which help to calculate the 5- and 10-year survival in patients with PBC. Because many of the traditional prognostic scores describing UDCA response were calculated at 12 and 24 months after initiation of UDCA therapy, there is now a move to define response to therapy sooner, as early as 3 or 6 months after treatment. This has the benefit of moving to a second-line agent sooner, without allowing patients to progress for months, on an ineffective treatment.

An important complication of PBC is HCC, which has an incidence of as high as 13 per 1000 person-years in patients with PBC cirrhosis, and 2.7 per 1000 person-years among patients with PBC without cirrhosis. HCC in PBC is more common among men, as well as among those with cirrhosis, with some studies suggesting that treatment with UDCA and UDCA response may reduce risk. While some guidelines recommend HCC surveillance in men with PBC in the absence of cirrhosis, there are limited data currently to support this recommendation.

While UDCA remains the first-line agent for PBC, obeticholic acid and bezafibrate are both evolving as alternative second-line agents. Bezafibrate may have an additional benefit of reducing pruritus, and studies combining bezafibrate and obeticholic acid are currently ongoing. As pruritus is now being recognized as an important and disabling symptom in PBC, efforts are underway to develop newer agents to treat this debilitating symptom. In addition to bezafibrate, alternative treatments for pruritus include anion exchangers, rifampin, selective-serotonin receptor uptake inhibitors, and opioid receptor antagonists. Newer agents, such as the apical sodium-dependent bile acid transporter inhibitors, that act by decreasing bile acid accumulation and thereby reducing bile toxicity are now being investigated.

Clinical trials in the field of PBC treatment have expanded greatly, with a number of agents, chiefly PPAR agonists and NOX 1/4 inhibitors, holding the most promise to prevent disease progression and in the improvement of symptoms.

There are a number of PPAR agonists with varying activity against the different isoforms. While fenofibrate predominantly binds to PPAR-alpha, bezafibrate binds to the alpha, gamma, and delta isoforms, seladelpar binds only to the delta isoform. Elafibranor is a dual PPAR-alpha and -gamma agonist, and saroglitazar binds primarily to alpha and gamma isoforms. Several of these agents, having shown promising results in phase II studies, are currently in phase III studies. There is much to look forward to in patients with PBC, as our understanding of genetics, pathophysiology, and immunology improves, and a large number of potential treatments are being investigated in clinical trials.

I would like to thank the authors, who are leading experts in the field of PBC, assembled from 10 institutions in six different countries in the United States and Europe. It is my hope that readers will find this issue comprehensive, state-of-the-art, clinically relevant, and useful, to better manage their patients with PBC.

Binu V. John, MD, MPH, FACG, FAASLD
University of Miami
Miami VA Health System
1201 NW 16th Street
Miami, FL 33125, USA

E-mail address:
Binu.John@va.gov

Contemporary Epidemiology of Primary Biliary Cholangitis

Francesca Colapietro, MD[a,b], Arianna Bertazzoni, MD[a,b],
Ana Lleo, MD, PhD[a,b],*

KEYWORDS

- Primary biliary cholangitis • Epidemiology • Incidence • Prevalence • Sex
- Mortality • Rare diseases

KEY POINTS

- Primary biliary cholangitis (PBC) is a rare disease, mainly affecting middle aged women worldwide.
- Increasing prevalence is reported across Europe, North America, and the Asia-Pacific region due to advances in diagnostic tools, research strategies, and management of the disease.
- Age at diagnosis and sex play a key role in response to treatment and clinical outcomes.
- Improved awareness of the disease both in Western countries and in unexplored areas of South America and Asia is expected to influence epidemiologic trends of PBC in the next decades.

INTRODUCTION

Primary biliary cholangitis (PBC) is an immune-mediated cholestatic liver disease mainly diagnosed in middle-aged women, with a female-to-male ratio between 4 to 5:1 and 9 to 10:1.[1,2] It is characterized by progressive inflammation and injury of the intrahepatic bile ducts, leading to cholestasis, development of fibrosis, and eventually liver cirrhosis. The natural history of the disease consists of slow but relentless progression to cirrhosis and eventually its complications, including hepatocellular carcinoma (HCC) and the need for liver transplantation (LT). First-line treatment ursodeoxycholic acid (UDCA) and recently introduced second-line therapy obeticholic acid (OCA) aim to manage symptoms and obtain biochemical response, slowing down

[a] Division of Internal Medicine and Hepatology, Department of Gastroenterology, IRCCS Humanitas Research Hospital, Via A. Manzoni 56, Rozzano 20089, Italy; [b] Department of Biomedical Sciences, Humanitas University, Pieve Emanuele, Milan, Italy
* Corresponding author.
E-mail address: ana.lleo@humanitas.it

Clin Liver Dis 26 (2022) 555–570
https://doi.org/10.1016/j.cld.2022.06.001
1089-3261/22/

Abbreviations	
HLA	human leukocyte antigen
DRB1	
DQB1	
DPB1	
OR	odds ratio
CMV	cytomegalovirus
EBV	Epstein-Barr Virus
AILD	Autoimmune Liver Disease

disease progression.[3,4] However, a significant number of patients with PBC still fail to respond to available therapies; further strategies are strongly needed, but research is limited due to epidemiologic features.[1]

According to the Orphanet report on the prevalence of rare diseases in January 2022, PBC shows an average incidence rate of 3.0 cases per 100,000 individuals per year and a prevalence rate of 21.05 cases/100,000 individuals;[5] thus, it is still considered a rare disease. However, PBC affects all ethnic groups and nationalities and epidemiologic studies have demonstrated an increasing trend in the past decades.[2,6–8] This could be imputable to several factors, including better knowledge and awareness of the disease; increased patient's survival in light of UDCA treatment; and improved clinical research, based on electronic medical records mostly collected at referral centers.

The aim of this review was to analyze meaningful changes in PBC epidemiology, highlighting currently observed global trends and possible geographic variations.

Gender and Sex Differences

As already mentioned, PBC is characterized by a striking sex divergence, with a reported female-to-male ratio up to 9 to 10:1 in historical cohorts.[9] Even if lower ratios were recently observed in population-based studies,[10] female predominance still represents a key feature of the disease, with prevalence and incidence being fivefold and fourfold increased, respectively, in women than men in European and Asian countries.[9,11,12]

The reasons behind this strong difference are varied and not fully understood so far. Sex hormones, fetal microchimerism, and genetic factors might play a determinant role, also confirmed by the fact that PBC may present along with other autoimmune diseases, most commonly scleroderma, thyroid diseases, and Sjögren syndrome.[13] No loci on the X chromosome have been clearly associated with PBC so far, although major genetic abnormalities in sex chromosomes were demonstrated in the disease[14]; interestingly, the Y chromosome carries genes involved in immune function and thus in autoimmune and neoplastic diseases. Thus, further research based on novel approaches is needed to shed a light on this genetic implication. The age- and sex-standardized incidence of PBC reflect female predominance despite variable ratios across different decades of age, as observed in population-based studies from England.[15] However, several elements suggest under-reporting and underdiagnosis of PBC among males. First of all, the F:M ratio of 2:1 observed for antimitochondrial antibody (AMA) positivity among the general population is highly different from F:M ratios observed in PBC itself, and this is scarcely covered for by the cases of AMA-negative PBC.[7] Furthermore, male patients tend to be diagnosed at more advanced stages of liver disease, with higher alkaline phosphatase (ALP) levels, decreased response to UDCA therapy, increased incidence of HCC, and worse overall prognosis.[16–18]

Moreover, delayed diagnosis could be accounted for by an inherent bias in medical practice, as autoimmunity examinations are requested more promptly in females with respect to male patients, hence generating time loss before the actual initiation of therapy.[7]

Geographic Variability in the Incidence and Prevalence of Primary Biliary Cholangitis

As already mentioned, PBC epidemiology showed a changing trend during the past years, likely imputable to higher-quality studies, improved case-finding techniques, and increased disease awareness.[2] In support of this, the proportion of patients diagnosed at an early stage raised from 41% in the seventies to 72% in the nineties, as elucidated by Registry data from the PBC Study Group.[19]

More recently, global incidence rates grew constantly until the year 2000 and then reached a plateau; in 2011 to 2020 incidence rates ranged from 0.86 in the Asia-Pacific region to 2.61 and 2.75 in Europe and North America, versus 0.69, 2.28, and 3.51, respectively, in the previous decade.[2] Similarly, prevalence of PBC is increasing across the world and is estimated at 14.6 per 100,000 inhabitants, ranging from 1.91 to 40.2, with North America having the highest prevalence (pooled estimates: 21.8).[8]

In the following paragraphs, we report data on incidence and prevalence of PBC according to the different geographic areas.

Europe

Epidemiologic studies published before the mid-eighties were carried out almost exclusively on European populations (**Table 1**) and reported an average incidence rate of 0.6 to 13.7 cases/million/year and a point prevalence ranging from 1.1 to 12.8 cases per 100,000 individuals.[20] More recent data have shown that the prevalence has almost doubled, with an overall value of 22.27 cases per 100,000 inhabitants and a pooled incidence rate of 1.7 new cases per 100,000 inhabitants per year.[12]

The increasing prevalence across Europe during the last decades may be explained by emerging data from territories such as Greece (40.8/100,000 inhabitants per year)[21] and Iceland (38.4 of 100,000 inhabitants per year for the years 2001–2010; 41.0/ 100,000 inhabitants per year for the years 1991–2015),[22,23] areas which had not been previously investigated. On the other hand, age-standardized incidence in Iceland increased only slightly from 20 every million inhabitants per year for a period spanning 1991 to 2000, to 25/million/year for the years 2001 to 2010.

Of note, consistent differences between European countries, and even within regions of the same country, have been reported by several studies, with a certain North-to-South gradient.[12,24,25] Indeed, incidence varies between Western Europe (2.26/100,000 inhabitants per year), Eastern Europe (0.77/100,000 inhabitants per year), Southern Europe (2.09/100,000 inhabitants per year), and Northern Europe (1.83/100,000 inhabitants per year), with a prevalence rate as high as 30/100,000 individuals in northern European countries.[8]

Reports from the United Kingdom constitute a clear example of this trend, with a disease prevalence of 20 cases per 100,000 subjects in South Wales versus 33.46 in Northern England, as reported in the late nineties.[26,27] Some of the highest incidence rates were reported in the geographic area of Newcastle upon Tyne, with values as high as 5.8 cases/100 000 individuals/y in 1994, suggesting one or more environmental triggers for disease development. Similar increasing trends were reported for Tayside, Scotland, where incidence and prevalence rates increased from 4.8 to 5.5

Table 1
Studies reporting primary biliary cholangitis incidence and prevalence from 2014 onward across Europe

Authors, Publication Year	Study Country	Number of Patients with PBC Included	Incidence/ 100,000/year (CI 95%)	Prevalence/ 100,000 (CI 95%)	F:M Ratio	Mean Age at Diagnosis (Years, SD)	Other Investigated Outcomes
Koulentaki et al.,[21] 2014	Greece	222	2.1 (0.4–3.6)	36.5	7.2:1	58 (24–87)	Map the spatial distribution of patients with PBC
Boonstra et al.,[74] 2014	Netherlands	992	1.1	13.2[a]	7.2:1	♂ (61 ± 12) ♀ (57 ± 13)	Association with smoking, age at menarche, age at first pregnancy or number of pregnancies
McNally et al.,[15] 2014	England	482 (years span 1987–1994) 500 (years span 1995–2003)	5.4 (4.9–5.8)[d] 4.5 (4.1–4.)[d]		9.3:1	65	Spatial clusters
Lleo et al.,[10] 2016	Italy Sweden	2970 (Italy) 722 (Sweden)	1.67 (Italy) 1.14 (Sweden)	16 (Italy) 11.5 (Sweden)	2.3:1 (Italy) 4.2:1 (Sweden)	61 (Italy) 62 (Sweden)	Male prevalence, all-cause mortality
Örnolfsson et al.,[23] 2018	Iceland	222	—	41	4.5:1	62 (13–92)	Familial RR Average KC
Terziroli Beretta-Piccoli et al.,[47] 2018	Switzerland	474	Not reported	Not reported	5.5:1	53 (45–63)	Clinical phenotype Disease course including LT and death

Marzioni et al.,[84] 2019	Italy	412	5.3	27.90	4.6:1	64.7 ± 14.4	Link to treatment patterns
Marschall et al.,[31] 2019	Sweden	5350	2.6	34.6[b]	4.0:1	64 (15–94)	Survival, comorbidities, link to treatment patterns
Drazilova et al.,[85] 2020	Slovakia	256	0.7–1.5	10.2–14.9	22.3:1	56.3 ± 10.9	Natural course, response to UDCA, treatment and natural course differences according to sex and age
Webb et al.,[25] 2021	United Kingdom	1314	2.47 (2.33–2.60)	39.62 (37.50–41.74)[c]	6.6:1	63 (53–72)	Relationship between latitude and incidence of AILD

Abbreviations: KC, kinship coefficient; LT, liver transplantation; NA, not available; RR, relative risk; SD, standard deviation.
[a] In 2018.
[b] In 2014.
[c] In 2015.
[d] ASR, age-standardized incidence rates.

cases and from 18.6 to 37.9 cases per 100,000 inhabitants, respectively, between 1986 and 1996.[28]

Increasing trends have been reported also in Scandinavian countries: although reports from Sweden during the late nineties assessed a point-prevalence of 128 to 151 cases/million individuals, a nationwide population-based study demonstrated a prevalence of 350 cases/million inhabitants in 2014.[29–31]

Furthermore, in 2018 results of the Delphy study were published by Parés and colleagues[32]; the authors investigated the epidemiology of PBC among the Spanish population and identified a mean prevalence rate of 20.2 per 100,000 inhabitants and an estimated annual incidence of 2.2, in line with other European countries and previous studies.

North America

The epidemiology of PBC in North America does not change consistently with respect to European countries (**Table 2**). In a study carried out in the United States encompassing the years from 2003 to 2014, the incidence rate remained quite stable, with values of 4.2 per 100,000 inhabitants per year, whereas the prevalence rose from 21.7 to 39.2 cases per 100,000 individuals.[33] These values parallel the aforementioned incidence and prevalence rates in the UK and Sweden.

Localized clusters of PBC have been observed in the United States, similar to that described from Newcastle upon Tyne in the UK. Firstly, data from Olmsted County, Minnesota, report a high prevalence rate of 40 cases/100 000 individuals, suggesting the presence of an unknown environmental trigger.[34] Moreover, clustering of PBC cases has been reported in some areas of New York City in proximity to toxic waste sites.[35] A similar concept was brought up by identification of clusters in highly polluted areas, such as Los Angeles and cities of the Great Lakes, with a 1.92-fold to 2.12-fold increased relative risk for PBC.[36]

Asia

Studies from the Middle East are scarce and report variable incidence and prevalence rates (see **Table 2**). Data from Israel demonstrated a mean incidence rate of PBC from 1.0 in the 1990 to 1999 years to 2.0 cases per 100, 000 individuals in the 2000 to 2010 year span, whereas prevalence rates were reported to vary from 13.5 to 45.0 cases/100 000 people, with lower values detected in subjects born in Israel and higher values reported in individuals of Russian and Eastern European origin.[37]

Until recently, the epidemiology and natural history of PBC in the Asia-Pacific region had not been studied thoroughly. However, a recent meta-analysis demonstrated incidence and prevalence rates in the Asia-Pacific region to be higher than expected. The authors reported an overall prevalence of 15.9 cases/100 000 individuals in the 2009 to 2019 timeframe, with subregional analysis highlighting markedly increased rates for East Asia (15.6) versus Oceania (5.3).[38]

High prevalence rates have been observed in Japan (22.1 cases per 100,000 individuals), similar to that observed in the West.[11,38] Intermediate prevalence (9.9 cases per 100,000) and incidence rates have been encountered in New Zealand, where it has remained relatively stable since 2001[38,39]; on the other hand, Australia reported an increasing prevalence from 1.9 per 100,000 in the last decade of the twentieth century to 18.9 per 100,000 in the years 2011 to 2020. Australian studies report higher prevalence rates in European immigrants (18.3 per 100,000) based on their country of birth, particularly among individuals of English, Italian and Greek origin, thus confirming strong genetic predisposing factors.[8] Lastly, the lowest prevalence values in the Pacific region were reported in South Korea,[40] where several population-based studies

Table 2
Studies reporting primary biliary cholangitis incidence and prevalence from 2014 onward worldwide except Europe

Author, Publication Year	Study Country	Number of Patients with PBC Included	Incidence/ 100,000/year (CI 95%)	Prevalence/ 100,000 (CI 95%)	F:M Ratio	Mean Age at Diagnosis (Years) (SD, IQR, or Range)	Other Outcomes
Kim et al.,[86] 2016	South Korea	2824	0.86[a]	4.8[b]	6.2:1	57.4	Liver-related morbidity and mortality
Cheung et al.,[59] 2017	China	1016	0.84[a]	5.6[b]	3.7:1	60.6 (51.8–72.6)	Liver-related morbidity and mortality
Kanth et al.,[87] 2017	United States	79	4.9[a]	NA	18.7:1	58 (27–93)	Survival
Yoshida et al.,[88] 2018	Canada	8680	NA	31.8 (30.9–32.7)	4:1	NA	LT trends
French et al.,[89] 2019	Australia	1012	Not reported	18.9	4.7:1	Not reported	–
Tanaka et al.,[11] 2019	Japan	10,847	Not reported	33.8 (33.0–34.6)[c]	3.9:1	Not reported	–
Lamba et al.,[90] 2021	New Zealand	26	0.51	9.33 (7.12–12.05)[c]	3.3:1	57.9	–

Abbreviations: IQR, interquartile range; LT, liver transplantation; NA, not available; SD, standard deviation.
[a] Average age- and sex-adjusted incidence rate.
[b] Average age- and sex-adjusted prevalence.
[c] In 2016.

were carried out from 2000 to 2015 reporting estimated incidence rates of 0.84 to 0.86 cases/100 000 population per year and an average prevalence of 4.75 to 5.64 cases per 100,000 inhabitants. However, also these studies confirm the increasing trend in PBC epidemiology during the past decades.

NATURAL HISTORY AND TREATMENT BENEFIT

AMAs represent the hallmark of PBC, being present in more than 90% of patients[41]; indeed, diagnosis of the disease relies on AMA detection together with elevation of ALP levels and typical histology obtained through liver biopsy.[4] However, AMA positivity is not specific to PBC and can be found in up to 1/1000 individuals in the general population. Moreover, almost 5% to 10% of patients result negative to AMA testing with routine methods. Finally, despite having a strong diagnostic value, AMA does not display any prognostic significance, nor the title is associated with clinical outcome.[42] In a study comparing AMA-negative and AMA-positive recipients with cirrhosis, AMA-negative PBC cirrhosis was associated with similar rates of liver-related death (sub-Hazard Ratio [sHR] 1.27, 95% confidence interval [CI] 0.71 to 2.28, $P = .42$, death [sHR] 1.24, 95% CI 0.81–1.90, $P = .32$), decompensation (sHR 1.05, 95% CI 0.56–1.98, $P = .87$) and HCC (sHR 0.48, 95% CI 0.11–2.10, $P = .33$) to AMA-positive patients.[43,44]

In 1996 *Metcalf and colleagues* analyzed a series of 29 AMA-positive subjects and observed up to 75% of them developing PBC after 18 years from first antibody detection[45]; these reports were further confirmed in Chinese[46] and Swiss[47] case series, in which even emerged that histologic involvement appears earlier than the elevation of ALP or impairment of liver tests. On the other hand, data coming from French[48] and Austrian[49] cohorts showed lower rates of PBC development in AMA-positive subjects but with a shorter mean follow-up (4.0 ± 1.8 years and 5.8 ± 5.6 years, respectively).

If left untreated, PBC leads to liver cirrhosis and eventually death. Furthermore, significant liver-related morbidity was reported for patients with PBC, with an incidence of HCC as high as 3.4/1000 patients/y [50,51] This highlights the relevance of prompt diagnosis and treatment, as well as periodic HCC screening in cirrhotic patients with PBC. LT should also be evaluated in end-stage liver disease, as it yields survival rates as high as 90% to 95% at 1 year and 77% to 83% at 5 years, and a risk of PBC recurrence of 21% to 37% after 10 years.[52,53]

As highlighted by a historical cohort before the universal use of UDCA, the median survival of patients after diagnosis was of 6 to 10 years and about one-fourth of untreated patients was at risk of liver failure during such timeframe.(1, 48) For decades, UDCA at a daily dose of 13 to 15 mg/kg has represented the first-line treatment of PBC[4,54] and, until 2016, the only officially Food and Drug Administration (FDA)-approved therapy. Response to UDCA is associated with better liver transplant-free survival; this association is significant, irrespective of age, sex, or stage of the disease. Importantly, the survival benefit is confirmed also in patients with an incomplete response to UDCA, supporting the universal treatment with UDCA for patients with PBC.[54] For patients not responding to UDCA after 1 year of treatment, farnesoid X receptor agonist OCA has been proven to reduce ALP levels.[55]

Several studies have highlighted that the clinical impact of PBC differs according to age and sex.[56] Male patients, although more frequently asymptomatic, are more likely to present with advanced disease and portal hypertension,[16,57] present an increased risk for HCC,[50] and have significantly shorter transplant-free survival.[10,58] Male sex has also been associated to non-response to UDCA,[16] with a lower age-related influence with respect to females; this feature is likely but not only imputable to the fact that PBC tends to be more advanced in male individuals at presentation due to delayed diagnosis, with an increased risk of HCC development. These results were underscored also by several studies analyzing the variability of UDCA response across countries.[24,31,32,59] Interestingly, age at presentation is associated with the clinical course of the disease, with younger patients being more symptomatic (fatigue, pruritus, asthenia).[16,59] *Griffiths and colleagues* confirmed in a cohort from the UK the inverse relationship between age and response to UDCA treatment, as well as the lower responses in the male population. Indeed, they reported a 90% response for patients older than 70, a rate that falls less than 50% in individuals younger than 40 years of age. In the latter cohort, up to 50% of patients had already undergone LT or were at high risk for needing it.[24] Data from Sweden showed a similar trend, reporting a 41.3% decrease in ALP levels after 1 year, as well as a 19% overall cancer mortality rate.[31] Finally, in a Spanish cohort the rate of non-responders was estimated to be 35% to 40%, with consistent liver-related morbidity and mortality.[32]

Finally, the role of ethnicity in PBC remains poorly investigated. Recent data have identified black race as a risk factor for all-cause mortality in untreated PBC (HR compared with white subjects: 1.34, 95% CI 1.08–1.67), although this association reverses when UDCA is administered (aHR = 0.67, 95% CI 0.51–0.86).[60] A study from Canada including 1538 patients with PBC (82% White patients, 4.7% Indigenous, 5.5% East Asian, 2.6% South Asian, and 5.1% miscellaneous) demonstrated that indigenous patients were the only ethnic group with impaired liver transplant-free and event-free survival compared with White patients (HR 3.66, 95%CI 2.23–6.01; HR 3.09, 95%CI 1.94–4.92).[61]

RISK FACTORS

PBC is an autoimmune disease with a complex and not yet fully understood etiology, where an interplay of genetics and environmental factors leads to loss of self-tolerance and immune-mediated damage of small intrahepatic bile ducts.[1,13,62] Heritable features of PBC are evident from concordance observed among monozygotic twins which is more than 60%, as well as family history of PBC in first-degree relatives emerged as a significant risk factor for disease development (OR 6.8, 95% CI 2.8–16.4).[63,64] To note, an average of 11% of first-degree relatives testing positive for AMA detection, show no evolution to overt PBC after an average of 9 years of observation.[65]

PBC is characterized by a strong genetic predisposition where the strongest association is shown by the major histocompatibility complex class II haplotypes (primarily HLA-DRB1, DQB1, and DPB1).[66,67] In addition, genome-wide association studies have identified a high number of non-MHC loci significant to the disease risk; mostly genes that contribute to cell-mediated immune mechanisms.[62,67–70] Despite some degree of locus heterogeneity, these studies highlight an overlap in susceptibility loci between East Asian and European populations. Further, an extensive analysis of chromosome X has demonstrated additional genes that possibly contribute to PBC heritability and to its female preponderance.[14] However, only a small fraction of PBC heritability (approximately 15%) has been explained. All in all, such studies and reports warrant for a more in-depth analysis of the interplay of genetics and environmental factors.

Evidences of environmental factors involved in PBC development come from disease clusters observed in areas receiving pollutants and toxic waste in the city of New York,[35] as well as distribution differences observed between rural and industrialized regions in the UK (prevalence 3.7 vs 14.4 per 100,000 population).[71] Reports of increased PBC prevalence among Nagasaki bomb survivors could also suggest an association with radiations; however, such findings require further validation and analysis.[72]

Xenobiotics, including cosmetics such as nail polish or hair dyes, as well as smoking represent other well-identified risk factors for the diseases.[13] The latter seems to have a strong relationship with the development of PBC (OR ranging from 1.5 to 3),[64] not only in qualitative but also quantitative terms. Indeed, the amount of tobacco consumed seemed to be directly related to the degree of histologic damage on liver biopsies.[73,74] Furthermore, latitude seems to have a role in the incidence of PBC, with increases of more than two-fold for every 7° in latitude.[25] The proposed mechanism seems to be related to sun exposure, vitamin D and its interactions with the immune system.[75]

Like other autoimmune diseases, infections seem to play a key role in loss of tolerance, via molecular mimicry and cross-reactivity mechanisms. Most common instances include *E. coli* urinary tract infections in women (OR 2.7; 95% CI 2.0–3.7),[76] but other putative bacterial (ie, *S. aureus*, *P. mirabilis*, *K. pneumoniae* and *N. meningitides*), viral (ie, CMV, EBV), parasitic, and fungal infections have been proposed to trigger autoimmune mechanisms in PBC.[77]

PRECISION MEDICINE IN PRIMARY BILIARY CHOLANGITIS

Precision medicine (PM) is a patient-based approach that considers the genotypic and phenotypic characteristics correlated to a particular treatment response or disease outcome. The major aim of PM is to address medical interventions to those who will benefit, sparing those who will not.[78]

For many years the "one-size-fits-all" approach has been the only one available to manage and treat patients affected by PBC. The introduction of OCA in 2016 as a second-line treatment, the evidence of the beneficial effect of fibrates,[79] and the creation and validation of biochemically based risk scores to stratify the risk of progressive disease[80–82] have highlighted the need to redefine the actual paradigm. Importantly, current guidelines recommend stratifying patients with PBC according to their risk of critical outcomes and, consequently, their potential need for additional treatments.[4,83]

Mostly using epidemiologic data, it is possible to recognize variant syndromes and to stratify patients with PBC according to their risk of critical outcomes, such as chronic liver failure, variceal hemorrhage, and HCC. Further, the use of multi-omics technologies for a deeper definition of disease molecular and genetic pathways will help to translate this knowledge into new therapeutic opportunities.

SUMMARY AND FUTURE PROSPECTIVE

Prevalence and incidence trends of PBC have been strongly influenced by the improvement of diagnostic methods and therapeutic options during the last decades, together with a higher quality of clinical research mainly relying on registry-based studies, which overcame limitations associated with rare diseases. However, in contrast to Western countries, African regions, South America, and most of South-East nations lack of robust epidemiologic statistical so far. Future research should focus on covering the gap, as distribution of socioeconomic factors having role of concomitant risk factors for liver diseases has a typical geographic feature. Coexistence of metabolic-associated liver disease should be considered to integrate epidemiologic data, and improve diagnosis and management of patients. Moreover, recent introduction of OCA, together with new target molecules currently investigated in clinical trials for PBC, should encourage constant update of dataset-based registry and re-evaluation of outcomes.

Because the clinical phenotype differs among patients with PBC, it is essential to better define the prognosis of clinical variants of PBC. Further, we are convinced that the study of PBC epidemiology cannot be complete without a careful evaluation of the disease among males, including a deep genetic and epigenetic characterization. Indeed, the study of sex differences in PBC will help toward a deeper understanding of the mechanisms beneath the different clinical features and risk, allowing a clear identification of cases more likely to progress and to develop novel therapeutic approaches and a personalized management of the single patient.

FINANCIAL SUPPORT

The authors did not receive any financial support to complete the study or write the article.

CLINICS CARE POINTS

- Primary Biliary Cholangitis (PBC) is a rare disease with increasing prevalence worldwide.
- PBC has a substantial impact on quality of life and survival of affected patients.
- Young age at diagnosis and male sex are associated to worse response to treatment and clinical outcomes.
- Female prevalence characterizes the disease; however, smoothing sex differences are being reported.
- Using epidemiologic data, it is possible to recognize variant syndromes and to stratify patients with PBC according to their risk of clinical outcomes.

CONFLICT OF INTEREST

A. Lleo has received consulting fees from Intercept Pharma, AlfaSigma, and Takeda, lecture fees from AbbVie, Gilead, Takeda, AlfaSigma and MSD and travel expenses from Intercept Pharma, AlfaSigma, and AbbVie. F. Colapietro and A. Bertazzoni reported no conflict of interest.

REFERENCES

1. Lleo A, Wang GQ, Gershwin ME, et al. Primary biliary cholangitis. Lancet 2020; 396(10266):1915–26.
2. Trivedi PJ, Hirschfield GM. Recent advances in clinical practice: epidemiology of autoimmune liver diseases. Gut 2021;70(10):1989–2003.
3. Lammers WJ, van Buuren HR, Hirschfield GM, et al. Levels of alkaline phosphatase and bilirubin are surrogate end points of outcomes of patients with primary biliary cirrhosis: an international follow-up study. Gastroenterology 2014;147(6): 1338–49, e1335; quiz e1315.
4. European Association for the Study of the Liver. Electronic address eee, European Association for the Study of the L. EASL Clinical Practice Guidelines: the diagnosis and management of patients with primary biliary cholangitis. J Hepatol 2017;67(1):145–72.

5. Orphanet report series - prevalence and incidence of rare diseases: Bibliographic data. 2022. Available at: http://www.orpha.net/orphacom/cahiers/docs/GB/Prevalence_of_rare_diseases_by_alphabetical_list.pdf. Accessed February 10 2022.

6. Jepsen P, Gronbaek L, Vilstrup H. Worldwide incidence of autoimmune liver disease. Dig Dis 2015;33(Suppl 2):2–12.

7. Podda M, Selmi C, Lleo A, et al. The limitations and hidden gems of the epidemiology of primary biliary cirrhosis. J Autoimmun 2013;46:81–7.

8. Lv T, Chen S, Li M, et al. Regional variation and temporal trend of primary biliary cholangitis epidemiology: a systematic review and meta-analysis. J Gastroenterol Hepatol 2021;36(6):1423–34.

9. Schwinge D, Schramm C. Sex-related factors in autoimmune liver diseases. Semin Immunopathol 2019;41(2):165–75.

10. Lleo A, Jepsen P, Morenghi E, et al. Evolving trends in female to male incidence and male mortality of primary biliary cholangitis. Sci Rep 2016;6:25906.

11. Tanaka A, Mori M, Matsumoto K, et al. Increase trend in the prevalence and male-to-female ratio of primary biliary cholangitis, autoimmune hepatitis, and primary sclerosing cholangitis in Japan. Hepatol Res 2019;49(8):881–9.

12. Gazda J, Drazilova S, Janicko M, et al. The epidemiology of primary biliary cholangitis in European countries: a systematic review and meta-analysis. Can J Gastroenterol Hepatol 2021;2021:9151525.

13. Gershwin ME, Selmi C, Worman HJ, et al. Risk factors and comorbidities in primary biliary cirrhosis: a controlled interview-based study of 1032 patients. Hepatology 2005;42(5):1194–202.

14. Asselta R, Paraboschi EM, Gerussi A, et al. X chromosome contribution to the genetic Architecture of primary biliary cholangitis. Gastroenterology 2021;160(7):2483–2495 e2426.

15. McNally RJ, James PW, Ducker S, et al. No rise in incidence but geographical heterogeneity in the occurrence of primary biliary cirrhosis in North East England. Am J Epidemiol 2014;179(4):492–8.

16. Carbone M, Mells GF, Pells G, et al. Sex and age are determinants of the clinical phenotype of primary biliary cirrhosis and response to ursodeoxycholic acid. Gastroenterology 2013;144(3):560–9, e567; quiz e513-564.

17. John BV, Aitcheson G, Schwartz KB, et al. Male sex is associated with higher rates of liver-related mortality in primary biliary cholangitis and cirrhosis. Hepatology 2021;74(2):879–91.

18. John BV, Khakoo NS, Schwartz KB, et al. Ursodeoxycholic acid response is associated with reduced mortality in primary biliary cholangitis with Compensated cirrhosis. Am J Gastroenterol 2021;116(9):1913–23.

19. Murillo Perez CF, Goet JC, Lammers WJ, et al. Milder disease stage in patients with primary biliary cholangitis over a 44-year period: a changing natural history. Hepatology 2018;67(5):1920–30.

20. Prince MI, James OF. The epidemiology of primary biliary cirrhosis. Clin Liver Dis 2003;7(4):795–819.

21. Koulentaki M, Mantaka A, Sifaki-Pistolla D, et al. Geoepidemiology and space-time analysis of Primary biliary cirrhosis in Crete, Greece. Liver Int 2014;34(7):e200–7.

22. Baldursdottir TR, Bergmann OM, Jonasson JG, et al. The epidemiology and natural history of primary biliary cirrhosis: a nationwide population-based study. Eur J Gastroenterol Hepatol 2012;24(7):824–30.

23. Ornolfsson KT, Olafsson S, Bergmann OM, et al. Using the Icelandic genealogical database to define the familial risk of primary biliary cholangitis. Hepatology 2018;68(1):166–71.

24. Griffiths L, Dyson JK, Jones DE. The new epidemiology of primary biliary cirrhosis. Semin Liver Dis 2014;34(3):318–28.

25. Webb GJ, Ryan RP, Marshall TP, et al. The epidemiology of UK autoimmune liver disease varies with geographic latitude. Clin Gastroenterol Hepatol 2021;19(12):2587–96.

26. Kingham JG, Parker DR. The association between primary biliary cirrhosis and coeliac disease: a study of relative prevalences. Gut 1998;42(1):120–2.

27. James OF, Bhopal R, Howel D, et al. Primary biliary cirrhosis once rare, now common in the United Kingdom? Hepatology 1999;30(2):390–4.

28. Steinke DT, Weston TL, Morris AD, et al. The epidemiology of liver disease in Tayside database: a population-based record-linkage study. J Biomed Inform 2002;35(3):186–93.

29. Lofgren J, Jarnerot G, Danielsson D, et al. Incidence and prevalence of primary biliary cirrhosis in a defined population in Sweden. Scand J Gastroenterol 1985;20(5):647–50.

30. Danielsson A, Boqvist L, Uddenfeldt P. Epidemiology of primary biliary cirrhosis in a defined rural population in the northern part of Sweden. Hepatology 1990;11(3):458–64.

31. Marschall HU, Henriksson I, Lindberg S, et al. Incidence, prevalence, and outcome of primary biliary cholangitis in a nationwide Swedish population-based cohort. Sci Rep 2019;9(1):11525.

32. Pares A, Albillos A, Andrade RJ, et al. Primary biliary cholangitis in Spain. Results of a Delphi study of epidemiology, diagnosis, follow-up and treatment. Rev Esp Enferm Dig 2018;110(10):641–9.

33. Lu M, Zhou Y, Haller IV, et al. Increasing prevalence of primary biliary cholangitis and reduced mortality with treatment. Clin Gastroenterol Hepatol 2018;16(8):1342–1350 e1341.

34. Kim WR, Lindor KD, Locke GR 3rd, et al. Epidemiology and natural history of primary biliary cirrhosis in a US community. Gastroenterology 2000;119(6):1631–6.

35. Ala A, Stanca CM, Bu-Ghanim M, et al. Increased prevalence of primary biliary cirrhosis near Superfund toxic waste sites. Hepatology 2006;43(3):525–31.

36. Gross RG, Odin JA. Recent advances in the epidemiology of primary biliary cirrhosis. Clin Liver Dis 2008;12(2):289–303, viii.

37. Delgado J, Sperber AD, Novack V, et al. The epidemiology of primary biliary cirrhosis in southern Israel. Isr Med Assoc J 2005;7(11):717–21.

38. Zeng N, Duan W, Chen S, et al. Epidemiology and clinical course of primary biliary cholangitis in the Asia-Pacific region: a systematic review and meta-analysis. Hepatol Int 2019;13(6):788–99.

39. Ngu JH, Gearry RB, Wright AJ, et al. Low incidence and prevalence of primary biliary cirrhosis in Canterbury, New Zealand: a population-based study. Hepatol Int 2012;6(4):796–800.

40. Jeong SH. Current epidemiology and clinical characteristics of autoimmune liver diseases in South Korea. Clin Mol Hepatol 2018;24(1):10–9.

41. Colapietro F, Lleo A, Generali E. Antimitochondrial antibodies: from Bench to Bedside. Clin Rev Allergy Immunol 2021;Sep 29:1–12.

42. Invernizzi P, Crosignani A, Battezzati PM, et al. Comparison of the clinical features and clinical course of antimitochondrial antibody-positive and -negative primary biliary cirrhosis. Hepatology 1997;25(5):1090–5.

43. John BV, Dahman B, Deng Y, et al. Rates of decompensation, hepatocellular carcinoma and mortality in AMA-negative primary biliary cholangitis cirrhosis. Liver Int 2022;42(2):384–93.

44. Cancado GGL, Braga MH, Ferraz MLG, et al. Anti-mitochondrial antibody-negative primary biliary cholangitis is part of the same Spectrum of Classical primary biliary cholangitis. Dig Dis Sci 2022 Jul;67(7):3305–12.

45. Metcalf JV, Mitchison HC, Palmer JM, et al. Natural history of early primary biliary cirrhosis. Lancet 1996;348(9039):1399–402.

46. Sun C, Xiao X, Yan L, et al. Histologically proven AMA positive primary biliary cholangitis but normal serum alkaline phosphatase: is alkaline phosphatase truly a surrogate marker? J Autoimmun 2019;99:33–8.

47. Terziroli Beretta-Piccoli B, Stirnimann G, Mertens J, et al. Primary biliary cholangitis with normal alkaline phosphatase: a neglected clinical entity challenging current guidelines. J Autoimmun 2021;116:102578.

48. Dahlqvist G, Gaouar F, Carrat F, et al. Large-scale characterization study of patients with antimitochondrial antibodies but nonestablished primary biliary cholangitis. Hepatology 2017;65(1):152–63.

49. Zandanell S, Strasser M, Feldman A, et al. Low rate of new-onset primary biliary cholangitis in a cohort of anti-mitochondrial antibody-positive subjects over six years of follow-up. J Intern Med 2020;287(4):395–404.

50. Trivedi PJ, Lammers WJ, van Buuren HR, et al. Stratification of hepatocellular carcinoma risk in primary biliary cirrhosis: a multicentre international study. Gut 2016;65(2):321–9.

51. Natarajan Y, Tansel A, Patel P, et al. Incidence of hepatocellular carcinoma in primary biliary cholangitis: a systematic review and meta-analysis. Dig Dis Sci 2021; 66(7):2439–51.

52. Montano-Loza AJ, Hansen BE, Corpechot C, et al. Factors associated with recurrence of primary biliary cholangitis after liver transplantation and effects on Graft and patient survival. Gastroenterology 2019;156(1):96–107 e101.

53. Corpechot C, Chazouilleres O, Belnou P, et al. Long-term impact of preventive UDCA therapy after transplantation for primary biliary cholangitis. J Hepatol 2020;73(3):559–65.

54. Harms MH, van Buuren HR, Corpechot C, et al. Ursodeoxycholic acid therapy and liver transplant-free survival in patients with primary biliary cholangitis. J Hepatol 2019;71(2):357–65.

55. Nevens F, Andreone P, Mazzella G, et al. A Placebo-controlled trial of Obeticholic acid in primary biliary cholangitis. N Engl J Med 2016;375(7):631–43.

56. Boonstra K, Beuers U, Ponsioen CY. Epidemiology of primary sclerosing cholangitis and primary biliary cirrhosis: a systematic review. J Hepatol 2012;56(5): 1181–8.

57. Rubel LR, Rabin L, Seeff LB, et al. Does primary biliary cirrhosis in men differ from primary biliary cirrhosis in women? Hepatology 1984;4(4):671–7.

58. Myers RP, Shaheen AA, Fong A, et al. Epidemiology and natural history of primary biliary cirrhosis in a Canadian health region: a population-based study. Hepatology 2009;50(6):1884–92.

59. Cheung AC, Lammers WJ, Murillo Perez CF, et al. Effects of age and sex of response to ursodeoxycholic acid and transplant-free survival in patients with primary biliary cholangitis. Clin Gastroenterol Hepatol 2019;17(10):2076–2084 e2072.

60. Gordon SC, Wu KH, Lindor K, et al. Ursodeoxycholic acid treatment Preferentially improves overall survival among African Americans with primary biliary cholangitis. Am J Gastroenterol 2020;115(2):262–70.

61. Roberts SB, Hirschfield GM, Worobetz LJ, et al. Ethnicity, disease severity and survival in Canadian patients with Primary Biliary Cholangitis. Hepatology 2022; Feb 26. https://doi.org/10.1002/hep.32426. Online ahead of print.

62. Liu X, Invernizzi P, Lu Y, et al. Genome-wide meta-analyses identify three loci associated with primary biliary cirrhosis. Nat Genet 2010;42(8):658–60.

63. Selmi C, Mayo MJ, Bach N, et al. Primary biliary cirrhosis in monozygotic and dizygotic twins: genetics, epigenetics, and environment. Gastroenterology 2004;127(2):485–92.

64. Corpechot C, Chretien Y, Chazouilleres O, et al. Demographic, lifestyle, medical and familial factors associated with primary biliary cirrhosis. J Hepatol 2010; 53(1):162–9.

65. Gulamhusein AF, Juran BD, Atkinson EJ, et al. Low incidence of primary biliary cirrhosis (PBC) in the first-degree relatives of PBC probands after 8 years of follow-up. Liver Int 2016;36(9):1378–82.

66. Invernizzi P, Selmi C, Poli F, et al. Human leukocyte antigen polymorphisms in Italian primary biliary cirrhosis: a multicenter study of 664 patients and 1992 healthy controls. Hepatology 2008;48(6):1906–12.

67. Hirschfield GM, Liu X, Xu C, et al. Primary biliary cirrhosis associated with HLA, IL12A, and IL12RB2 variants. N Engl J Med 2009;360(24):2544–55.

68. Mells GF, Floyd JA, Morley KI, et al. Genome-wide association study identifies 12 new susceptibility loci for primary biliary cirrhosis. Nat Genet 2011;43(4):329–32.

69. Juran BD, Hirschfield GM, Invernizzi P, et al. Immunochip analyses identify a novel risk locus for primary biliary cirrhosis at 13q14, multiple independent associations at four established risk loci and epistasis between 1p31 and 7q32 risk variants. Hum Mol Genet 2012;21(23):5209–21.

70. Nakamura M, Nishida N, Kawashima M, et al. Genome-wide association study identifies TNFSF15 and POU2AF1 as susceptibility loci for primary biliary cirrhosis in the Japanese population. Am J Hum Genet 2012;91(4):721–8.

71. Probert PM, Leitch AC, Dunn MP, et al. Identification of a xenobiotic as a potential environmental trigger in primary biliary cholangitis. J Hepatol 2018;69(5): 1123–35.

72. Ohba K, Omagari K, Kinoshita H, et al. Primary biliary cirrhosis among atomic bomb survivors in Nagasaki, Japan. J Clin Epidemiol 2001;54(8):845–50.

73. Corpechot C, Gaouar F, Chretien Y, et al. Smoking as an independent risk factor of liver fibrosis in primary biliary cirrhosis. J Hepatol 2012;56(1):218–24.

74. Boonstra K, Kunst AE, Stadhouders PH, et al. Rising incidence and prevalence of primary biliary cirrhosis: a large population-based study. Liver Int 2014;34(6): e31–8.

75. Ebadi M, Ip S, Lytvyak E, et al. Vitamin D is associated with clinical outcomes in patients with primary biliary cholangitis. Nutrients 2022;14(4).

76. Yang Y, Choi J, Chen Y, et al. E. coli and the etiology of human PBC: antimitochondrial antibodies and spreading determinants. Hepatology 2022;75(2):266–79.

77. Zhang H, Carbone M, Lleo A, et al. Geoepidemiology, genetic and environmental risk factors for PBC. Dig Dis 2015;33(Suppl 2):94–101.

78. Di Sanzo M, Cipolloni L, Borro M, et al. Clinical Applications of personalized medicine: a new paradigm and Challenge. Curr Pharm Biotechnol 2017;18(3): 194–203.

79. Corpechot C, Chazouilleres O, Rousseau A, et al. A Placebo-controlled trial of Bezafibrate in primary biliary cholangitis. N Engl J Med 2018;378(23):2171–81.

80. Lammers WJ, Hirschfield GM, Corpechot C, et al. Development and validation of a scoring system to Predict outcomes of patients with primary biliary cirrhosis receiving ursodeoxycholic acid therapy. Gastroenterology 2015;149(7): 1804–1812 e1804.

81. Carbone M, Sharp SJ, Flack S, et al. The UK-PBC risk scores: Derivation and validation of a scoring system for long-term prediction of end-stage liver disease in primary biliary cholangitis. Hepatology 2016;63(3):930–50.

82. Goet JC, Murillo Perez CF, Harms MH, et al. A Comparison of prognostic scores (Mayo, UK-PBC, and GLOBE) in primary biliary cholangitis. Am J Gastroenterol 2021;116(7):1514–22.

83. Lindor KD, Bowlus CL, Boyer J, et al. Primary biliary cholangitis: 2018 practice guidance from the American association for the study of liver diseases. Hepatology 2019;69(1):394–419.

84. Marzioni M, Bassanelli C, Ripellino C, et al. Epidemiology of primary biliary cholangitis in Italy: evidence from a real-world database. Dig Liver Dis 2019;51(5): 724–9.

85. Drazilova S, Babinska I, Gazda J, et al. Epidemiology and clinical course of primary biliary cholangitis in Eastern Slovakia. Int J Public Health 2020;65(5): 683–91.

86. Kim KA, Ki M, Choi HY, et al. Population-based epidemiology of primary biliary cirrhosis in South Korea. Aliment Pharmacol Ther 2016;43(1):154–62.

87. Kanth R, Shrestha RB, Rai I, et al. Incidence of primary biliary cholangitis in a rural Midwestern population. Clin Med Res 2017;15(1–2):13–8.

88. Yoshida EM, Mason A, Peltekian KM, et al. Epidemiology and liver transplantation burden of primary biliary cholangitis: a retrospective cohort study. CMAJ Open 2018;6(4):E664–70.

89. French J, van der Mei I, Simpson S Jr, et al. Increasing prevalence of primary biliary cholangitis in Victoria, Australia. J Gastroenterol Hepatol 2020;35(4): 673–9.

90. Lamba M, Ngu JH, Stedman CAM. Trends in incidence of autoimmune liver diseases and increasing incidence of autoimmune hepatitis. Clin Gastroenterol Hepatol 2021;19(3):573–9.e1.

Genetics of Primary Biliary Cholangitis

Alessio Gerussi, MD, PhD[a,b],*, Rosanna Asselta, PhD[c,d], Pietro Invernizzi, MD, PhD[a,b],*

KEYWORDS

- Complex trait • GWAS • Liver • HLA • Autoimmunity

KEY POINTS

- Genome-wide association studies have shed a light on the genetic architecture of Primary biliary cholangitis (PBC) but several open questions still remain
- The two pathogenetic theories in PBC-induced need to be reconciled in a unitary model
- Despite the great progress in risk stratification modeling, no genetic variants have been incorporated in clinical risk models predicting treatment response
- The study of the X chromosome, neglected for too long, may inform both PBC pathogenesis and the genetic determinants of its female predominance

Abbreviations	
HLA	human leukocyte antigen
IL	interleukin

INTRODUCTION

Primary biliary cholangitis (PBC) is a rare autoimmune disease of the small bile ducts of the liver.[1] Despite the etiologic agent, it is still unknown, two phases of its pathogenesis have recently been described: the initiation phase and the progression phase.[2] The former is driven by perturbations in the biliary homeostasis that, together with a genetic predisposition to abnormal antigen presentation, lead to liver autoimmunity; the latter moves around the progression of the liver damage due to cholestasis (ie, toxic retention of bile acids).[2] Several drugs are now available to treat PBC, but no

[a] Division of Gastroenterology and Center for Autoimmune Liver Diseases, Department of Medicine and Surgery, University of Milano-Bicocca, Via Cadore 48, 20900 Monza (MB), Italy; [b] European Reference Network on Hepatological Diseases (ERN RARE-LIVER), San Gerardo Hospital, Monza, Italy; [c] Department of Biomedical Sciences, Humanitas University, Via Rita Levi Montalcini 4, Pieve Emanuele 20072, Italy; [d] Humanitas Clinical and Research Center, IRCCS, Via Manzoni 56, Rozzano 20089, Italy
* Corresponding authors.
E-mail addresses: alessio.gerussi@unimib.it (A.G.); pietro.invernizzi@unimib.it (P.I.)

Clin Liver Dis 26 (2022) 571–582
https://doi.org/10.1016/j.cld.2022.06.002
1089-3261/22/© 2022 Elsevier Inc. All rights reserved.

agent is predicted to work on the initiation phase.[3] The dissection of the genetic basis of PBC can pinpoint candidate genes and druggable downstream pathways that may hopefully fill this gap.[3]

In addition, genetic variants can be used as risk stratifiers both in subjects affected by PBC, as prognostic and predictive biomarkers of disease progression and treatment, and in first-degree relatives, to assess their inherent genetic risk to develop the disease and, consequently, set up a tailored follow-up.

A large portion of PBC heritability still remains to be explained, likely due to the underrepresentation of non-European populations in genome-wide association studies (GWAS), the neglect of sexual chromosomes in analytical pipelines, and the lack of exome- and whole-genome sequencing studies to detect rare variants at large effect size. Remarkably, no studies are still available linking genetic variability to (1) disease progression and (2) treatment response.

This review outlines the state-of-the-art regarding the genetic architecture of PBC and thoughtful reflections on the limitations of current genetic methods. It also discusses how the growing body of information derived from genetic studies can be leveraged in the clinic.

DISCUSSION
Primary Biliary Cholangitis Is a Complex Heritable Trait

In genetic terminology, PBC is a complex trait, which means that the interplay of environmental agents with an unfavorable set of gene variants shapes the susceptibility to the disease.[4] There is established evidence that some environmental triggers (e.g., recurrent urinary tract infections, tobacco, hair dyes) have a not negligible role in the etiopathogenesis of the disease.[5] Interestingly, a recent report from the UK has shown the presence of a geographic cluster, which further stresses the concept that an environmental agent may trigger the onset of PBC.[6]

PBC has a heritable component: the argument that supports this concept derives from the observation that there is a familiar predisposition to the disease. More specifically, patients with a positive family history comprise comprise 1.3% to 9.0% of cases, which is higher than the expected risk in the general population.[7] In addition, if a subject with PBC has a first-degree relative affected, there is an increase in the risk to develop PBC in another first-degree relative estimated to be around 6.8 to 10.7 (Odds ratio).[8] Finally, the concordance rate in homozygous twins is 0.63.[9]

Genetic Studies in Primary Biliary Cholangitis: Pre- and Post-Genome-Wide Association Studies Eras

On top of the epidemiologic evidence showing disease aggregation within families, there is direct evidence of the genetic predisposition of PBC. Before the coming of GWAS, the candidate gene approach was the most common method of investigation. Several groups showed that the HLA region harbors a genetic signal specific for PBC. Yet, the lack of power of pre-GWAS studies hampered the study of non-HLA regions.[10]

The GWAS revolution has allowed the dissection of the genetic architecture of the disease, not only in subjects of European ancestry but also in Japanese and Chinese individuals.[11–19]

HLA molecules are involved in both physiologic immune response and disease-causing autoimmunity.[20] Most autoimmune diseases have been associated with genetic variation in this genetic region.[21] HLA associations with PBC are presented in **Table 1**. In line with other autoimmune conditions, HLA associations represent a large

Table 1
Main HLA haplotypes associated with primary biliary cholangitis

HLA Associations	Cases A1/N	%	Controls A1/N	%	OR	P-Value	Country
DQB1*0301	109/412	26.0	80/236	34.0	0.70	.045	UK
DQB1*0402	44/412	11.0	9/236	4.0	3.02	.002	UK
DRB1*0405	126/668	18.9	68/516	13.2	1.53	.005	Japan
DRB1*08	50/412	12.1	10/236	4.2	3.05	8.70E-04	UK
DRB1*08	48/664	7.2	46/1992	2.3	3.32	4.00E-32	Italy
DRB1*0803	89/668	13.3	33/516	6.4	2.24	1.00E-04	Japan
DRB1*11	7/668	1.0	19/516	3.7	0.28	.002	Japan
DRB1*1101	7/668	1.0	19/516	3.7	0.28	.002	Japan
DRB1*13	57/412	14.0	47/236	20.0	0.65	.042	UK
DRB1*13	57/664	8.6	319/1992	16.0	0.70	3.60E-06	Italy
DRB1*1302	15/668	2.2	29/516	5.6	0.38	.003	Japan
DRB1*1501	46/668	6.9	60/516	11.6	0.56	.005	Japan
DQA1*0401/DQB1*0402	44/824	5.3	9/472	1.9	2.90	.003	UK
DRB1*0405/DQB1*0401	373/1199	31.1	277/1193	23.2	1.49	1.44E-05	Japan
DRB1*0801/DQA1*0401/DQB1*0402	44/824	5.3	9/472	1.9	2.90	.003	UK
DRB1*0803/DQB1*0601	278/1199	23.2	174/1193	14.6	1.77	7.82E-08	Japan
DRB1*1302/DQB1*0604	36/1199	3.0	169/1193	14.2	0.19	1.84E-22	Japan
DRB1*1403/DQB1*0301	7/1199	0.6	32/1193	2.7	0.21	5.1E-05	Japan
Not(DRB1*1403)/DQB1*0301	137/1199	11.4	224/1193	18.8	0.54	8.54E-08	Japan

Only studies with at least 300 PBC cases were included.
Abbreviation: OR, odds ratio.

portion of the explained heritability of PBC and should be incorporated into integrative risk models. As compared to other diseases like autoimmune hepatitis[22] or celiac disease,[23] HLA evaluation is not part of the clinical diagnostic pathway in PBC. Moreover, the strong linkage disequilibrium is an obstacle to determine a functional link between variants and disease pathogenesis.[21]

Fig. 1 enlists in detail the 44 genetic variants outside the Major Histocompatibility Complex (MHC) region that have been associated with PBC. For a thorough description of the possible role of each of these variants, which is beyond the scope of this review, see Mells *and colleagues,*[24] and Gerussi *and colleagues,*.[25]

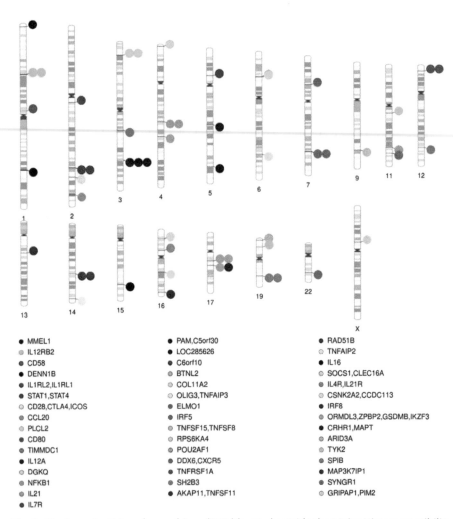

● MMEL1	● PAM,C5orf30	● RAD51B
◑ IL12RB2	● LOC285626	◯ TNFAIP2
● CD58	● C6orf10	● IL16
● DENN1B	◑ BTNL2	◑ SOCS1,CLEC16A
● IL1RL2,IL1RL1	◯ COL11A2	● IL4R,IL21R
● STAT1,STAT4	◯ OLIG3,TNFAIP3	◑ CSNK2A2,CCDC113
◯ CD28,CTLA4,ICOS	● ELMO1	● IRF8
◑ CCL20	● IRF5	◑ ORMDL3,ZPBP2,GSDMB,IKZF3
◑ PLCL2	◑ TNFSF15,TNFSF8	● CRHR1,MAPT
● CD80	◑ RPS6KA4	◑ ARID3A
● TIMMDC1	◑ POU2AF1	◑ TYK2
● IL12A	◑ DDX6,CXCR5	● SPIB
◯ DGKQ	● TNFRSF1A	● MAP3K7IP1
◑ NFKB1	● SH2B3	● SYNGR1
◑ IL21	● AKAP11,TNFSF11	◯ GRIPAP1,PIM2
● IL7R		

Fig. 1. Single nucleotide polymorphisms (SNPs) located outside the Major Histocompatibility Complex locus are associated with Primary Biliary Cholangitis. If multiple SNPs tagging the same locus have been identified in different studies, this has been made visible by the presence of multiple dots of the same color along the chromosome.

Missing Heritability in Primary Biliary Cholangitis: Just a Matter of Sample Size?

The proportion of heritability clarified by a set of variants is the ratio of the heritability because of these variants (ie, the numerator), typically estimated directly from their effect sizes, to the total heritability (ie, the denominator), inferred in an indirect way from studies on twins. Teri Manolio introduced the notion of "missing heritability" to stress the fact that the explained ratio is for many diseases below 0.5.[26] Despite greater than 40 variants identified so far, the largest portion of PBC heritability is still to be investigated. The only estimate available about explained heritability in PBC dates back to 2015 when it has been scored in 5.3%.[27] Several factors may account for this large gap in PBC: the sample size is too small leading to underpowered GWAS, lack of whole-genome and exome studies, neglect of X chromosome (chrX), and lack of epistatic studies.

The common disease-common variant hypothesis postulates that most of the missing heritability is in common variants that still need to be identified (**Fig. 2**). The most important evidence to support this concept is the finding that when all the single nucleotide polymorphisms (SNPs) are fitted altogether instead of testing one-by-one and adopting a stringent threshold for multiple testing, the variance of a highly polygenic trait—such as height - goes from less than 10% to around 45%.[28] One could argue that by massively increasing the number of subjects with PBC sequenced around the world the number of variants would increase and so the explained heritability.

Rare Variants and Primary Biliary Cholangitis: A Story Still to Be Written

Conversely, the common disease-rare variant hypothesis focuses its attention on rare variants. It postulates that rare variants that are mildly deleterious are key players in the susceptibility to complex traits.[29] Detection of rare variants with small effects

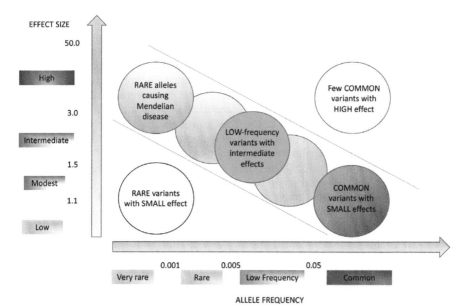

Fig. 2. Types of genetic variants by risk allele frequency and strength of the genetic effect. (*Adapted from* Manolio TA, Collins FS, Cox NJ, et al. Finding the missing heritability of complex diseases. *Nature.* 2009;461(7265):747-753. https://doi.org/10.1038/nature08494.)

and ultrarare (allele frequency 1 in 100,000 subjects) variants is inherently impossible with GWAS.[30] Arrays used to perform genotyping studies do not commonly capture these variants, and this would explain missing heritability (see **Fig. 1**).

Whole-exome and whole-genome sequencing have identified new variants in several complex traits, including rare diseases.[31,32] A recent study from China has found an association between 10 variants located in the *HLA-DRB1* gene with PBC in three PBC families.[33] Another report from China has shown that the transcription factor *Myocyte Enhancer Factor 2D* (*MEF2D*) and the DNA repair gene *Poly(ADP-Ribose) Polymerase 2* (*PARP2*) are hub genes involved in the pathogenesis of PBC; this evidence has been derived from whole-exome sequencing of 90 subjects, including 30 PBC cases.[34] To date, no other data are available from whole-exome sequencing studies outside China, representing an important gap that needs to be covered.

Variation Within the X Chromosome Influence Genetic Predisposition and Female Predominance in Primary Biliary Cholangitis

The study of the chrX can be valuable in PBC for two important reasons: variation within the chrX can be associated with the risk of developing the disease but also could explain the reason why PBC is much more frequent in women than men. Although evidence linking chrX and female bias has been historically generated,[35] the identification of genetic variants on chrX at a genome-wide level of significance has been only recently reported.[36]

As regards sex bias, gene expression is widely modulated by sex, at a greater magnitude than autosomes.[37] Remarkably, immune-related tissues show high levels of gene expression of X-related gene variants that have been linked with autoimmunity and autoimmune conditions.[38]

Since females carry two copies of chrX, to balance allele dosage random chrX inactivation (XCI) does occur in mammals.[39] Yet, recent estimates report that up to 23% of genes located on chrX undergo incomplete XCI, contributing to phenotypic diversity.[40] One theory behind sex bias in autoimmunity is that females may be more predisposed to autoimmune phenomena because of the action of some immune-related genes that escape XCI and cause an enhanced activity of the immune system. An indirect proof of this concept is the higher frequency of Systemic Lupus Erythematosus (SLE) in patients with the Klinefelter's syndrome (XXY)[41] and the overexpression of chrX-related genes with immune functions in patients of female sex affected by SLE.[42,43] A paradigmatic example pertains to the *Toll-like receptor 7* (*TLR7*) locus, which is located on chrX; the encoded protein acts as a pivotal component of the innate antiviral response. In subjects with the Klinefelter's syndrome, the *TLR7* gene escapes silencing in immune cells, and this has been associated with an augmented tendency to immunoglobulin G class switch in biallelic B lymphocytes.[44]

Another theory postulates somehow the opposite: the observation that patients with autoimmune diseases have higher rates of chrX monosomy in peripheral blood mononuclear cells — also known as somatic loss of chrX— may support functional haploinsufficiency. Turner's syndrome represents an interesting model because it is characterized by germinal widespread loss of chrX (X0 karyotype).[45] Patients with Turner's syndrome have higher rates of some autoimmune diseases.[46] Likewise, female patients with the isochromosome-Xq syndrome, where the short arm of chrX is completely deleted, are more prone to develop autoimmune thyroid and inflammatory bowel diseases.[47] Yet, it is still a matter of debate that genes would be functionally lost and consequently predisposing to autoimmunity. For instance, some genes located in the pseudoautosomal region (PAR) 1 of chrX have been linked to immunity.[47] Another theoretic explanation might be that monosomy would cause the loss of function of genes that permanently escape XCI.[47,48]

To sum up, despite reliable theoretic postulations, there is still a need for a comprehensive theory and more experimental data in support to dissect the role of chrX in shaping sex bias of autoimmunity.

Gene-Gene Interactions: The Conundrum of Statistical Genetics

When heritability is calculated, the assumption is that no genetic interactions (epistasis) are present. After including epistatic effects, it has been proved that the denominator can be overinflated, exaggerating the missing heritability issue.[49] All in all, even in that case, a gap still remains. Whether gene–gene interactions may account for a part of this gap is still a matter of hot debate.

Molecular biology studies clearly show that gene–gene interactions are common in nature, although quantitative genetics falls short in showing the non-additive effects to phenotypic variation.[50] Although the presence of non-additive interactions, inside and outside the HLA region, has been shown in autoimmune diseases,[51,52] a recent work from the group of Peter Visscher has partly sung the "requiem" for the quantitative epistasis.[53] The authors created a new method to estimate heritability that is less biased than classical ones and validated that on the UK Biobank cohort, showing that most of the heritability of complex traits is due to additive effects and that dominance and epistatic interactions seem quite negligible. Investigators conclude that to reach precise estimates of epistatic variance millions of unrelated subjects are needed.

Therefore, we can derive two statements: epistasis is a natural phenomenon that is pervasive in nature and it is typically well modeled in model organisms such as *Drosophila melanogaster*, since environmental forces and allele frequencies can be easily controlled.[54] However, higher-order interactions between genetic variants, the so-called statistical epistasis, are very challenging to study and its variance seems only to add on additive variance for complex traits.[53]

A possible aid can derive from the evolutionary approach to genetics, allowing to better target the analysis: regulatory variants that are under positive selection show epistatic interactions with their partners. By looking for signatures of positive selection, researchers can select a restricted list of variants to study.[55]

How Genetic Variants Informs Primary Biliary Cholangitis Pathogenesis

Interestingly, no predisposing genes involved in biliary physiology have been discovered so far, which contrasts with data derived from animal models suggesting that biliary epithelium abnormalities might be a primer of the disease.[2]

This discrepancy may be partly explained by the different methodology used to investigate the cause of PBC: on one hand genetic epidemiology (GWAS), on the other hand, preclinical experiments in the lab (in vitro/in vivo models). Furthermore, to reconcile the two aspects of the disease, we could suggest that GWAS data inform about the predisposing background on which abnormalities described in cellular and animal models may occur following the action of an environmental trigger.

Have Genome-Wide Association Studies Failed in Primary Biliary Cholangitis in Guiding Drug Discovery?

Some authors have stated the failure of GWAS in PBC after the unsatisfactory results of clinical trials where compounds targeting proteins encoded by allegedly causal genes had been evaluated.

The most famous case is that of Ustekinumab, a monoclonal antibody targeting IL-12/IL-23, which did not meet the primary endpoint of alkaline phosphatase reduction.[56]

Methods have pros and cons, and perform well in specific contexts and less well in others. It is not that GWAS have failed: GWAS have limitations and should be asked what they can provide and not beyond. Several strategies to dissect tagged loci and avoid simplistic inferences from associations to causality have been progressively proposed.[57] Other fields of medicine have elegantly shown that the relationship between tagged loci and downstream pathways is far more complex than initially thought. For example, the *FTO* region is associated with the risk of obesity but there is no link between this locus and homeostasis of fat. The causal variant *rs1421085* acts on a repressor binding site, which, in turn, modulates two genes involved in adipocyte differentiation located far from the *FTO* locus.[58] Dissection of GWAS signals would probably require the integration of several layers of information, as elegantly reported by recent studies.[59] We should also keep in mind the difference between disease susceptibility and disease progression, so that a good therapeutic target should not necessarily be found immediately downstream the susceptibility genetic locus. The evaluation of immunomodulators in PBC would also likely require a modification in clinical trial design, adopting different endpoints than those used for anticholestatic medications and different selection criteria.[60]

Genetic Variants and Risk Stratification: Still a Long Road to Go

The availability of a novel second-line therapy in PBC (obeticholic acid) together with several other compounds close to registration has paved the way for several multi-center, international studies in the field of risk stratification.[61] The definition of prognostic endpoints has dominated the research agenda over the last decade, with solid evidence supporting the role of total bilirubin and alkaline phosphatase,[62,63] together with other biomarkers.[64,65] Yet, in contrast with other liver diseases like Non-Alcoholic Fatty Liver Disease,[66] no genetic variants have been incorporated in clinical risk models. Some preliminary evidence has been generated in the field of liver transplantation, where *rs62270414* (tagging the *IL-12* locus) has been associated with the risk of PBC recurrence.[67]

To our knowledge, there is no published evidence linking specific SNPs and treatment response; similarly, there is a lack of evidence associating genetic variation and disease progression. Single cohorts might represent a starting point, but to address these research issues we foresee that an international endeavor will be necessary; the presence of a large consortium that already dissected its pathogenesis represents the common ground from which researchers should start working.[68]

SUMMARY

The genetic basis underlying PBC has been progressively better understood, with remarkable contribution provided by GWAS. The *MHC* locus remains the most significant genomic region despite its dissection is is still difficult; in addition, specific HLA haplotypes are not assessed in clinical practice. Many non-HLA loci have been discovered, with a large overlap of signals with other non-liver-related autoimmune diseases, reinforcing the strong autoimmune identity of the disease. The major effort of the genetic community interested in PBC is now focused on the dissection of the downstream pathways for the identification of causal genes and druggable targets. The translation to clinical practice remains complex, due to the historical adoption of clinical endpoints related to cholestasis, which poorly correlate with immunologic pathways pinpointed by GWAS signals. The study of the chrX has recently gained more traction, because it is predicted to bring information on both the genetic architecture and the female predominance. Open questions remain about the lack of genetic signals related to cholangiocyte physio(patho)logy, the role of genetic variants in shaping treatment response, and the discovery of rare and ultrarare variants associated with PBC.

DISCLOSURE

A. Gerussi and P. Invernizzi are members of the European Reference Network on Hepatological Diseases (ERN RARE LIVER). The authors thank AMAF Monza ONLUS and AIRCS for the unrestricted research funding.

REFERENCES

1. Lleo A, Wang G-Q, Gershwin ME, et al. Primary biliary cholangitis. Lancet 2020; 396(10266):1915–26.
2. Rodrigues PM, Perugorria MJ, Santos-Laso A, et al. Primary biliary cholangitis: a tale of epigenetically-induced secretory failure? J Hepatol 2018. https://doi.org/10.1016/j.jhep.2018.08.020.
3. Gerussi A, Lucà M, Cristoferi L, et al. New therapeutic targets in autoimmune Cholangiopathies. Front Med 2020;7:117. Available at: https://www.frontiersin.org/article/10.3389/fmed.2020.00117.
4. Gerussi A, Carbone M, Asselta R, et al. In: Gershwin ME, Vierling JM, Tanaka A, et al, editors. Genetics of autoimmune liver diseases BT - liver immunology : principles and practice. Cham: Springer International Publishing; 2020. p. 69–85. https://doi.org/10.1007/978-3-030-51709-0_5.
5. Selmi C. Environmental factors in primary biliary cirrhosis. Hepatol Res 2007; 37(Suppl 3):S370–6.
6. Dyson JK, Blain A, Foster Shirley MD, et al. Geo-epidemiology and environmental co-variate mapping of primary biliary cholangitis and primary sclerosing cholangitis. JHEP Rep 2021;3(1). https://doi.org/10.1016/j.jhepr.2020.100202.
7. Boonstra K, Beuers U, Ponsioen CY. Epidemiology of primary sclerosing cholangitis and primary biliary cirrhosis: a systematic review. J Hepatol 2012;56(5): 1181–8.
8. Corpechot C, Chrétien Y, Chazouillères O, et al. Demographic, lifestyle, medical and familial factors associated with primary biliary cirrhosis. J Hepatol 2010; 53(1):162–9.
9. Selmi C, Mayo MJ, Bach N, et al. Primary biliary cirrhosis in monozygotic and dizygotic twins: genetics, epigenetics, and environment. Gastroenterology 2004;127(2):485–92.
10. Mells GF, Kaser A, Karlsen TH. Novel insights into autoimmune liver diseases provided by genome-wide association studies. J Autoimmun 2013;46:41–54.
11. Hirschfield GM, Liu X, Xu C, et al. Primary biliary cirrhosis associated with HLA, IL12A, and IL12RB2 variants. N Engl J Med 2009;360(24):2544–55.
12. Hirschfield GM, Liu X, Han Y, et al. Variants at IRF5-TNPO3, 17q12-21 and MMEL1 are associated with primary biliary cirrhosis. Nat Genet 2010;42:655. https://doi.org/10.1038/ng.631.
13. Liu X, Invernizzi P, Lu Y, et al. Genome-wide meta-analyses identify three loci associated with primary biliary cirrhosis. Nat Genet 2010;42(8):658–60.
14. Mells GF, Floyd JAB, Morley KI, et al. Genome-wide association study identifies 12 new susceptibility loci for primary biliary cirrhosis. Nat Genet 2011;43:329.

15. Nakamura M, Nishida N, Kawashima M, et al. Genome-wide association study identifies TNFSF15 and POU2AF1 as susceptibility loci for primary biliary cirrhosis in the Japanese population. Am J Hum Genet 2012;91(4):721–8.
16. Qiu F, Tang R, Zuo X, et al. A genome-wide association study identifies six novel risk loci for primary biliary cholangitis. Nat Commun 2017;14828. https://doi.org/10.1038/ncomms14828.
17. Juran BD, Hirschfield GM, Invernizzi P, et al. Immunochip analyses identify a novel risk locus for primary biliary cirrhosis at 13q14, multiple independent associations at four established risk loci and epistasis between 1p31 and 7q32 risk Variants. Hum Mol Genet 2012;21(23):5209–21.
18. Liu JZ, Almarri MA, Gaffney DJ, et al. Dense fine-mapping study identifies new susceptibility loci for primary biliary cirrhosis. Nat Genet 2012;44:1137. https://doi.org/10.1038/ng.2395.
19. Cordell HJ, Han Y, Mells GF, et al. International genome-wide meta-analysis identifies new primary biliary cirrhosis risk loci and targetable pathogenic pathways. Nat Commun 2015;6:8019. https://doi.org/10.1038/ncomms9019.
20. Dendrou CA, Petersen J, Rossjohn J, et al. HLA variation and disease. Nat Rev Immunol 2018;18(5):325–39.
21. Dendrou CA, Petersen J, Rossjohn J, et al. HLA variation and disease. Nat Rev Immunol 2018;18:325. https://doi.org/10.1038/nri.2017.143.
22. Alvarez F, Berg PA, Bianchi FB, et al. International autoimmune hepatitis group report: review of criteria for diagnosis of autoimmune hepatitis. J Hepatol 1999; 31(5):929–38.
23. Fasano A, Catassi C. Celiac disease. N Engl J Med 2012;367(25):2419–26.
24. Mells GF, Hirschfield GM. Genetics of primary biliary cirrhosis. eLS 2013. https://doi.org/10.1002/9780470015902.a0024406.
25. Gerussi A, Carbone M, Corpechot C, et al. The genetic architecture of primary biliary cholangitis. Eur J Med Genet 2021;64(9):104292.
26. Manolio TA, Collins FS, Cox NJ, et al. Finding the missing heritability of complex diseases. Nature 2009;461(7265):747–53.
27. Tang R, Chen H, Miao Q, et al. The cumulative effects of known susceptibility variants to predict primary biliary cirrhosis risk. Genes Immun 2015;16:193. https://doi.org/10.1038/gene.2014.76.
28. Yang J, Benyamin B, McEvoy BP, et al. Common SNPs explain a large proportion of the heritability for human height. Nat Genet 2010;42(7):565–9.
29. Pritchard JK. Are rare variants responsible for susceptibility to complex diseases? Am J Hum Genet 2001;69(1):124–37.
30. Tam V, Patel N, Turcotte M, et al. Benefits and limitations of genome-wide association studies. Nat Rev Genet 2019;20(8):467–84.
31. Turro E, Astle WJ, Megy K, et al. Whole-genome sequencing of patients with rare diseases in a national health system. Nature 2020;583(July). https://doi.org/10.1038/s41586-020-2434-2.
32. Thaventhiran JED, Lango Allen H, Burren OS, et al. Whole-genome sequencing of a sporadic primary immunodeficiency cohort. Nature 2020. https://doi.org/10.1038/s41586-020-2265-1.
33. Li Y, Liu X, Wang Y, et al. Novel HLA-DRB1 alleles contribute risk for disease susceptibility in primary biliary cholangitis. Dig Liver Dis Off J Ital Soc Gastroenterol Ital Assoc Study Liver 2022;54(2):228–36.
34. Wang L, Li J, Wang C, et al. Mapping of de novo mutations in primary biliary cholangitis to a disease-specific co-expression network underlying homeostasis and metabolism. J Genet Genomics 2021. https://doi.org/10.1016/j.jgg.2021.07.019.

35. Invernizzi P, Miozzo M, Battezzati PM, et al. Frequency of monosomy X in women with primary biliary cirrhosis. Lancet 2004;363(9408):533–5.
36. Asselta R, Paraboschi EM, Gerussi A, et al. X chromosome contribution to the genetic architecture of primary biliary cholangitis. Gastroenterology 2021;2483–95.
37. Kukurba KR, Parsana P, Balliu B, et al. Impact of the X chromosome and sex on regulatory variation. Genome Res 2016;26(6):768–77.
38. Chang D, Gao F, Slavney A, et al. Accounting for eXentricities: analysis of the X Chromosome in GWAS reveals X-linked genes implicated in autoimmune diseases. PLoS One 2014;9(12):1–31.
39. Deng X, Berletch JB, Nguyen DK, et al. X chromosome regulation: Diverse patterns in development, tissues and disease. Nat Rev Genet 2014;15(6):367–78.
40. Tukiainen T, Villani A-C, Yen A, et al. Landscape of X chromosome inactivation across human tissues. Nature 2017;550:244. https://doi.org/10.1038/nature24265.
41. Scofield RH, Bruner GR, Namjou B, et al. Klinefelter's syndrome (47,XXY) in male systemic lupus erythematosus patients: support for the notion of a gene-dose effect from the X chromosome. Arthritis Rheum 2008;58(8):2511–7.
42. Lu Q, Wu A, Tesmer L, et al. Demethylation of CD40LG on the inactive X in T cells from women with lupus. J Immunol 2007;179(9):6352 LP–6358.
43. Hewagama A, Gorelik G, Patel D, et al. Overexpression of X-linked genes in T cells from women with lupus. J Autoimmun 2013;41:60–71.
44. Souyris M, Cenac C, Azar P, et al. TLR7 escapes X chromosome inactivation in immune cells. Sci Immunol 2018;3(19). https://doi.org/10.1126/sciimmunol.aap8855.
45. Sybert VP, Mccauley E. Turner's syndrome. N Engl J Med 2004;1227–38.
46. Lleo A, Moroni L, Caliari L, et al. Autoimmunity and Turner's syndrome. Autoimmun Rev 2012;11(6–7):A538–43.
47. Libert C, Dejager L, Pinheiro I. The X chromosome in immune functions: when a chromosome makes the difference. Nat Rev Immunol 2010;10(8):594–604.
48. Invernizzi P, Miozzo M, Selmi C, et al. X chromosome monosomy: a common Mechanism for autoimmune diseases. J Immunol 2005;175(1):575–8.
49. Zuk O, Hechter E, Sunyaev SR, et al. The mystery of missing heritability: genetic interactions create phantom heritability. Proc Natl Acad Sci 2012;109(4):1193–8.
50. Wray NR, Wijmenga C, Sullivan PF, et al. Common disease is more complex than Implied by the Core gene Omnigenic model. Cell 2018;173(7):1573–80.
51. Gregersen JW, Kranc KR, Ke X, et al. Functional epistasis on a common MHC haplotype associated with multiple sclerosis. Nature 2006;443(7111):574–7.
52. Lenz TL, Deutsch AJ, Han B, et al. Widespread non-additive and interaction effects within HLA loci modulate the risk of autoimmune diseases. Nat Genet 2015;47(9):1085–90.
53. Hivert V, Sidorenko J, Rohart F, et al. Estimation of non-additive genetic variance in human complex traits from a large sample of unrelated individuals. Am J Hum Genet 2021;108(5):786–98.
54. Phillips PC. Epistasis - the essential role of gene interactions in the structure and evolution of genetic systems. Nat Rev Genet 2008;9(11):855–67.
55. Sadee W, Hartmann K, Seweryn M, et al. Missing heritability of common diseases and treatments outside the protein-coding exome. Hum Genet 2014;133(10):1199–215.
56. Hirschfield GM, Gershwin ME, Strauss R, et al. Ustekinumab for patients with primary biliary cholangitis who have an inadequate response to ursodeoxycholic acid: a proof-of-concept study. Hepatology 2016;64(1):189–99.

57. Cano-Gamez E, Trynka G. From GWAS to function: using functional genomics to identify the Mechanisms underlying complex diseases. Front Genet 2020;1–21.

58. Claussnitzer M, Dankel SN, Kim K-H, et al. FTO obesity variant circuitry and adipocyte Browning in Humans. N Engl J Med 2015;373(10):895–907.

59. Boix CA, James BT, Park YP, et al. Regulatory genomic circuitry of human disease loci by integrative epigenomics. Nature 2021;590. https://doi.org/10.1038/s41586-020-03145-z.

60. Bowlus CL, Yang G-X, Liu CH, et al. Therapeutic trials of biologics in primary biliary cholangitis: an open label study of abatacept and review of the literature. J Autoimmun 2019;101:26–34. https://doi.org/10.1016/j.jaut.2019.04.005.

61. Nevens F, Andreone P, Mazzella G, et al. A Placebo-controlled trial of obeticholic acid in primary biliary cholangitis. N Engl J Med 2016;375(7):631–43.

62. Lammers WJ, Van Buuren HR, Hirschfield GM, et al. Levels of alkaline phosphatase and bilirubin are surrogate end points of outcomes of patients with primary biliary cirrhosis: an international follow-up study. Gastroenterology 2014;147(6):1338–49.e5.

63. Carbone M, Sharp SJ, Flack S, et al. The UK-PBC risk scores: Derivation and validation of a scoring system for long-term prediction of end-stage liver disease in primary biliary cholangitis. Hepatology 2016;63(3):930–50.

64. Gerussi A, Bernasconi DP, O'Donnell SE, et al. Measurement of Gamma Glutamyl Transferase to determine risk of liver transplantation or Death in patients with primary biliary cholangitis. Clin Gastroenterol Hepatol 2020. https://doi.org/10.1016/j.cgh.2020.08.006.

65. Carbone M, Mells GF, Pells G, et al. Sex and age are determinants of the clinical phenotype of primary biliary cirrhosis and response to ursodeoxycholic acid. Gastroenterology 2013;144(3):560–9.

66. Bianco C, Jamialahmadi O, Pelusi S, et al. Non-invasive stratification of hepatocellular carcinoma risk in non-alcoholic fatty liver using polygenic risk scores. J Hepatol 2020;1–8. https://doi.org/10.1016/j.jhep.2020.11.024.

67. Carbone M, Mells GF, Alexander GJ, et al. Calcineurin inhibitors and the IL12A locus influence risk of recurrent primary biliary cirrhosis after liver transplantation. Am J Transpl Off J Am Soc Transpl Am Soc Transpl Surg 2013;13(4):1110–1.

68. Cordell HJ, Fryett JJ, Ueno K, et al. An international genome-wide meta-analysis of primary biliary cholangitis: novel risk loci and candidate drugs. J Hepatol 2021. https://doi.org/10.1016/j.jhep.2021.04.055.

Immunologic Responses and the Pathophysiology of Primary Biliary Cholangitis

Ruiling Chen, PhD[a], Ruqi Tang, PhD[a], Xiong Ma, MD[a,*],
M. Eric Gershwin, MD[b,*]

KEYWORDS

- Immune tolerance • Biliary epithelial cell • Apoptosis • Senescence • Bile acids
- X chromosome • Microbiome

KEY POINTS

- Selective destruction of small bile ducts is mediated by multilineage immune responses with the loss of immune tolerance to the E2 component of pyruvate dehydrogenase complex (PDC-E2).
- Biliary epithelial cells (BECs) act not only as passive targets undergoing apoptosis, followed by the presentation of immunologically intact autoantigen PDC-E2 recognized by antimitochondrial antibodies, but also as active participants undergoing senescence to recruit immune cells.
- Destruction of the protective bicarbonate-rich umbrella is attributed to the decreased expression of membrane transporters in BECs, leading to the accumulation of hydrophobic bile acids and sensitizing BECs to apoptosis.
- A recent X-wide association study reveals a novel risk locus on the X chromosome, which reiterates the importance of Treg cells. Epigenetic alterations of the X chromosome may be helpful for filling the missing heritability gap and unraveling the biology of female predisposition.
- Emerging data on compositional and functional changes of the microbiome highlight a close relationship between the microbiome and primary biliary cholangitis.

[a] Division of Gastroenterology and Hepatology, Key Laboratory of Gastroenterology and Hepatology, Ministry of Health, State Key Laboratory for Oncogenes and Related Genes, Renji Hospital, School of Medicine, Shanghai JiaoTong University, Shanghai Institute of Digestive Disease, 145 Middle Shandong Road, Shanghai, China; [b] Division of Rheumatology-Allergy and Clinical Immunology, University of California at Davis, 451 Health Sciences Drive, Suite 6510, Davis, CA 95616, USA
* Corresponding authors.
E-mail addresses: maxiongmd@hotmail.com (X.M.); megershwin@ucdavis.edu (M.E.G.)

Clin Liver Dis 26 (2022) 583–611
https://doi.org/10.1016/j.cld.2022.06.003
1089-3261/22/© 2022 Elsevier Inc. All rights reserved.

liver.theclinics.com

INTRODUCTION

Primary biliary cholangitis (PBC) is an autoimmune liver disease with a striking female predisposition and selective destruction of intrahepatic small bile ducts leading to nonsuppurative destructive cholangitis.[1–3] It is characterized by seropositivity of anti-mitochondrial antibodies (AMAs) or PBC-specific antinuclear antibodies (ANAs), progressive cholestasis, and typical liver histologic manifestations.[4] PBC was originally termed "primary biliary cirrhosis," and the histologic manifestations in the liver can progress through lymphocytic cholangitis to progressive ductopenia, cholestasis and biliary cirrhosis if left untreated.[5,6] There are only two licensed agents for PBC treatment, namely, ursodeoxycholic acid (UDCA) and obeticholic acid (OCA).[7,8] Both of these drugs are choleretics that can efficiently ameliorate cholestasis.

The major immunodominant mitochondrial antigen is well defined and identified as the E2 component of pyruvate dehydrogenase complex (PDC-E2), which is located on the inner membrane of mitochondria. Despite the ubiquitous nature of mitochondria, the selective destruction of small bile ducts is mediated by multilineage immune responses with the loss of immune tolerance to PDC-E2. Cholangiocytes act not only as passive targets undergoing apoptosis, followed by the presentation of immunologically intact autoantigen PDC-E2 recognized by AMAs, but also as active participants undergoing senescence to recruit immune cells. Destruction of the protective bicarbonate-rich umbrella is attributed to the decreased expression of membrane transporters in biliary epithelial cells (BECs) thus leading to the accumulation of hydrophobic bile acids and sensitizing BECs to apoptosis. Genome-wide association studies demonstrate several important immunoregulatory pathways, key among them being IL-12 and IFN-γ, whereas a recent X-wide association study (XWAS) reveals a novel risk locus on the X chromosome, which reiterates the importance of Treg cells. Emerging data on compositional and functional changes of the microbiome have highlighted a close relationship between microbiome and PBC despite hitherto only limited data being available on the molecular mechanisms. Targeting the gut–liver–immune axis has overwhelmingly emerged as a prospective treatment strategy in PBC. Epigenetic alterations of the X chromosome may be helpful for filling the missing heritability gap and illuminating the biology of female predisposition.

A widely accepted consensus about PBC etiopathogenesis is that multiple factors mutually interact and synergistically promote the initiation and progression of PBC.[9–13] In this review, we aim to overview our current understanding of the immunology and pathophysiology in the initiation and progression of PBC with an ultimate aim of improving clinical therapies (**Fig. 1**).

AUTOANTIBODY
Antimitochondrial Antibodies

PBC is considered an archetypal autoimmune disease with regard to a striking female predisposition and well-defined autoantigens. AMA is highly specific and detected in the sera in up to 95% of PBC patients, which was first reported in 1965.[14] A landmark article by Gershwin in 1987 reported the identification and cloning of the major AMA target antigen, PDC-E2.[15] Increasing evidence confirms that AMAs react against conserved autoantigens that belong to 2-oxoacid dehydrogenase complexes (2-OADCs) of the oxidative phosphorylation pathway and are located on the inner membrane of mitochondria, including PDC-E2, the E2 subunit of the 2-oxoglutarate dehydrogenase complex (OGDC-E2), the E2 subunit of the branched-chain 2-oxoacid dehydrogenase complex (BCOADC-E2) and the E3-binding protein (E3BP).[16–18] Intriguingly, one theme in common among these mitochondrial antigens is the

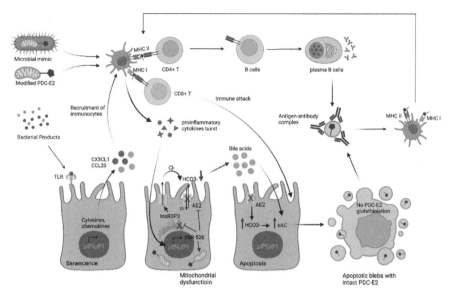

Fig. 1. Immunology and pathophysiology of PBC. Exposures to a microbial mimic or PDC-E2 modified by xenobiotics leads to production of AMAs and multilineage immune responses targeting BECs. Bacterial products from portal circulation activate BECs via TLRs and facilitate the production of cytokines and chemokines in BECs, including CX3CL1 and CCL20, which further promote the migration and recruitment of immunocytes. APCs produce a burst of proinflammatory cytokines in the coexistence of AMAs and BEC apotopes, which upregulate the expression of miR-506 in BECs, leading to a reduction of AE2 and InsP$_3$R$_3$, and mitochondrial dysfunction. Destruction of protective bicarbonate-rich umbrella leads to accumulation of hydrophobic bile acids and sensitizes BECs to apoptosis. The immunologically intact PDC-E2 without glutathiolation exists in apoptotic blebs, which can be recognized and targeted by circulating AMAs. The antigen–antibody complexes further facilitate dysregulated immune responses, contributing to perpetual biliary inflammation, progressive cholestasis, and biliary cirrhosis.

covalent attachment of lipoic acid cofactors to the lysine residue at position 173.[19,20] All these immunodominant epitopes contain a highly conserved sequence motif that is essential for antigen recognition.[21] Epitope-mapping studies of AMAs were performed; the epitope for autoreactive CD4 T, CD8 T and B cells contained lipoylated lysine. The PDC-E2-specific autoreactive CD4 and CD8 T cells are extensively enriched in the liver and hilar lymph nodes as compared with peripheral blood.[22,23]

Several established spontaneous or inducible PBC murine models have been reported to recapitulate the phenotypes of human PBC, especially the characteristic presence of AMA-targeting PDC-E2.[24,25] Hitherto the most commonly used PBC model is the dominant negative TGF-β receptor II (dnTGFβRII) mice, with an overexpression of a dominant negative form of TGF-β receptor II under the control of the CD4 promoter, causing almost complete abolition of TGF-β signaling.[26] This model provides a platform on which numerous functional and mechanistic studies on PBC pathogenesis are based.[27–29] AMAs are not pathogenic *per se* but a burst of proinflammatory cytokines may be evoked in the coexistence of AMAs, such as BEC apotopes and macrophages from PBC patients.[30]

Antinuclear Antibodies

Although ANAs are commonly found in many autoimmune diseases, including systemic lupus erythematosus, PBC-specific ANAs are identified and have diagnostic and prognostic values in PBC.[31] About 50% of PBC patients have seropositivity of ANAs, and up to 85% of AMA-negative PBC patients have positive detection of ANAs in serum.[32,33] As shown by indirect immunofluorescence, a nuclear rim pattern is identified by ANAs directed at glycoprotein 210 (gp210) and nucleoporin 62 (p62), which are located in the nuclear pore complex, and a multinuclear dot pattern is identified by ANAs directed against nuclear body proteins including speckled 100 kDa (sp100) promyelocytic leukemia (PML) cells and sp140.[34-38] Another PBC-specific ANA is identified to target centromeric proteins (CENPs).[39] Approximately 20% of AMA-negative PBC patients have positive detection of serum ANAs targeting gp210 or sp100.[32] The seropositivity of anti-gp210 and anti-sp100 antibodies is helpful for the diagnosis of PBC whereas the seropositivity of anti-CENP antibody is not listed as a diagnostic criterion of PBC.[3] The positive detection of anti-gp210 and anti-CENP antibodies appears associated with disease progression and worse prognosis.[40] However, the generation of PBC-specific nuclear antigens and the potential pathogenic roles of ANAs remain to be further investigated.

BILIARY EPITHELIAL CELL
Passive Target and Apoptosis

Despite accounting for only 5% of the total liver cell mass, cholangiocytes possess crucial physiologic functions and are involved in diverse pathologic states of bile ducts.[41,42] Once under exposure of stimuli, quiescent cholangiocytes become activated and gain the ability to proliferate in order to compensate for the anatomic loss of biliary cells as well as sustain the secretory functions.[43] Apoptosis of cholangiocytes gradually becomes prevalent accompanied by the decrease of cell proliferation as diseases progress. As a result, the development of ductopenia occurs when apoptotic events prevail on proliferation.[44]

Apoptosis is a basic biological phenomenon occurring in cells, and clearance of apoptotic cells is normally under a tight regulation of the immune system. However, impairment in the clearance of apoptotic cell debris is deemed to cause the development of autoimmunity.[45] Apoptosis and formation of apoptotic blebs are considered essential events in the initiation and progression of PBC.[30,46,47] Increased apoptosis as evidenced by the occurrence of DNA fragmentation is observed in cholangiocytes from PBC patients as compared with healthy controls.[48] A higher expression of death receptor 5 is found in BECs from PBC patients.[49] Treatment of an agonistic antibody targeting death receptor 5 significantly induces apoptosis of cholangiocytes, cholangitis, and cholestasis, which indicates the important role of apoptosis in mediating cholestatic liver injury.[49]

Generally, mitochondrial PDC-E2 is modified by covalent binding of glutathione in apoptotic cells. However, this modification disappears in PBC and the immunologically intact PDC-E2 with the attachment of lipoic acid exists in apoptotic blebs, which can be recognized and targeted by circulating AMAs.[30] As a result, the antigen–antibody complexes further promote the activation of immune responses and apoptosis of cholangiocytes, leading to unremitting inflammation. Despite the ubiquitous existence of mitochondria in all cells, the selective damage of small bile ducts is a unique phenomenon in PBC, which is consistent with the observation of intense and PBC-specific staining at the apical surface of small bile ducts using monoclonal antibodies against PDC-E2.[50,51] This observation firmly supports the mainstream hypothesis that the excessive immune responses targeting BECs with the loss of tolerance to PDC-E2 is the central culprit of PBC pathogenesis.

Active Participant and Senescence

BECs are more than simply innocent victims but also actively participate in disease progression or resolution in response to stimuli. Cholangiocytes are heterogenous in response to stimuli with a subpopulation acquiring a proliferative phenotype reflected as ductular reaction and another subpopulation undergoing senescence characterized by permanent cell cycle arrest.[52] Other hallmarks of cellular senescence include resistance to apoptosis, hypersecretion of proinflammatory and profibrotic molecules, and attaining the senescence-associated secretory phenotype (SASP).[53] The current view is that cholangiocyte senescence exerts a deleterious role in immune-mediated cholangiopathies by mediating inflammation and recruitment of immune cells.[53,54]

Senescent cholangiocytes are found to accumulate in the damaged bile ducts in PBC livers, but they exhibit senescence-associated secretory phenotypes releasing inflammatory chemokines, including CX3CL1, CCL20, IL6, and interferons.[55,56] Of note, the secretion amounts of cytokines in BECs are comparable between PBC patients and non-PBC patients whereas BECs from PBC patients produce more amount of CX3CL1 as compared with non-PBC patients.[57,58] In PBC livers, increased expression of CX3CL1 is observed in the injured BECs whereas increased expression of CX3CR1 is observed in both monocytes located in the portal tracts and intraepithelial lymphocytes situated in injured bile ducts.[59] Intriguingly, the elevated serum level of CX3CL1 coexists with the increased expression of CX3CR1 in liver infiltrating mononuclear cells in PBC patients.[59] It is indicated that the high production of CX3CL1 in BECs is responsible for the migration and recruitment of liver-infiltrating monocytes and lymphocytes that express their corresponding receptor CX3CR1 into portal tracts and biliary epithelia. Higher expressions of CCL20 and its receptor CCR6 are observed in PBC livers particularly around the inflamed bile ducts, responsible for the infiltration of pathogenic Th17 in PBC livers.[60] Of note, *CCL20* gene is also identified as a susceptibility locus in PBC from a meta-analysis of genome-wide association studies.[61]

BECs express many surface proteins allowing their direct interaction with immune cells. In response to stimuli, BECs can act as antigen-presenting cells (APC) by upregulating the expression of major histocompatibility complex (MHC) class I and II, CD80, CD86 and CD40.[62] For example, BECs are demonstrated to increase membrane expression of HLA-DR and CD40 in culture with hydrophobic bile acid glycochenodeoxycholic acid.[63] The interaction between BECs and T cells further amplifies the immune responses and promotes the disease progression.[64,65] Besides, the phagocytic function of BECs acting as APC to remove apoptopes is impaired, leading to the accumulation of apoptotic cells and concomitant peribiliary inflammation.[66] BECs also interact with NKT cells by expressing CD1d, and mucosal-associated invariant T (MAIT) cells by expressing class I-related molecule (MR1).[67,68]

In conclusion, BECs *per se* also actively participate in immune responses targeting BECs, mainly through undergoing senescence or interaction with other immune cells, which promotes the development of chronic peribiliary inflammation in PBC.

Cytotoxic Bile Acids

The important physiologic function of cholangiocytes is to secret bicarbonate into bile via the involvement of membrane transporters to modify bile volume and composition. There are various transporters located on the apical and basolateral membrane of cholangiocytes, whose functional impairment could contribute to a pathologic state, namely cholestasis.[69] Under normal conditions, secretin recognizes and binds to the secretin receptor (SR) on the basolateral membrane of cholangiocytes, and then induces the generation of adenosine 3',5'-cyclic monophosphate (cAMP) and protein kinase A (PKA), followed by the PKA-dependent phosphorylation of the cystic fibrosis transmembrane conductance regulator (CFTR) that is located on the apical membrane of cholangiocytes. CFTR is responsible for the excretion of Cl^- into the lumen of bile ducts to form a Cl^- concentration gradient across plasma membrane, which subsequently activates another apical membrane transporter, the $Cl^-/HCO3^-$ exchanger (AE2), and ultimately causes a net excretion of bicarbonate into the bile along with passive efflux of water.[44,69] Secreted bicarbonate acting as an alkaline barrier, deprotonates apolar hydrophobic bile acids, preventing their transmembrane permeability into BECs.[70] Protonated hydrophobic bile acids can directly enter BECs without transporters, inducing cell apoptosis.[70] Therefore, BECs are considered to functionally form a membrane-protective bicarbonate-rich umbrella in the lumen of bile ducts. The intracellular pH homeostasis of cholangiocytes is under the tight regulation of AE2 as well.[71,72]

In PBC patients, decreased expression and activity of AE2 in BECs have been demonstrated as also the impairment in secretin-induced biliary secretion of bicarbonate.[70,71,73,74] Hydrophobic bile acids inhibit AE2 expression via the induction of reactive oxygen species.[63] Reduction of AE2 activates intracellular soluble adenylyl cyclase (sAC), which is a conserved intracellular bicarbonate sensor and mediated by intrinsic apoptotic pathway. Thus it sensitizes human BECs to bile salt-induced apoptosis.[71,75] Intriguingly, UDCA restores the secretin-induced choleresis and upregulates AE2 expression in combination with steroids.[73,76] It is known that UDCA is a choleretic bile acid licensed for PBC treatment by supporting the important role of bile composition in PBC pathogenesis.[77,78]

Gene knockout murine models were subsequently established to further explore PBC pathogenesis. Most AE2a,b−/− mice develop AMAs, cholestasis, and portal inflammation with infiltration of immune cells surrounding inflamed bile ducts resembling human PBC.[79] Destruction of the bicarbonate-rich umbrella is also observed in cystic fibrosis, which is a monogenic disease caused by a defect of CFTR in BECs.[80,81] Mouse with CFTR deficiency is an accepted PSC murine model without a PBC-like immune phenotype.[25]

Increasing evidence suggests that immune-mediated BEC injury occurs early in PBC concurrent with an impairment of physiologic functions of BECs, leading to progressive cholestasis.[82] Destruction of the protective bicarbonate-rich umbrella is attributed to decreased expression of membrane transporters in BECs, leading to accumulation of hydrophobic bile acids and sensitizing BECs to apoptosis. BECs act not only as passive targets undergoing apoptosis followed by the presentation of immunologically intact autoantigen PDC-E2 recognized by AMAs but also active participants undergoing senescence to recruit immune cells. Immune-mediated BEC injury and bile acid-mediated BEC injury reflect a triangular relationship between immunity, BECs, and cholestasis, leading to progressive and perpetual biliary inflammation and eventually cirrhosis.[4] (**Fig. 2**) The current controversy is that whether PBC is initially triggered by a defect of the biliary bicarbonate umbrella, challenging the hypothesis that the breakdown of biliary homeostasis is secondary to immune dysregulation. Based on current observations and understandings, the answer to this question requires more data.

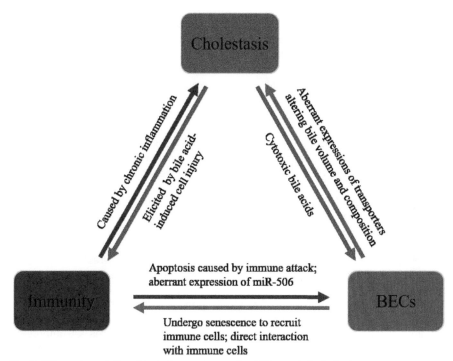

Fig. 2. Triangular relationship between immunity, BECs, and cholestasis.

ABERRANT IMMUNOREGULATION
Adaptive Immunity

The involvement of adaptive immunity has long been investigated in PBC pathogenesis, given that antigen-specific autoreactive CD4 and CD8 T cells are extensively enriched in the portal tracts of PBC livers.[83] The chemokine receptors, such as CX3CR1, CXCR3, and CCR6, are highly expressed in PBC livers and responsible for T cell trafficking and differentiation.[60,84] Notably, CCR6 was recently identified as a novel PBC risk gene from an international genome-wide meta-analysis.[85] CD8+ T cells enriched in portal tracts of PBC livers are believed to play an important role in selective biliary destruction in both human PBC and murine models.[28,86,87] Increasing evidence confirms the participation of different T cell subpopulations in PBC pathogenesis, including Th1, Th17, regulatory T cells (Treg), follicular helper T (Tfh) cells, and follicular regulatory T (Tfr) cells.

Proinflammatory Th1 and Th17 subsets are pathogenic and accumulated in the damaged interlobular bile ducts of PBC livers.[88] It has been demonstrated that the immune pattern skews from IL12-dominated Th1 signaling toward IL23-dominated Th17 signaling in advanced PBC patients.[89] Reduction of immunoregulatory Treg is demonstrated in both peripheral blood and liver of PBC patients explaining for the loss of self-tolerance.[90,91] Besides, Treg cells from PBC patients show an increased sensitivity to a low dose of IL-12, driving their differentiation into IFN-γ secreting cells as compared with that from PSC patients and healthy controls.[92] In isolated liver mononuclear cells, a significantly higher proportion of IL-12Rβ2+ Treg cells was detected.[92] This observation indicates the importance of the IL12- IL-12Rβ2-STAT4 pathway in PBC pathogenesis. Tfh and Tfr cells are critical for the development and maintenance of the geminal center. Tfh cells interact with B cells to facilitate their maturation and antibody production, which is regulated by Tfr cells.[93] The enrichment of Tfh cells is observed in circulation and the liver of PBC patients.[94,95] The circulating Tfr/Tfh ratio is demonstrated to be dramatically decreased in PBC as compared with healthy controls and negatively associated with serum IgM level.[96] However, whether Tfr cells' role in PBC requires further investigations.[97]

Innate Immunity

PBC is mediated by excessive multilineage immune responses specifically targeting BECs. Innate immune responses are increasingly considered active participants in PBC pathogenesis and not simply because of the presence of granuloma and polyclonal IgM.[98]

Macrophages from PBC patients cultured with BEC apotopes in the presence of AMAs could produce overwhelming proinflammatory cytokines, including IL12, and upregulate their expression of tumor necrosis factor-related apoptosis-inducing ligand (TRAIL).[30,99] This observation indicates the potential roles of macrophages in the process of immune-mediated BECs injury.[100] Chemokines released by BECs are responsible for the infiltration of monocytes and macrophages expressing corresponding receptors in PBC livers, including chemokine (C-C motif) receptor 2 (CCR2) recognized by chemokine (C-C motif) ligand 2 (CCL2), and CX3CR1 recognized by CX3CL1.[56,58,101,102] In a 2-octynoic acid-bovine serum albumin (2OA-BSA)-immunized PBC murine model, liver inflammation and fibrosis are improved by knockout of CCR2 gene, or treatment with cenicriviroc, a CCR2/CCR5 antagonist.[103] Notably, this compound has been investigated in a clinical trial (NCT02653625) in primary sclerosing cholangitis (PSC).[104] However, no expected benefits are observed. A recent study demonstrates that IL-23 produced by hepatic monocyte-derived macrophages is responsible for liver inflammation in 2OA-BSA-immunized mice.[105] The underlying mechanisms of monocytes and macrophages in PBC pathogenesis still remain unclear and require further investigations.

Myeloid-derived suppressor cells (MDSC) are significantly expanded in both peripheral blood and liver of PBC patients. The frequency of circulating MDSCs is positively correlated with serum alkaline phosphatase (ALP) and total bilirubin levels and are upregulated in UDCA-responding PBC patients.[106] Elevated expression of CCN1 is detected in the portal tracts of PBC livers as compared with healthy controls and is responsible for the expansion and immunosuppressive function of MDSCs.[106]

Natural killer (NK) cells account for approximately 30% of hepatic lymphocytes, actively participating in the innate responses in liver. Generally, NK cells distinguish self from nonself through expressing inhibitory receptors that recognize MHC class I molecules present on autologous cells.[107] NK cells are enriched in the portal tracts in PBC as compared with disease controls and healthy controls, and hepatic NK cells from PBC patients possess enhanced cytotoxic activity against autologous BECs upon stimulation.[108] At a high NK/BEC ratio, NK cells isolated from PBC livers attack autologous BECs and the release of autoantigen further activates autoreactive T cells in the presence of APCs. In contrast, at a low NK/BEC ratio, IFN-γ is secreted from NK cells and upregulates expression of MHC I and MHC II molecules on BECs to protect them from attack by NK cells. Autologous BECs are subsequently targeted by cytopathic autoreactive T cells that are exposed to IFN-γ.[109] Circulating NK cells from PBC patients are sensitive to a low dose of IL-12, inducing a significant upregulation of liver-homing marker CXCR6, as compared with that from disease controls and healthy controls.[110] These observations indicate that NK cells may play an essential role in the initiation and progression of PBC.

MAIT cells are a subset of innatelike T cells expressing a semi-invariant T cell receptor (TCR) and restricted by MR1, which presents bacterial vitamin B metabolites. MAIT cells can be activated in an antigen-dependent or independent way and produce proinflammatory cytokines.[111,112] The roles of MAIT cells in the liver are believed to be bidirectional, that is, protective in antimicrobial immunity and deleterious in chronic peribiliary inflammation.[113] Circulating MAIT cells are reduced in PBC patients as compared with healthy controls with aberrant function of cytokine production.[114,115] In contrast, MAIT cells accumulate in PBC livers possibly through CXCL12-CXCR4-mediated chemotaxis.[116] Whether and how MAIT cells participate in the pathogenesis of PBC remain unclear.[117]

In conclusion, the immune responses involve multilineage cells in both human and murine models, which is complicated but essential in the pathogenesis of PBC. Therefore, immunomodulation remains a potential treatment target for PBC.[118]

GENETIC SUSCEPTIBILITY

The phenomena of familial clustering and high concordance rate in monozygotic twins emphasize the importance of genetic susceptibility.[119,120] At present, the genome-wide association study (GWAS) provides great benefits for our better understanding of the genetic architecture of PBC.[121] Indeed, genetic variants play an important but not deterministic role in the development of PBC, principally by modulating important biologic processes. Until now, several GWAS and meta-analyses of PBC have been performed in individuals from Europe, North America, Japan and China.[61,85,122–129] HLA loci show the strongest association with PBC, concurrent with more than 40 non-HLA risk loci identified at a genome-wide level of significance.[121] Twenty novel risk loci are revealed in a second international meta-analysis published recently pointing to a total of 22 genes.[85] According to pathway-based analysis, these identified risk loci, including both HLA and non-HLA loci, point to several immunoregulatory pathways, including antigen presentation and production of IL-12, activation of T cells and IFN-γ production, and activation of B cells and production of immunoglobulins.[121]

Existing insights underscore that IL-12 and IFN-γ are two key drivers of immune-mediated lymphocytic cholangitis, as evidenced by observations demonstrated in human and animal models. Enhanced expression of IL12 subunits, the cognate receptor IL12RB2 and IFN-γ are observed around damaged interlobular bile ducts in the portal tracts of PBC liver sections, as compared with hepatitis disease controls.[89] IL12p40 deficiency in dnTGFβRII mice (IL12p40(−/−) dnTGFβRII) demonstrates the dramatic amelioration of lymphocytic cholangitis and a significant reduction in cytokine production.[26,130] Chronic expression of IFN-γ drives murine autoimmune cholangitis resembling human PBC, particularly with a female predominance that was first demonstrated in murine models, highlighting the critical role of IFN-γ in PBC pathogenesis.[131]

In recent years, several studies on clinical transformation have been conducted based on genetic observations and functional investigations. A proof-of-concept phase II study examined the effect of a monoclonal antibody targeting IL12 and IL23, called ustekinumab, in PBC patients with an inadequate response to UDCA, which demonstrated no significant benefits.[132] Treatment with cytotoxic T lymphocyte antigen 4-immunoglobulin (CTLA-4-Ig) demonstrated significant therapeutic benefits in 2OA-BSA-immunized PBC model, as evidenced by the amelioration of autoimmune cholangitis.[133] Thereafter, an open-label trial was performed to test the effect of CTLA-4-Ig abatacept in PBC patients with an incomplete response to UDCA, which demonstrated no benefits in achieving biochemical responses.[134]

It is worth mentioning that no signals located on the X chromosome have been reported at a genome-wide level of significance in studies mentioned above. Actually, genetic alterations identified hitherto poorly explain for the female predominance in PBC. Given that much data on the X chromosome have been neglected in existing GWAS analyses, conducting an XWAS will be helpful not only for digging out novel risk loci but also for illuminating the biology of the female predisposition in autoimmune diseases.[135] A recent landmark article by Rosanna and his colleagues was the first to report the contribution of the X chromosome to the genetic architecture of PBC, unraveling a novel PBC-related genome-wide significant locus.[136] This polymorphism locus is characterized by the presence of 7 different genes and a superenhancer that targets all these genes as well as FOXP3. This work reiterates the importance of Treg cells in PBC pathogenesis. On that note, it is inevitable to mention scurfy mice, a well-known PBC-like murine model with a complete deficiency of Treg cells by Foxp3 gene mutation.[137] Of note, 100% of mice manifest disease features at 3 to 4 weeks of age and die by 4 weeks of age, showing no differences in sexes, which indicates that the complete abolition of Treg cells should be blamed for the unremitting and lethal inflammation. Besides, adoptive transfer of Foxp3+ Treg cells from wild-type mice to recombinant activating gene (Rag)1−/− recipients successfully ameliorates autoimmune cholangitis, as compared with that from dnTGFβRII mice.[138]

In conclusion, despite immense progress made in our understanding of the genetic architecture of PBC, the functional validations of these genetic variants require more efforts. Actually, these single nucleotide polymorphism loci identified in PBC are also reported in other autoimmune diseases, indicating that a genetic variant predisposing an individual to autoimmunity has pleiotropic effects.[121]

ENVIRONMENTAL TRIGGER
Molecular Mimicry and Xenobiotics

Several epidemiologic observations, including disease clustering and disparities in regional prevalence, prompt us to link environmental exposure to the occurrence of PBC. Epidemiologic studies have consistently reported that PBC has significant associations with a history of urinary tract infections (UTI), cigarette smoke, residence close to toxic waste sites, and use of nail polish. These exposure conditions as well as the proposed mechanisms have been robustly investigated so far.[139,140]

Molecular mimicry hypothesis suggests that cross-reactive molecular mimics are recognized by T and/or B cells, causing loss of self-tolerance to mitochondrial autoantigens PDC-E2 and subsequent autoimmunity.[141,142] PBC patients are reported to have a higher rate of incident and recurrent UTI and an increased frequency of bacteriuria as compared with controls, first linking bacteria to the risk of PBC.[143] In fact, the sequence motifs essential for antigen recognition by PDC-E2-specific T cells are highly conserved across species as evidenced by the strong cross-reactivity of PBC sera with PDC-E2 from Escherichia coli and Novosphingobium aromaticivorans.[144,145] PBC is associated with residence adjacent to toxic waste sites because of exposure to volatile organic compounds that are considered mimickers of lipoylated PBC autoantigens.[146,147] Risks of PBC are increased among individuals exposed to cigarette smoke, possibly due to the direct exposure to aromatic hydrocarbons acting as mimickers of autoantigens, or indirect influences by dysregulated immune responses.[148,149]

Xenobiotics are exogenous chemicals that can alter autologous proteins, having been investigated in PBC pathogenesis.[150] A frequent use of nail polish is associated with increased PBC susceptibility.[143] Further investigations demonstrate that 2-octy-noic acid (2OA) is abundantly present in cosmetics and food additives and show enhanced reactivity with PBC sera by modifying the inner lipoyl domain of PDC-E2.[151,152] Furthermore, 2OA-BSA-immunized murine models have established and reported to manifest a PBC-like phenotype characterized by the presence of serum AMAs and lymphocytic cholangitis.[153] 2-Nonyamide is another xenobiotic present in cosmetics possessing an optimal structure for the modification of PDC-E2 contributing to enhanced reactivity with PBC sera.[154] A common electrophilic agent acetaminophen is immunoreactive with AMAs by the electrophilic modification of lipoic acid in PDC-E2.[155,156] An ionic liquid 3-methyl-1-octyl-1H-imidazole-3-ium (M8OI), present at high levels in soils around landfill waste sites, can be metabolized by human hepatocytes into a carboxylic acid bearing structural similarity to lipoic acid.[157]

Microbiome

The microbiome has attracted increasing attentions in recent years.[158–160] It has been reported that the use of the oral antibiotic rifampin in PBC patients has therapeutic benefits for symptoms of pruritus, which supports the involvement of the microbiome in PBC pathogenesis.[161,162] Microbial compositional and functional changes have recently been described in PBC (**Table 1**). A cross-sectional study in China demonstrated alterations in the gut microbiome with a decrease in some potentially beneficial bacteria in early-stage PBC patients as compared with healthy controls.[163] Several altered bacterial taxa have associations with altered metabolism, immunity, and liver function indexes of PBC patients.[163] Our group further revealed a significant reduction of microbial diversity and alterations in 12 genera by comparing UDCA treatment-naïve PBC patients with matched healthy controls, which can be partially reverted by UDCA treatment.[164] Subsequently, our group analyzed the bile acid compositions in serum and feces, as well as the linkage between bile acids and gut microbiota.[165] Ratios of conjugated/unconjugated bile acids in both serum and feces are increased in treatment-naïve PBC as compared with controls, which can be reverted after UDCA treatment resulting from a decreased level of taurine-conjugated bile acids, concurrent with an increase of taurine-metabolizing bacteria *Bilophila spp.*[165] The level of serum secondary bile acids, which is lower in treatment-naïve PBC, is negatively correlated with PBC-enriched bacteria such as *Veillonella* and *Klebsiella*, and positively correlated with control-enriched bacteria such as *Faecalibacterium* and *Oscillospira*.[165] Our group then demonstrated beneficial effects of cholestyramine in icteric PBC patients as reflected by alterations in gut microbiota and metabolites.[166] A Japanese study analyzed the microbial composition in the mucosa of the terminal ileum, demonstrating a reduction in diversity and overgrowth of *Sphingomonadaceae* and *Pseudomonas* in PBC patients as compared with healthy controls.[167] Another Japanese study confirmed the lower bacterial diversity in PBC and demonstrated that the abundance of *Faecalibacterium* is significantly decreased in UDCA nonresponders, indicating its predictive potential in disease prognosis.[168] A study from an American group demonstrated higher levels of fecal acetate and short-chain fatty acids, as well as lower bacterial diversity in PBC patients with advanced fibrosis.[169] A recent study from China reported that serum total bilirubin level is associated with altered gut microbiota in PBC patients treated with UDCA for 12 months.[170]

Researchers also focus on exploring gut microbial profiles in murine models. Significant differences in gut microbiota are observed between NOD.c3c4 mice, which develop spontaneous biliary inflammation, and NOD control mice.[171] After rederivation, germ-free NOD.c3c4 mice exhibit a milder biliary affection as compared with conventionally raised NOD.c3c4 mice.[171] Intriguingly, another study demonstrates

Table 1
Studies of microbiome in PBC

Study	Country	Treatment	Cohort	Material	Method	Diversity	Increased Taxa in Disease Group	Decreased Taxa in Disease Group
Lv et al,[163] 2016	China	/	PBC (42) vs HC (30)	Stool	16S rRNA	NS	Proteobacteria, Enterobacteriaceae, Neisseriaceae, Spirochaetaceae, Veillonella, Streptococcus, Klebsiella, Actinobacillus, Anaeroglobus, Enterobacter, Haemophilus, Megasphaera, Paraprevotella	Acidobacteria, Lachnobacterium, Bacteroides and Ruminococcus
Tang et al,[164] 2018	China	Naïve	PBC (79) vs HC (114)	Stool	16S rRNA	↓	Hemophilus, Veillonella, Clostridium, Lactobacillus, Streptococcus, Pseudomonas, Klebsiella, Enterobacteriaceae	Oscillospira, Faecalibacterium, Sutterlla and Bacteroides
		UDCA for 6 mo	treatment-naïve PBC vs UDCA-treated PBC (37)	Stool	16S rRNA	NS	Bacteroidetes spp, Sutterella spp and Oscillospira sp	Haemophilus spp, Streptococcus spp and Pseudomonas spp
Abe et al,[212] 2018	Japan	/	PBC (39) vs HC (15)	Saliva	16S rRNA	/	Eubacterium and Veillonella	Fusobacterium

Study	Country	Treatment	Comparison	Sample	16S rRNA		
Hegade et al,[213] 2019	UK	Autotaxin for 2 wk	PBC with pruritus_2 wk (22) vs PBC with pruritus_baseline (31)	Stool	16S rRNA /	Clostridia, Clostridiales	Bacteroidia, Bacteroidales
Furukawa et al,[168] 2020	Japan	UDCA for over 12 mo	PBC (76) vs HC (23)	Stool	16S rRNA ↓	Lactobacillales	Clostridiales Faecalibacterium
			[a] non-responder (30) vs responder (43)	Stool	16S rRNA /	/	/
Liwinski et al,[214] 2020	Germany	/	PBC (99) vs HC (95)	Stool	16S rRNA ↓	Proteobacteria Bifidobacterium	Firmicutes Faecalibacterium
		/	PBC (99) vs AIH (72)	Stool	16S rRNA NS		
Lammert et al,[169] 2021	USA	UDCA	Advanced fibrosis PBC (8) vs non-advanced fibrosis PBC (15)	Stool	16S rRNA ↓	Weisella	/
Lv et al,[215] 2021	China	/	PBC (39) vs HC (37)	Saliva	16S rRNA ↓	Bacteroidetes, Campylobacter, Prevotella and Veillonella	Enterococcaceae, Granulicatella, Rothia and Streptococcus
Li et al,[166] 2021	China	Cholestyramine for 16 wk	[b]SR PBC_16 wk vs SR PBC_Baseline (14)	Stool	16S rRNA NS	Lachnospiraceae 3146FAA, Lachnospiraceae 1157FAA	Roseburia intestinalis
		Cholestyramine for 16 wk	[b]IR PBC_16 wk vs IR PBC_Baseline (14)	Stool	16S rRNA NS	Klebsiella pneumoniae /	/
Kitahata et al,[167] 2021	Japan	/	PBC (34) vs HC (21)	Mucosa	16S rRNA ↓	Sphingomonas, Pseudomonas, Methylobacterium, Carnobacterium, Acinetobacter, Curvibacter, and Clostridiaceae	Leptotrichia, Morganella, Lautropia, Mogibacterium, Atopobium, Bulleidia, Eikenella, Paludibacter, an unknown genus belonging to the class TM7_3, and F16.g

(continued on next page)

Table 1
(continued)

Study	Country	Treatment	Cohort	Material	Method	Diversity	Increased Taxa in Disease Group	Decreased Taxa in Disease Group
Han et al,[170] 2022	China	UDCA for 12 mo	[c]TB(+) PBC (20) vs TB(−) PBC (27)	Stool	16S rRNA	↓	/	Gemmiger, Blautia, Anaerostipes and Coprococcus genera, Holdemania

[a] PBC patients with UDCA treatment are divided into two different subgroups according to the Nara criteria (reduction rate of gamma-glutamyl transpeptidase ≥69% after 1 y).

[b] PBC patients are stratified according to the median decrease of bilirubin at 16 wk: group with superior remission of cholestasis (SR) and group with inferior remission (IR).

[c] PBC patients are divided into the TB (+) (TB > 1 × upper limit of the normal range [ULN]) and TB (−) (TB ≤ 1 × ULN) groups.

Data from Refs.[163–170,212–215]

that oral antibiotics markedly reduce the sexual differences with regard to lymphocytic infiltration and cytokines in dnTGFβRII mice, and further compares the gut microbial composition between the male and female groups.[172]

Emerging data on compositional and functional changes of microbiome have highlighted a close relationship between microbiome and PBC, despite hitherto limited data on the molecular mechanisms (causality) linking microbiome to autoimmunity. Significant attention has been paid to whether these PBC-associated genera can be noninvasive biomarkers for disease diagnosis or prognosis, and whether dysbiosis of gut microbiome is a cause or a consequence of PBC pathogenesis. In conclusion, it is nonnegligible that the microbiome integrally participates in PBC pathogenesis, as evidenced by a consensus that PBC occurs in genetically predisposed individuals with environmental triggers (microbiota and xenobiotics), but further mechanistic studies remain to be explored.

Gut–Liver Axis

Attention has been focused on the gut–liver axis linking gut microbiome to hepatic autoimmunity, in light of its anatomic and physiologic connections that exist naturally. Putative mechanisms whereby gut microbiome contributes to PBC development include molecular mimicry, translocation of gut commensals to distal organs, and migration of gut immune cells to distal organs.[173–175] The physiologic interplay naturally exists between the hosts and the microbiome, as reflected by the enterohepatic circle of bile acids. Primary bile acids conjugated with taurine or glycine are secreted by hepatocytes into the gut, where intestinal bacteria metabolize and modify primary conjugated bile acids by dihydroxylation and removal of taurine or glycine, producing secondary bile acids and subsequently reabsorbed by the liver.[176] Bile acids can inversely shape microbial composition by acting as energy sources or exerting anti- or probacterial effects.[4]

The liver is present in an unfriendly environment in light of small quantities of bacterial products reaching the liver via portal circulation despite the limitation of gut barrier for the translocation of these compounds.[177] These bacterial components including pathogen-associated molecular patterns and lipopolysaccharides are promptly removed by hepatocytes and Kupffer cells, which also activate BECs via toll-liker receptors (TLRs) and facilitate the production of adherent molecules, cytokines and chemokines in BECs.[62,178] In physiologic conditions, immune tolerance mechanisms in the body suffice to inhibit excessive immune responses against exogenous insults.[177,179,180]

The integrity of the intestinal epithelium is essential in maintaining the physiologic interplay between the hosts and the gut microbiome.[173] Dysbiosis of the gut microbiome, either as a cause or a consequence of diseases, might influence nutrient digestion and destroy intestinal barriers, leading to so-called "leaked gut" with increased intestinal permeability.[181] On this occasion, the translocation of gut pathobionts to the liver through portal circulation occurs and drives hepatic immune responses in humans and mice.[182] Besides, immune cells activated in the gut by bacteria, including dendritic cells, macrophages, MAIT cells, and Th17 cells partially enter into the hepatic microenvironment via portal circulation, leading to liver inflammation and fibrosis.[183–186] Under cholestatic conditions, a complex triangular relationship between bile acids, intestinal microbiota, and cholestasis is hypothesized to explain PBC pathogenesis, causing immune-mediated cholangiocyte damage and facilitating the progression of diseases.[4,187–189] Based on existing insights, targeting the gut–liver–immune axis has emerged as a prospective treatment strategy in hepatobiliary diseases.[183,190] Novel therapeutic drugs for PBC at present are focused on bile acid

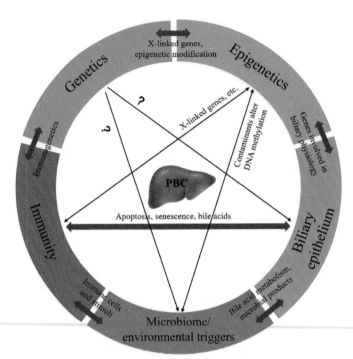

Fig. 3. Multiple factors mutually interact and synergistically promote the development of PBC. Thick lines represent a well-accepted interplay relationship whereas thin lines represent a weak relationship based on some emerging concepts.

synthetic pathways by modulating the gut–liver axis, as reflected by drugs targeting farnesoid X receptor and peroxisome proliferator-activated receptor.[118]

Epigenetics in X Chromosome

Genetic alterations are unable to fully explain phenotypic variability present in PBC, in light of the disconcordance in familial first-degree relatives and monozygotic twins, which indicates the involvement of epigenetic factors.[119,191] Current concerns about epigenetics in PBC mainly focus on architecture of the X chromosome, DNA methylation, and microRNAs. A significant higher frequency of X monosomy in peripheral leukocytes, particularly T and B cells, is observed in women with PBC than in controls.[192–194] X chromosome inactivation (XCI) randomly happens in diploid cells during embryogenesis, representing a natural feature in females, and physiologically can be preferentially chosen, which is more frequent in older subjects.[195] In PBC, XCI occurs in a random manner whereas X chromosome loss occurs not only frequently but also in a preferential fashion.[196] Although not restricted to women, haploinsufficiency for specific X-linked genes underlines the potential roles of the X chromosome in autoimmunity and female predisposition of PBC, considering that many immunotolerance-related genes are located on the X chromosome, including *FOXP3, TNFSF5, IL2RG.*[195,197,198]

Aberrant DNA methylation has been described and most differentially methylated regions are mapped to the X chromosome.[199] CD40 L, another well-known X-linked gene, is expressed on activated T cells to provide costimulatory signals for humoral immune responses by recognizing its receptor CD40 expressed primarily on B cells.[200] The interaction between CD40 and CD40 L is essential for IgM production, which is elevated in PBC, whereas no significant association signals on CD40-CD40 L system have been revealed in GWAS hitherto. In PBC patients, the level of CD40 L expression in liver infiltration T cells is elevated, but not that of soluble CD40 L in plasma.[201,202] DNA methylation level of the CD40 L promoter in CD4+ T cells is reduced in PBC patients as compared with healthy controls, which is negatively associated with CD40 L expression and serum IgM level.[203] A clinical trial of CD40 monoclonal antibody (NCT2193360) is approved but fails to complete. A hypomethylation level is also observed in the promoter of CXCR3 in CD4+ T cells, concurrent with an increase of CXCR3 expression.[204] Increased expression of CXCR3 in the portal tracts and a higher frequency of CXCR3-expressing cells in peripheral blood are observed in PBC as compared with healthy controls.[205]

Although increasing number of studies have reported that microRNAs (miRNAs) have great value in PBC diagnosis and prognosis, there is a substantial lack of functional investigations of miRNAs in the immunopathology of PBC, with one exception of miR-506.[206] Intriguingly, the X chromosome has a higher density of miRNAs as compared with the autosomes and Y chromosome.[207] MiR-506 located on the X chromosome, is upregulated in intrahepatic bile ducts of PBC livers as compared with normal and PSC livers, and regulates AE2 expression by directly binding to the 3'-untranslated region (3'-UTR) of AE2.[71] Proinflammatory cytokines upregulate the expression of miR-506 in human BECs leading to a reduction of AE2 and aberrant mitochondrial metabolism whereas activation and proliferation of PBC immunocytes, in turn, are induced by the coculture of immunocytes with miR-506 overexpressing BECs.[208] As mentioned above, BECs can interact with immune cells to actively participate in immune responses.[65] Downregulation of miR-506 expression in PBC cholangiocytes improves AE2 activity, indicating that miR-506 may be a potential therapeutic target.[71] Type III inositol 1,4,5-triphosphage receptor (InsP$_3$R$_3$), identified as another direct target of miR-506, is an important component located in the endoplasmic reticulum of BECs, activated by extracellular acetylcholine and facilitate biliary bicarbonate secretion by regulating Ca^{2+} signaling.[209] A reduction of InsP$_3$R$_3$ is observed specifically in cholangiocytes in both human PBC and cholestatic murine models, leading to impairment of intracellular Ca^{2+} signaling and biliary bicarbonate secretion, and eventually cholestasis.[210] Therefore, the upregulation of miR-506 in BECs of PBC reduces expression of AE2 and InsP$_3$R$_3$, leading to a failure of bicarbonate secretion.[71]

As miR-506 directly targets both AE2 and InsP$_3$R$_3$, two important transporters involved in biliary secretion, immense interest has been generated in the treatment potential of miR-506. Genes involved in biliary physiology have not been reported to be significantly associated in GWAS, possibly attributed to the paucity of much data on the X chromosome. In conclusion, a better understanding the epigenetic alterations of the X chromosome would greatly broaden our knowledge of PBC etiopathology, including biology of sex differences, and shed light on the missing heritability.

SUMMARY

Current insights into the complex etiopathogenesis of PBC suggest that the central culprit of pathogenesis is the excessive multilineage immune responses against biliary epithelial cells (BECs) with the loss of immune tolerance to PDC-E2, which is synergistically influenced by genetic background, environmental triggers and epigenetic alterations (**Fig. 3**). Immunogenetics and study of biliary epithelium have become two major research directions. One current controversy is whether PBC is initially triggered by a defect of the biliary bicarbonate umbrella, challenging the hypothesis that the breakdown of biliary homeostasis is secondary to immune dysregulation. PBC is an autoimmune disease as evidenced by GWAS and clinical data. Although an overlap of risky loci does exist between PBC and PSC, shared genetic loci seem not to play a substantial role in the pathogenesis of PBC, including *SH2B3*, *TNFRF14*, *CD28*, and *IL21*.[211] Knowledge about the contribution of the X chromosome in PBC pathogenesis is poorly understood but intriguing. Emerging data on compositional and functional changes of the microbiome have highlighted a close relationship between microbiome and PBC. Whether dysbiosis of gut microbiome is a cause or a consequence of PBC pathogenesis remains ambiguous.

FUNDING

This work was supported by the National Natural Science Foundation of China grants (#81830016, 81771732 and 81620108002 to XM, #81922010,81873561 and 81570469 to RT).

REFERENCES

1. Kaplan MM, Gershwin ME. Primary biliary cirrhosis. N Engl J Med 2005;353: 1261–73.
2. Selmi C, Bowlus CL, Gershwin ME, et al. Primary biliary cirrhosis. Lancet 2011; 377:1600–9.
3. Lleo A, Wang G-Q, Gershwin ME, et al. Primary biliary cholangitis. Lancet 2020; 396:1915–26.
4. Terziroli Beretta-Piccoli B, Mieli-Vergani G, Vergani D, et al. The challenges of primary biliary cholangitis: what is new and what needs to be done. J Autoimmun 2019;105:102328.
5. Beuers U, Gershwin ME, Gish RG, et al. Changing nomenclature for PBC: from 'cirrhosis' to 'cholangitis. J Hepatol 2015;63:1285–7.
6. Rice S, Albani V, Minos D, et al. Effects of primary biliary cholangitis on Quality of Life and Health Care Costs in the United Kingdom. Clin Gastroenterol Hepatol 2021;19:768–776 e10.
7. European Association for the Study of the Liver. Electronic address eee and European Association for the Study of the L. EASL Clinical Practice Guidelines: the diagnosis and management of patients with primary biliary cholangitis. J Hepatol 2017;67:145–72.
8. Lindor KD, Bowlus CL, Boyer J, et al. Primary biliary cholangitis: 2018 Practice Guidance from the American association for the study of liver diseases. Hepatology 2019;69:394–419.
9. Carbone M, Milani C, Gerussi A, et al. Primary biliary cholangitis: a multifaceted pathogenesis with potential therapeutic targets. J Hepatol 2020;73:965–6.
10. Martin EM, Fry RC. Environmental influences on the Epigenome: exposure-associated DNA methylation in human Populations. Annu Rev Public Health 2018;39:309–33.
11. Xu F, Fu Y, Sun TY, et al. The interplay between host genetics and the gut microbiome reveals common and distinct microbiome features for complex human diseases. Microbiome 2020;8:145.
12. Marzorati S, Lleo A, Carbone M, et al. The epigenetics of PBC: the link between genetic susceptibility and environment. Clin Res Hepatol Gastroenterol 2016;40: 650–9.

13. Zhang P, Lu Q. Genetic and epigenetic influences on the loss of tolerance in autoimmunity. Cell Mol Immunol 2018;15:575–85.

14. Walker JG, Doniach D, Roitt IM, et al. Serological tests in diagnosis of primary biliary cirrhosis. Lancet 1965;1:827–31.

15. Gershwin ME, Mackay IR, Sturgess A, et al. Identification and specificity of a cDNA encoding the 70 kd mitochondrial antigen recognized in primary biliary cirrhosis. J Immunol 1987;138:3525–31.

16. Yeaman SJ, Fussey SP, Danner DJ, et al. Primary biliary cirrhosis: identification of two major M2 mitochondrial autoantigens. Lancet 1988;1:1067–70.

17. Coppel RL, McNeilage LJ, Surh CD, et al. Primary structure of the human M2 mitochondrial autoantigen of primary biliary cirrhosis: dihydrolipoamide acetyl-transferase. Proc Natl Acad Sci U S A 1988;85:7317–21.

18. Fussey SP, Guest JR, James OF, et al. Identification and analysis of the major M2 autoantigens in primary biliary cirrhosis. Proc Natl Acad Sci U S A 1988; 85:8654–8.

19. Bruggraber SF, Leung PS, Amano K, et al. Autoreactivity to lipoate and a conjugated form of lipoate in primary biliary cirrhosis. Gastroenterology 2003;125: 1705–13.

20. Mao TK, Davis PA, Odin JA, et al. Sidechain biology and the immunogenicity of PDC-E2, the major autoantigen of primary biliary cirrhosis. Hepatology 2004;40: 1241–8.

21. Shimoda S, Van de Water J, Ansari A, et al. Identification and precursor frequency analysis of a common T cell epitope motif in mitochondrial autoantigens in primary biliary cirrhosis. J Clin Invest 1998;102:1831–40.

22. Kita H, Matsumura S, He XS, et al. Quantitative and functional analysis of PDC-E2-specific autoreactive cytotoxic T lymphocytes in primary biliary cirrhosis. J Clin Invest 2002;109:1231–40.

23. Kita H, Lian ZX, Van de Water J, et al. Identification of HLA-A2-restricted CD8(+) cytotoxic T cell responses in primary biliary cirrhosis: T cell activation is augmented by immune complexes cross-presented by dendritic cells. J Exp Med 2002;195:113–23.

24. Li H, Guan Y, Han C, et al. The pathogenesis, models and therapeutic advances of primary biliary cholangitis. Biomed Pharmacother 2021;140:111754.

25. Trzos K, Pydyn N, Jura J, Kotlinowski J. Selected transgenic murine models of human autoimmune liver diseases. Pharmacol Rep 2022;74(2):263–72.

26. Oertelt S, Lian ZX, Cheng CM, et al. Anti-mitochondrial antibodies and primary biliary cirrhosis in TGF-beta receptor II dominant-negative mice. J Immunol 2006;177:1655–60.

27. Chuang YH, Lian ZX, Yang GX, et al. Natural killer T cells exacerbate liver injury in a transforming growth factor beta receptor II dominant-negative mouse model of primary biliary cirrhosis. Hepatology 2008;47:571–80.

28. Yang GX, Lian ZX, Chuang YH, et al. Adoptive transfer of CD8(+) T cells from transforming growth factor beta receptor type II (dominant negative form) induces autoimmune cholangitis in mice. Hepatology 2008;47:1974–82.

29. Moritoki Y, Lian ZX, Lindor K, et al. B-cell depletion with anti-CD20 ameliorates autoimmune cholangitis but exacerbates colitis in transforming growth factor-beta receptor II dominant negative mice. Hepatology 2009;50:1893–903.

30. Lleo A, Bowlus CL, Yang GX, et al. Biliary apotopes and anti-mitochondrial antibodies activate innate immune responses in primary biliary cirrhosis. Hepatology 2010;52:987–98.

31. Bogdanos DP, Invernizzi P, Mackay IR, et al. Autoimmune liver serology: current diagnostic and clinical challenges. World J Gastroenterol 2008;14:3374–87.

32. Leung KK, Deeb M, Hirschfield GM. Review article: pathophysiology and management of primary biliary cholangitis. Aliment Pharmacol Ther 2020;52: 1150–64.

33. Worman HJ, Courvalin JC. Antinuclear antibodies specific for primary biliary cirrhosis. Autoimmun Rev 2003;2:211–7.

34. Wesierska-Gadek J, Hohenauer H, Hitchman E, et al. Anti-gp210 antibodies in sera of patients with primary biliary cirrhosis. Identification of a 64 kD fragment of gp210 as a major epitope. Hum Antibodies Hybridomas 1996;7:167–74.

35. Courvalin JC, Worman HJ. Nuclear envelope protein autoantibodies in primary biliary cirrhosis. Semin Liver Dis 1997;17:79–90.

36. Szostecki C, Guldner HH, Will H. Autoantibodies against "nuclear dots" in primary biliary cirrhosis. Semin Liver Dis 1997;17:71–8.

37. Granito A, Yang WH, Muratori L, et al. PML nuclear body component Sp140 is a novel autoantigen in primary biliary cirrhosis. Am J Gastroenterol 2010;105: 125–31.

38. Nakamura M, Takii Y, Ito M, et al. Increased expression of nuclear envelope gp210 antigen in small bile ducts in primary biliary cirrhosis. J Autoimmun 2006;26:138–45.

39. Parveen S, Morshed SA, Nishioka M. High prevalence of antibodies to recombinant CENP-B in primary biliary cirrhosis: nuclear immunofluorescence patterns and ELISA reactivities. J Gastroenterol Hepatol 1995;10:438–45.

40. Nakamura M, Kondo H, Mori T, et al. Anti-gp210 and anti-centromere antibodies are different risk factors for the progression of primary biliary cirrhosis. Hepatology 2007;45:118–27.

41. Alpini G, McGill JM, Larusso NF. The pathobiology of biliary epithelia. Hepatology 2002;35:1256–68.

42. Strazzabosco M, Spirli C, Okolicsanyi L. Pathophysiology of the intrahepatic biliary epithelium. J Gastroenterol Hepatol 2000;15:244–53.

43. Lesage G, Glaser SS, Gubba S, et al. Regrowth of the rat biliary tree after 70% partial hepatectomy is coupled to increased secretin-induced ductal secretion. Gastroenterology 1996;111:1633–44.

44. Lazaridis KN, Strazzabosco M, Larusso NF. The cholangiopathies: disorders of biliary epithelia. Gastroenterology 2004;127:1565–77.

45. Lleo A, Selmi C, Invernizzi P, et al. The consequences of apoptosis in autoimmunity. J Autoimmun 2008;31:257–62.

46. Lleo A, Selmi C, Invernizzi P, et al. Apotopes and the biliary specificity of primary biliary cirrhosis. Hepatology 2009;49:871–9.

47. Rong G, Zhong R, Lleo A, et al. Epithelial cell specificity and apotope recognition by serum autoantibodies in primary biliary cirrhosis. Hepatology 2011;54: 196–203.

48. Koga H, Sakisaka S, Ohishi M, et al. Nuclear DNA fragmentation and expression of Bcl-2 in primary biliary cirrhosis. Hepatology 1997;25:1077–84.

49. Takeda K, Kojima Y, Ikejima K, et al. Death receptor 5 mediated-apoptosis contributes to cholestatic liver disease. Proc Natl Acad Sci U S A 2008;105: 10895–900.

50. Tsuneyama K, Van de Water J, Leung PS, et al. Abnormal expression of the E2 component of the pyruvate dehydrogenase complex on the luminal surface of biliary epithelium occurs before major histocompatibility complex class II and BB1/B7 expression. Hepatology 1995;21:1031–7.

51. Tsuneyama K, Van De Water J, Van Thiel D, et al. Abnormal expression of PDC-E2 on the apical surface of biliary epithelial cells in patients with antimitochondrial antibody-negative primary biliary cirrhosis. Hepatology 1995;22:1440–6.

52. Guicciardi ME, Trussoni CE, LaRusso NF, et al. The Spectrum of reactive cholangiocytes in primary sclerosing cholangitis. Hepatology 2020;71:741–8.

53. Trussoni CE, O'Hara SP, LaRusso NF. Cellular senescence in the cholangiopathies: a driver of immunopathology and a novel therapeutic target. Semin Immunopathol 2022. Online ahead of print.

54. Bogert PS, O'Hara SP, LaRusso NF. Cellular senescence in the cholangiopathies. Curr Opin Gastroenterol 2022;38:121–7.

55. Sasaki M, Ikeda H, Yamaguchi J, et al. Telomere shortening in the damaged small bile ducts in primary biliary cirrhosis reflects ongoing cellular senescence. Hepatology 2008;48:186–95.

56. Sasaki M, Miyakoshi M, Sato Y, et al. Modulation of the microenvironment by senescent biliary epithelial cells may be involved in the pathogenesis of primary biliary cirrhosis. J Hepatol 2010;53:318–25.

57. Shimoda S, Harada K, Niiro H, et al. Biliary epithelial cells and primary biliary cirrhosis: the role of liver-infiltrating mononuclear cells. Hepatology 2008;47:958–65.

58. Shimoda S, Harada K, Niiro H, et al. CX3CL1 (fractalkine): a signpost for biliary inflammation in primary biliary cirrhosis. Hepatology 2010;51:567–75.

59. Isse K, Harada K, Zen Y, et al. Fractalkine and CX3CR1 are involved in the recruitment of intraepithelial lymphocytes of intrahepatic bile ducts. Hepatology 2005;41:506–16.

60. Oo YH, Banz V, Kavanagh D, et al. CXCR3-dependent recruitment and CCR6-mediated positioning of Th-17 cells in the inflamed liver. J Hepatol 2012;57:1044–51.

61. Cordell HJ, Han Y, Mells GF, et al. International genome-wide meta-analysis identifies new primary biliary cirrhosis risk loci and targetable pathogenic pathways. Nat Commun 2015;6:8019.

62. Chuang YH, Lan RY, Gershwin ME. The immunopathology of human biliary cell epithelium. Semin Immunopathol 2009;31:323–31.

63. Hisamoto S, Shimoda S, Harada K, et al. Hydrophobic bile acids suppress expression of AE2 in biliary epithelial cells and induce bile duct inflammation in primary biliary cholangitis. J Autoimmun 2016;75:150–60.

64. Kamihira T, Shimoda S, Harada K, et al. Distinct costimulation dependent and independent autoreactive T-cell clones in primary biliary cirrhosis. Gastroenterology 2003;125:1379–87.

65. Kamihira T, Shimoda S, Nakamura M, et al. Biliary epithelial cells regulate autoreactive T cells: implications for biliary-specific diseases. Hepatology 2005;41:151–9.

66. Savill J, Dransfield I, Gregory C, et al. A blast from the past: clearance of apoptotic cells regulates immune responses. Nat Rev Immunol 2002;2:965–75.

67. Schrumpf E, Tan C, Karlsen TH, et al. The biliary epithelium presents antigens to and activates natural killer T cells. Hepatology 2015;62:1249–59.

68. Jeffery HC, van Wilgenburg B, Kurioka A, et al. Biliary epithelium and liver B cells exposed to bacteria activate intrahepatic MAIT cells through MR1. J Hepatol 2016;64:1118–27.

69. Lazaridis KN, LaRusso NF. The cholangiopathies. Mayo Clin Proc 2015;90:791–800.

70. Hohenester S, Wenniger LM, Paulusma CC, et al. A biliary HCO3- umbrella constitutes a protective mechanism against bile acid-induced injury in human cholangiocytes. Hepatology 2012;55:173–83.

71. Banales JM, Saez E, Uriz M, et al. Up-regulation of microRNA 506 leads to decreased Cl-/HCO3- anion exchanger 2 expression in biliary epithelium of patients with primary biliary cirrhosis. Hepatology 2012;56:687–97.

72. Banales JM, Arenas F, Rodriguez-Ortigosa CM, et al. Bicarbonate-rich choleresis induced by secretin in normal rat is taurocholate-dependent and involves AE2 anion exchanger. Hepatology 2006;43:266–75.

73. Melero S, Spirli C, Zsembery A, et al. Defective regulation of cholangiocyte Cl-/HCO3(-) and Na+/H+ exchanger activities in primary biliary cirrhosis. Hepatology 2002;35:1513–21.

74. Kennedy L, Francis H, Invernizzi P, et al. Secretin/secretin receptor signaling mediates biliary damage and liver fibrosis in early-stage primary biliary cholangitis. FASEB J 2019;33:10269–79.

75. Chang JC, Go S, de Waart DR, et al. Soluble adenylyl cyclase regulates bile salt-induced apoptosis in human cholangiocytes. Hepatology 2016;64:522–34.

76. Arenas F, Hervias I, Uriz M, et al. Combination of ursodeoxycholic acid and glucocorticoids upregulates the AE2 alternate promoter in human liver cells. J Clin Invest 2008;118:695–709.

77. Rodrigues PM, Perugorria MJ, Santos-Laso A, et al. Primary biliary cholangitis: a tale of epigenetically-induced secretory failure? J Hepatol 2018;69:1371–83.

78. Farooqui N, Elhence A, Shalimar. A current understanding of bile acids in chronic liver disease. J Clin Exp Hepatol 2022;12:155–73.

79. Salas JT, Banales JM, Sarvide S, et al. Ae2a,b-deficient mice develop antimitochondrial antibodies and other features resembling primary biliary cirrhosis. Gastroenterology 2008;134:1482–93.

80. Fiorotto R, Strazzabosco M. Pathophysiology of cystic fibrosis liver disease: a Channelopathy leading to alterations in innate immunity and in microbiota. Cell Mol Gastroenterol Hepatol 2019;8:197–207.

81. Dana J, Debray D, Beaufrere A, et al. Cystic fibrosis-related liver disease: clinical presentations, diagnostic and monitoring approaches in the era of CFTR modulator therapies. J Hepatol 2022;76:420–34.

82. Hirschfield GM, Gershwin ME. The immunobiology and pathophysiology of primary biliary cirrhosis. Annu Rev Pathol 2013;8:303–30.

83. Krams SM, Van de Water J, Coppel RL, et al. Analysis of hepatic T lymphocyte and immunoglobulin deposits in patients with primary biliary cirrhosis. Hepatology 1990;12:306–13.

84. Zhang W, Ono Y, Miyamura Y, et al. T cell clonal expansions detected in patients with primary biliary cirrhosis express CX3CR1. J Autoimmun 2011;37:71–8.

85. Cordell HJ, Fryett JJ, Ueno K, et al. An international genome-wide meta-analysis of primary biliary cholangitis: novel risk loci and candidate drugs. J Hepatol 2021;75:572–81.

86. Ma HD, Ma WT, Liu QZ, et al. Chemokine receptor CXCR3 deficiency exacerbates murine autoimmune cholangitis by promoting pathogenic CD8(+) T cell activation. J Autoimmun 2017;78:19–28.

87. Tsuda M, Ambrosini YM, Zhang W, et al. Fine phenotypic and functional characterization of effector cluster of differentiation 8 positive T cells in human patients with primary biliary cirrhosis. Hepatology 2011;54:1293–302.

88. Damsker JM, Hansen AM, Caspi RR. Th1 and Th17 cells: adversaries and collaborators. Ann N Y Acad Sci 2010;1183:211–21.

89. Yang CY, Ma X, Tsuneyama K, et al. IL-12/Th1 and IL-23/Th17 biliary microenvironment in primary biliary cirrhosis: implications for therapy. Hepatology 2014; 59:1944–53.
90. Lan RY, Cheng C, Lian ZX, et al. Liver-targeted and peripheral blood alterations of regulatory T cells in primary biliary cirrhosis. Hepatology 2006;43:729–37.
91. Wang D, Zhang H, Liang J, et al. CD4+ CD25+ but not CD4+ Foxp3+ T cells as a regulatory subset in primary biliary cirrhosis. Cell Mol Immunol 2010;7:485–90.
92. Liaskou E, Patel SR, Webb G, et al. Increased sensitivity of Treg cells from patients with PBC to low dose IL-12 drives their differentiation into IFN-gamma secreting cells. J Autoimmun 2018;94:143–55.
93. Chung Y, Tanaka S, Chu F, et al. Follicular regulatory T cells expressing Foxp3 and Bcl-6 suppress germinal center reactions. Nat Med 2011;17:983–8.
94. Wang L, Sun Y, Zhang Z, et al. CXCR5+ CD4+ T follicular helper cells participate in the pathogenesis of primary biliary cirrhosis. Hepatology 2015;61: 627–38.
95. Webb GJ, Hirschfield GM. Follicles, germinal centers, and immune mechanisms in primary biliary cirrhosis. Hepatology 2015;61:424–7.
96. Zheng J, Wang T, Zhang L, et al. Dysregulation of circulating Tfr/Tfh ratio in primary biliary cholangitis. Scand J Immunol 2017;86:452–61.
97. Adam L, Zoldan K, Hofmann M, et al. Follicular T helper cell Signatures in primary biliary cholangitis and primary sclerosing cholangitis. Hepatol Commun 2018;2:1051–63.
98. Selmi C, Lleo A, Pasini S, et al. Innate immunity and primary biliary cirrhosis. Curr Mol Med 2009;9:45–51.
99. Lleo A, Invernizzi P. Apotopes and innate immune system: novel players in the primary biliary cirrhosis scenario. Dig Liver Dis 2013;45:630–6.
100. Bruneau A, Guillot A, Tacke F. Macrophages in cholangiopathies. Curr Opin Gastroenterol 2022;38:114–20.
101. Sasaki M, Miyakoshi M, Sato Y, et al. Chemokine-chemokine receptor CCL2-CCR2 and CX3CL1-CX3CR1 axis may play a role in the aggravated inflammation in primary biliary cirrhosis. Dig Dis Sci 2014;59:358–64.
102. Serbina NV, Pamer EG. Monocyte emigration from bone marrow during bacterial infection requires signals mediated by chemokine receptor CCR2. Nat Immunol 2006;7:311–7.
103. Reuveni D, Gore Y, Leung PSC, et al. The critical role of chemokine (C-C motif) receptor 2-positive monocytes in autoimmune cholangitis. Front Immunol 2018; 9:1852.
104. Eksteen B, Bowlus CL, Montano-Loza AJ, et al. Efficacy and Safety of cenicriviroc in patients with primary sclerosing cholangitis: PERSEUS study. Hepatol Commun 2021;5:478–90.
105. Reuveni D, Brezis MR, Brazowski E, et al. Interleukin 23 produced by hepatic monocyte-derived macrophages is essential for the development of murine primary biliary cholangitis. Front Immunol 2021;12:718841.
106. Zhang H, Lian M, Zhang J, et al. A functional characteristic of cysteine-rich protein 61: Modulation of myeloid-derived suppressor cells in liver inflammation. Hepatology 2018;67:232–46.
107. Hudspeth K, Pontarini E, Tentorio P, et al. The role of natural killer cells in autoimmune liver disease: a comprehensive review. J Autoimmun 2013;46:55–65.
108. Shimoda S, Harada K, Niiro H, et al. Interaction between Toll-like receptors and natural killer cells in the destruction of bile ducts in primary biliary cirrhosis. Hepatology 2011;53:1270–81.

109. Shimoda S, Hisamoto S, Harada K, et al. Natural killer cells regulate T cell immune responses in primary biliary cirrhosis. Hepatology 2015;62:1817–27.

110. Hydes TJ, Blunt MD, Naftel J, et al. Constitutive activation of natural killer cells in primary biliary cholangitis. Front Immunol 2019;10.

111. Treiner E, Duban L, Bahram S, et al. Selection of evolutionarily conserved mucosal-associated invariant T cells by MR1. Nature 2003;422:164–9.

112. Ussher JE, Bilton M, Attwod E, et al. CD161++ CD8+ T cells, including the MAIT cell subset, are specifically activated by IL-12+IL-18 in a TCR-independent manner. Eur J Immunol 2014;44:195–203.

113. Toubal A, Lehuen A. Lights on MAIT cells, a new immune player in liver diseases. J Hepatol 2016;64:1008–10.

114. Setsu T, Yamagiwa S, Tominaga K, et al. Persistent reduction of mucosal-associated invariant T cells in primary biliary cholangitis. J Gastroenterol Hepatol 2018;33:1286–94.

115. Jiang X, Lian M, Li Y, et al. The immunobiology of mucosal-associated invariant T cell (MAIT) function in primary biliary cholangitis: regulation by cholic acid-induced Interleukin-7. J Autoimmun 2018;90:64–75.

116. Chen Z, Liu S, He C, et al. CXCL12-CXCR4-Mediated chemotaxis supports accumulation of mucosal-associated invariant T cells into the liver of patients with PBC. Front Immunol 2021;12:578548.

117. Czaja AJ. Incorporating mucosal-associated invariant T cells into the pathogenesis of chronic liver disease. World J Gastroenterol 2021;27:3705–33.

118. Mayo MJ. Mechanisms & Molecules: what are the treatment targets for PBC? Hepatology 2022. Online ahead of print.

119. Selmi C, Mayo MJ, Bach N, et al. Primary biliary cirrhosis in monozygotic and dizygotic twins: genetics, epigenetics, and environment. Gastroenterology 2004;127:485–92.

120. Ornolfsson KT, Olafsson S, Bergmann OM, et al. Using the Icelandic genealogical database to define the familial risk of primary biliary cholangitis. Hepatology 2018;68:166–71.

121. Gerussi A, Carbone M, Corpechot C, et al. The genetic architecture of primary biliary cholangitis. Eur J Med Genet 2021;64:104292.

122. Hirschfield GM, Liu X, Xu C, et al. Primary biliary cirrhosis associated with HLA, IL12A, and IL12RB2 variants. N Engl J Med 2009;360:2544–55.

123. Hirschfield GM, Liu X, Han Y, et al. Variants at IRF5-TNPO3, 17q12-21 and MMEL1 are associated with primary biliary cirrhosis. Nat Genet 2010;42:655–7.

124. Liu X, Invernizzi P, Lu Y, et al. Genome-wide meta-analyses identify three loci associated with primary biliary cirrhosis. Nat Genet 2010;42:658–60.

125. Mells GF, Floyd JA, Morley KI, et al. Genome-wide association study identifies 12 new susceptibility loci for primary biliary cirrhosis. Nat Genet 2011;43:329–32.

126. Liu JZ, Almarri MA, Gaffney DJ, et al. Dense fine-mapping study identifies new susceptibility loci for primary biliary cirrhosis. Nat Genet 2012;44:1137–41.

127. Nakamura M, Nishida N, Kawashima M, et al. Genome-wide association study identifies TNFSF15 and POU2AF1 as susceptibility loci for primary biliary cirrhosis in the Japanese population. Am J Hum Genet 2012;91:721–8.

128. Qiu F, Tang R, Zuo X, et al. A genome-wide association study identifies six novel risk loci for primary biliary cholangitis. Nat Commun 2017;8:14828.

129. Juran BD, Hirschfield GM, Invernizzi P, et al. Immunochip analyses identify a novel risk locus for primary biliary cirrhosis at 13q14, multiple independent

associations at four established risk loci and epistasis between 1p31 and 7q32 risk variants. Hum Mol Genet 2012;21:5209–21.

130. Yoshida K, Yang GX, Zhang W, et al. Deletion of interleukin-12p40 suppresses autoimmune cholangitis in dominant negative transforming growth factor beta receptor type II mice. Hepatology 2009;50:1494–500.

131. Bae HR, Leung PS, Tsuneyama K, et al. Chronic expression of interferon-gamma leads to murine autoimmune cholangitis with a female predominance. Hepatology 2016;64:1189–201.

132. Hirschfield GM, Gershwin ME, Strauss R, et al. Ustekinumab for patients with primary biliary cholangitis who have an inadequate response to ursodeoxycholic acid: a proof-of-concept study. Hepatology 2016;64:189–99.

133. Dhirapong A, Yang GX, Nadler S, et al. Therapeutic effect of cytotoxic T lymphocyte antigen 4/immunoglobulin on a murine model of primary biliary cirrhosis. Hepatology 2013;57:708–15.

134. Bowlus CL, Yang GX, Liu CH, et al. Therapeutic trials of biologics in primary biliary cholangitis: an open label study of abatacept and review of the literature. J Autoimmun 2019;101:26–34.

135. Wise AL, Gyi L, Manolio TA. eXclusion: toward integrating the X chromosome in genome-wide association analyses. Am J Hum Genet 2013;92:643–7.

136. Asselta R, Paraboschi EM, Gerussi A, et al. Chromosome contribution to the genetic architecture of primary biliary cholangitis. Gastroenterology 2021;160:2483–2495 e26.

137. Zhang W, Sharma R, Ju ST, et al. Deficiency in regulatory T cells results in development of antimitochondrial antibodies and autoimmune cholangitis. Hepatology 2009;49:545–52.

138. Tanaka H, Zhang W, Yang GX, et al. Successful immunotherapy of autoimmune cholangitis by adoptive transfer of forkhead box protein 3(+) regulatory T cells. Clin Exp Immunol 2014;178:253–61.

139. Juran BD, Lazaridis KN. Environmental factors in primary biliary cirrhosis. Semin Liver Dis 2014;34:265–72.

140. Gulamhusein AF, Hirschfield GM. Primary biliary cholangitis: pathogenesis and therapeutic opportunities. Nat Rev Gastroenterol Hepatol 2020;17:93–110.

141. Oldstone MB. Molecular mimicry as a mechanism for the cause and a probe uncovering etiologic agent(s) of autoimmune disease. Curr Top Microbiol Immunol 1989;145:127–35.

142. Shimoda S, Nakamura M, Ishibashi H, et al. Molecular mimicry of mitochondrial and nuclear autoantigens in primary biliary cirrhosis. Gastroenterology 2003;124:1915–25.

143. Gershwin ME, Selmi C, Worman HJ, et al. Risk factors and comorbidities in primary biliary cirrhosis: a controlled interview-based study of 1032 patients. Hepatology 2005;42:1194–202.

144. Selmi C, Balkwill DL, Invernizzi P, et al. Patients with primary biliary cirrhosis react against a ubiquitous xenobiotic-metabolizing bacterium. Hepatology 2003;38:1250–7.

145. Shimoda S, Nakamura M, Ishibashi H, et al. HLA DRB4 0101-restricted immunodominant T cell autoepitope of pyruvate dehydrogenase complex in primary biliary cirrhosis: evidence of molecular mimicry in human autoimmune diseases. J Exp Med 1995;181:1835–45.

146. Ala A, Stanca CM, Bu-Ghanim M, et al. Increased prevalence of primary biliary cirrhosis near Superfund toxic waste sites. Hepatology 2006;43:525–31.

147. McNally RJ, James PW, Ducker S, et al. No rise in incidence but geographical heterogeneity in the occurrence of primary biliary cirrhosis in North East England. Am J Epidemiol 2014;179:492–8.

148. Corpechot C, Chretien Y, Chazouilleres O, et al. Demographic, lifestyle, medical and familial factors associated with primary biliary cirrhosis. J Hepatol 2010;53: 162–9.

149. Matsumoto K, Ohfuji S, Abe M, et al. Environmental factors, medical and family history, and comorbidities associated with primary biliary cholangitis in Japan: a multicenter case-control study. J Gastroenterol 2022;57:19–29.

150. Wang J, Yang G, Dubrovsky AM, et al. Xenobiotics and loss of tolerance in primary biliary cholangitis. World J Gastroenterol 2016;22:338–48.

151. Amano K, Leung PS, Rieger R, et al. Chemical xenobiotics and mitochondrial autoantigens in primary biliary cirrhosis: identification of antibodies against a common environmental, cosmetic, and food additive, 2-octynoic acid. J Immunol 2005;174:5874–83.

152. Shuai Z, Wang J, Badamagunta M, et al. The fingerprint of antimitochondrial antibodies and the etiology of primary biliary cholangitis. Hepatology 2017;65: 1670–82.

153. Wakabayashi K, Lian ZX, Leung PS, et al. Loss of tolerance in C57BL/6 mice to the autoantigen E2 subunit of pyruvate dehydrogenase by a xenobiotic with ensuing biliary ductular disease. Hepatology 2008;48:531–40.

154. Rieger R, Leung PS, Jeddeloh MR, et al. Identification of 2-nonynoic acid, a cosmetic component, as a potential trigger of primary biliary cirrhosis. J Autoimmun 2006;27:7–16.

155. Naiyanetr P, Butler JD, Meng L, et al. Electrophile-modified lipoic derivatives of PDC-E2 elicits anti-mitochondrial antibody reactivity. J Autoimmun 2011;37: 209–16.

156. Leung PS, Lam K, Kurth MJ, et al. Xenobiotics and autoimmunity: does acetaminophen cause primary biliary cirrhosis? Trends Mol Med 2012;18:577–82.

157. Probert PM, Leitch AC, Dunn MP, et al. Identification of a xenobiotic as a potential environmental trigger in primary biliary cholangitis. J Hepatol 2018;69: 1123–35.

158. Lynch SV, Pedersen O. The human intestinal microbiome in Health and disease. N Engl J Med 2016;375:2369–79.

159. Zhang X, Chen BD, Zhao LD, et al. The gut microbiota: emerging evidence in autoimmune diseases. Trends Mol Med 2020;26:862–73.

160. Wang R, Tang R, Li B, et al. Gut microbiome, liver immunology, and liver diseases. Cell Mol Immunol 2021;18:4–17.

161. Ghent CN, Carruthers SG. Treatment of pruritus in primary biliary cirrhosis with rifampin. Results of a double-blind, crossover, randomized trial. Gastroenterology 1988;94:488–93.

162. Bachs L, Pares A, Elena M, et al. Effects of long-term rifampicin administration in primary biliary cirrhosis. Gastroenterology 1992;102:2077–80.

163. Lv LX, Fang DQ, Shi D, et al. Alterations and correlations of the gut microbiome, metabolism and immunity in patients with primary biliary cirrhosis. Environ Microbiol 2016;18:2272–86.

164. Tang R, Wei Y, Li Y, et al. Gut microbial profile is altered in primary biliary cholangitis and partially restored after UDCA therapy. Gut 2018;67:534–41.

165. Chen W, Wei Y, Xiong A, et al. Comprehensive analysis of serum and fecal bile acid profiles and interaction with gut microbiota in primary biliary cholangitis. Clin Rev Allergy Immunol 2020;58:25–38.

166. Li B, Zhang J, Chen Y, et al. Alterations in microbiota and their metabolites are associated with beneficial effects of bile acid sequestrant on icteric primary biliary Cholangitis. Gut Microbes 2021;13:1946366.

167. Kitahata S, Yamamoto Y, Yoshida O, et al. Ileal mucosa-associated microbiota overgrowth associated with pathogenesis of primary biliary cholangitis. Sci Rep 2021;11:19705.

168. Furukawa M, Moriya K, Nakayama J, et al. Gut dysbiosis associated with clinical prognosis of patients with primary biliary cholangitis. Hepatol Res 2020;50: 840–52.

169. Lammert C, Shin A, Xu H, et al. Short-chain fatty acid and fecal microbiota profiles are linked to fibrosis in primary biliary cholangitis. FEMS Microbiol Lett 2021;368.

170. Han W, Huang C, Zhang Q, et al. Alterations in gut microbiota and elevated serum bilirubin in primary biliary cholangitis patients treated with ursodeoxycholic acid. Eur J Clin Invest 2022;52:e13714.

171. Schrumpf E, Kummen M, Valestrand L, et al. The gut microbiota contributes to a mouse model of spontaneous bile duct inflammation. J Hepatol 2017;66:382–9.

172. Huang MX, Yang SY, Luo PY, et al. Gut microbiota contributes to sexual dimorphism in murine autoimmune cholangitis. J Leukoc Biol 2021;110:1121–30.

173. Ruff WE, Greiling TM, Kriegel MA. Host-microbiota interactions in immune-mediated diseases. Nat Rev Microbiol 2020;18:521–38.

174. Chopyk DM, Grakoui A. Contribution of the intestinal microbiome and gut barrier to hepatic disorders. Gastroenterology 2020;159:849–63.

175. Tripathi A, Debelius J, Brenner DA, et al. The gut-liver axis and the intersection with the microbiome. Nat Rev Gastroenterol Hepatol 2018;15:397–411.

176. Dawson PA, Karpen SJ. Intestinal transport and metabolism of bile acids. J Lipid Res 2015;56:1085–99.

177. Tilg H, Cani PD, Mayer EA. Gut microbiome and liver diseases. Gut 2016;65: 2035–44.

178. Pinto C, Giordano DM, Maroni L, et al. Role of inflammation and proinflammatory cytokines in cholangiocyte pathophysiology. Biochim Biophys Acta Mol Basis Dis 2018;1864:1270–8.

179. Zhang H, Leung PSC, Gershwin ME, et al. How the biliary tree maintains immune tolerance? Biochim Biophys Acta Mol Basis Dis 2018;1864:1367–73.

180. Heymann F, Tacke F. Immunology in the liver–from homeostasis to disease. Nat Rev Gastroenterol Hepatol 2016;13:88–110.

181. Citi S. Intestinal barriers protect against disease. Science 2018;359:1097–8.

182. Manfredo Vieira S, Hiltensperger M, Kumar V, et al. Translocation of a gut pathobiont drives autoimmunity in mice and humans. Science 2018;359:1156–61.

183. Tranah TH, Edwards LA, Schnabl B, et al. Targeting the gut-liver-immune axis to treat cirrhosis. Gut 2021;70:982–94.

184. Li B, Selmi C, Tang R, et al. The microbiome and autoimmunity: a paradigm from the gut-liver axis. Cell Mol Immunol 2018;15:595–609.

185. Taniki N, Nakamoto N, Chu PS, et al. Th17 cells in the liver: balancing autoimmunity and pathogen defense. Semin Immunopathol 2022. Online ahead of print.

186. Bozward AG, Ronca V, Osei-Bordom D, et al. Gut-liver immune traffic: Deciphering immune-pathogenesis to Underpin translational therapy. Front Immunol 2021;12:711217.

187. Li Y, Tang R, Leung PSC, et al. Bile acids and intestinal microbiota in autoimmune cholestatic liver diseases. Autoimmun Rev 2017;16:885–96.

188. Maroni L, Ninfole E, Pinto C, et al. Gut-liver Axis and inflammasome activation in cholangiocyte pathophysiology. Cells 2020;9.

189. Giordano DM, Pinto C, Maroni L, et al. Inflammation and the gut-liver Axis in the pathophysiology of cholangiopathies. Int J Mol Sci 2018;19.

190. Cariello M, Gadaleta RM, Moschetta A. The gut-liver axis in cholangiopathies: focus on bile acid based pharmacological treatment. Curr Opin Gastroenterol 2022;38:136–43.

191. Gulamhusein AF, Juran BD, Atkinson EJ, et al. Low incidence of primary biliary cirrhosis (PBC) in the first-degree relatives of PBC probands after 8 years of follow-up. Liver Int 2016;36:1378–82.

192. Gerussi A, Cristoferi L, Carbone M, et al. The immunobiology of female predominance in primary biliary cholangitis. J Autoimmun 2018;95:124–32.

193. Invernizzi P, Miozzo M, Battezzati PM, et al. Frequency of monosomy X in women with primary biliary cirrhosis. Lancet 2004;363:533–5.

194. Invernizzi P, Miozzo M, Selmi C, et al. X chromosome monosomy: a common mechanism for autoimmune diseases. J Immunol 2005;175:575–8.

195. Libert C, Dejager L, Pinheiro I. The X chromosome in immune functions: when a chromosome makes the difference. Nat Rev Immunol 2010;10:594–604.

196. Miozzo M, Selmi C, Gentilin B, et al. Preferential X chromosome loss but random inactivation characterize primary biliary cirrhosis. Hepatology 2007;46:456–62.

197. Selmi C, Invernizzi P, Miozzo M, et al. Primary biliary cirrhosis: does X mark the spot? Autoimmun Rev 2004;3:493–9.

198. Pessach IM, Notarangelo LD. X-linked primary immunodeficiencies as a bridge to better understanding X-chromosome related autoimmunity. J Autoimmun 2009;33:17–24.

199. Selmi C, Cavaciocchi F, Lleo A, et al. Genome-wide analysis of DNA methylation, copy number variation, and gene expression in monozygotic twins discordant for primary biliary cirrhosis. Front Immunol 2014;5:128.

200. Elgueta R, Benson MJ, de Vries VC, et al. Molecular mechanism and function of CD40/CD40L engagement in the immune system. Immunol Rev 2009;229: 152–72.

201. Oertelt S, Invernizzi P, Selmi C, et al. Soluble CD40L in plasma of patients with primary biliary cirrhosis. Ann N Y Acad Sci 2005;1051:205–10.

202. Mayo MJ, Mosby JM, Jeyarajah R, et al. The relationship between hepatic immunoglobulin production and CD154 expression in chronic liver diseases. Liver Int 2006;26:187–96.

203. Lleo A, Liao J, Invernizzi P, et al. Immunoglobulin M levels inversely correlate with CD40 ligand promoter methylation in patients with primary biliary cirrhosis. Hepatology 2012;55:153–60.

204. Lleo A, Zhang W, Zhao M, et al. DNA methylation profiling of the X chromosome reveals an aberrant demethylation on CXCR3 promoter in primary biliary cirrhosis. Clin Epigenetics 2015;7:61.

205. Chuang YH, Lian ZX, Cheng CM, et al. Increased levels of chemokine receptor CXCR3 and chemokines IP-10 and MIG in patients with primary biliary cirrhosis and their first degree relatives. J Autoimmun 2005;25:126–32.

206. Afonso MB, Rodrigues CMP. MicroRevolution in understanding primary biliary cholangitis pathophysiology. Hepatology 2018;67:1213–5.

207. Bianchi I, Lleo A, Gershwin ME, et al. The X chromosome and immune associated genes. J Autoimmun 2012;38:J187–92.

208. Erice O, Munoz-Garrido P, Vaquero J, et al. MicroRNA-506 promotes primary biliary cholangitis-like features in cholangiocytes and immune activation. Hepatology 2018;67:1420–40.
209. Ananthanarayanan M, Banales JM, Guerra MT, et al. Post-translational regulation of the type III inositol 1,4,5-trisphosphate receptor by miRNA-506. J Biol Chem 2015;290:184–96.
210. Shibao K, Hirata K, Robert ME, et al. Loss of inositol 1,4,5-trisphosphate receptors from bile duct epithelia is a common event in cholestasis. Gastroenterology 2003;125:1175–87.
211. Liaskou E, Hirschfield GM. Genetic association studies and the risk factors for developing the "Immuno-bile-logic" disease primary biliary cholangitis. Hepatology 2018;67:1620–2.
212. Abe K, Takahashi A, Fujita M, et al. Dysbiosis of oral microbiota and its association with salivary immunological biomarkers in autoimmune liver disease. PLoS One 2018;13:e0198757.
213. Hegade VS, Pechlivanis A, McDonald JAK, et al. Autotaxin, bile acid profile and effect of ileal bile acid transporter inhibition in primary biliary cholangitis patients with pruritus. Liver Int 2019;39:967–75.
214. Liwinski T, Casar C, Ruehlemann MC, et al. A disease-specific decline of the relative abundance of Bifidobacterium in patients with autoimmune hepatitis. Aliment Pharmacol Ther 2020;51:1417–28.
215. Lv L, Jiang H, Chen X, et al. The salivary microbiota of patients with primary biliary cholangitis is Distinctive and pathogenic. Front Immunol 2021;12:713647.

Autoantibodies in Primary Biliary Cholangitis

Kristel K. Leung, MD, FRCPC, Gideon M. Hirschfield, MB BChir, FRCP (UK), PhD*

KEYWORDS

- Antimitochondrial antibodies • Autoantibodies • Diagnosis • Cholangitis
- Biliary liver disease

KEY POINTS

- Antimitochondrial antibodies (AMAs) have a significant role in the diagnosis of primary biliary cholangitis (PBC) and are highly specific and sensitive in the context of cholestasis.
- Patients with cholestasis who are AMA negative should have serology for PBC-specific antinuclear antibodies sent.
- Patterns of serology in patients with PBC are not only helpful diagnostically but can also provide prognostic and biologic insights into disease course.

Abbreviations	
AMA	antimitochondrial antibody
PBC	primary biliary cholangitis

INTRODUCTION

Primary biliary cholangitis (PBC) is a chronic immune-mediated liver disease with an estimated global prevalence of 14.6 per 100,000 population (range from 1.91 to 40.2).[1,2] Geographic variation is noted with North American prevalence at 21.8 per 100,000, Europe at 14.6 per 100,000 and the Asian-Pacific region at 9.8 per 100,000.[2] Most patients (85%) identify as women.[2,3] PBC is characterized by an immune-mediated destruction of small bile duct biliary epithelial cells, with a characteristic nonsuppurative destructive cholangitis and ductopenia. There is subsequent cholestasis, progressive liver fibrosis, and complications arise from end-stage liver disease.[4]

Department of Medicine, Division of Gastroenterology & Hepatology, University Health Network, University of Toronto, 200 Elizabeth Street, Eaton Building, 9th Floor, Toronto, Ontario M5G 2C4, Canada
* Corresponding author.
E-mail address: gideon.hirschfield@uhn.ca

Clin Liver Dis 26 (2022) 613–627
https://doi.org/10.1016/j.cld.2022.06.004
1089-3261/22/© 2022 Elsevier Inc. All rights reserved.

The diagnosis of PBC is generally based on 2 of 3 criteria being met: (1) an elevated alkaline phosphatase (ALP) as a marker of elevated cholestasis parameters, (2) positive autoantibodies for antimitochondrial antibody (AMA) with a minimum titer of 1:40, or specific antinuclear antibodies (ANAs) relating to PBC, and/or (3) liver histopathology consistent with PBC.[5] First-line treatment of PBC involves daily ursodeoxycholic acid (UDCA), a hydrophilic bile acid that improves cholestasis parameters and delays histologic and clinical progression to end-stage liver disease and its complications.[6] Second-line treatment options (obeticholic acid, fibrates, and clinical trial therapies) are available for those who have persistently elevated ALP and/or elevated conjugated bilirubin despite UDCA treatment.[7]

This review focuses on the role of autoantibodies in the diagnosis of PBC, as well as the relationship between autoantibodies with pathophysiology and prognostication, along with a discussion regarding novel and other related disease autoantibodies.

The Role of Antimitochondrial Antibodies in Primary Biliary Cholangitis

Mitochondria and their components are known to be recognized as damage-associated molecular patterns that activate the innate immune system and are implicated in signaling with both the innate and active immune response in many diseases.[8,9] Although this has yet to be directly demonstrated in PBC, AMAs have a clearly significant role in the diagnosis of PBC. Unlike most autoantibodies that are found in multiple diseases, AMA is unique in that it is both a highly specific and sensitive marker for PBC: more than 90% of patients with PBC have a positive AMA, whereas 0.5% of healthy individuals without PBC are AMA positive, and AMA can be found in up to 1% of individuals presenting with extrahepatic disorders.[10–13] AMA was discovered in initial investigations searching for autoantibodies associated with PBC. Walker and colleagues performed indirect immunofluorescence testing (IFT) on PBC-sera-stained human gastric mucosa and thyrotoxic human thyroid, and noted a granular cytoplasmic fluorescence pattern in these tissues that were especially rich in mitochondria.[14] The group then confirmed antimitochondrial reactivity of the sera to subcellular fractions of rat mitochondria and not other subcellular fractions.[14]

The target of AMA in PBC is a family of proteins called the 2-oxo-acid dehydrogenase complexes that participate in oxidative phosphorylation and decarboxylation of keto acid substrates along the inner mitochondrial matrix.[15] This includes the E2 subunits of the pyruvate dehydrogenase complex (PDC-E2), the branched-chain 2-oxo-acid dehydrogenase complex, the ketoglutaric acid dehydrogenase complex, and the anchoring dihydrolipoamide dehydrogenase-binding protein (E3) for PDC-E2.[15] The E2 subunits exhibit lipoyl domain homology, and several studies have demonstrated that the dominant epitope recognized by AMA is located within the lipoyl domain. Most patients with AMA reactivity react against PDC-E2, along with reactivity against the branched-chain 2-oxo acid dehydrogenase E2 complex, the ketoglutaric acid dehydrogenase E2 complex, or both.[15] AMA binding to epitopes within the lipoic acid binding domain disrupts the domain and inhibits enzymatic function.[16]

The role of molecular mimicry between pathogenic molecules and mitochondrial antigens is of particular interest in PBC because human E2 PDC subunits share similar epitope regions with those of Escherichia coli bacteria[17]. Notably, recurrent urinary tract infections in women are associated with PBC,[18] of which E. coli is a commonly detected pathogen. Thus, one concept (among many) involves E. coli PDC-E2 exposure leading to the development and production of AMA.[19,20] Although this may not be the only mechanism in the breakdown in immunologic tolerance in PBC (as other chemicals, infectious and drug triggers have been speculated about), AMA specificity to PDC-E2 hints at a potential contributory role of AMA and PDC-E2 in the immune-mediated pathophysiology of PBC. Notably, the destruction of biliary epithelial cells in PBC is mediated by infiltrative autoreactive T cells, of which some have found to be specific for PDC-E2.[21] Moreover, patients with PBC have abnormal expression of either PDC-E2 or cross-reacting molecules in the apical region of biliary epithelium.[22] However, the titer of AMA does not correlate with symptom duration, jaundice, or serum levels of ALP or immunoglobulins; the titer may fluctuate and fall with treatment, although without overt significance in terms of clinical outcomes.[23–26] Patients positive for immunoglobulin G (IgG) AMA may have significantly more severe disease (as defined by worse histology and elevated biochemical markers), whereas higher IgG and IgA AMA titers were associated with higher Mayo risk score; however, none of the isotypes or titer level was able to predict disease outcome.[26] Furthermore, mitochondria are present in all nucleated cells, including leukocytes and hepatocytes; yet the immune-mediated damage seen in PBC is focused on bile duct epithelial cells. Future research to further delineate the autoantigen and antibody interaction in bile duct epithelial ductal cells will be relevant to understanding the pathophysiology underpinning PBC.

Due to the specificity and sensitivity of AMA in PBC, AMA is an important criterion incorporated into diagnosing PBC. Thus, all patients being evaluated for unexplained chronic cholestasis or suspected PBC should have autoantibody testing for AMA (**Fig. 1**). Preferably, testing for AMA should be done using IFT on rodent kidney/liver tissue and confirmation of fluorescence pattern using human larynx epithelial cancer cell line (Hep-2) cells and solid-phase test systems such as enzyme-linked immunosorbent assays (ELISAs) using bovine or porcine heart mitochondrial fractions.[7] Confirmatory testing after IFT is usually required because other cytoplasmic antibodies (such as cardiolipin antibodies and anti-liver kidney muscle antibodies) can be misinterpreted for AMA.[27]

AMA may also be present for many years before the emergence of biochemical cholestasis and/or other PBC-associated symptoms. In the study by Dahlqvist and colleagues who followed AMA-positive patients without cholestasis or clinical evidence of liver disease, 9 of 92 patients developed clinical features of PBC (with a 5-year incidence rate of PBC of 16%).[28] Longitudinal follow-up of PBC patients with isolated AMA positivity demonstrate these patients often have less advanced histology compared with symptomatic patients at diagnosis, yet remain at risk for progression.[29] Notably, with increased availability of assays to evaluate for AMA, PBC-specific ANA, and other autoantibodies in the modern era, PBC is now often diagnosed at much earlier stages. Most recently, in the Swiss PBC Cohort Study, 24 of 30 patients (80%) with isolated positive PBC serology (with AMA and/or PBC-specific ANA) and normal ALP had histologic features of mild PBC, with 2 patients with Nakanuma stage 3 of 4 disease.[30] Notably, other liver enzymes were frequently mildly elevated. Initiation of UDCA treatment in early stage PBC may be beneficial, as evidenced by normalization of survival in early PBC patients to rates similar to the general population (including those with normal baseline ALP) with treatment.[31] Furthermore, a delay in starting UDCA treatment once PBC is diagnosed is associated with a lower probability of UDCA response, and thus, an increased risk for progression in disease.[32] These findings support the notion that patients who do not exhibit typical clinical cholestasis but have AMA positivity should be evaluated by a hepatologist with consideration for ultrasound and elastography (e.g., Fibroscan), as well as be evaluated for other cholestatic liver diseases (see **Fig. 1**). Thus, in patients with AMA positivity with normal liver enzymes, these patients usually remain with a mild PBC phenotype, but are at risk of PBC-associated complications and require risk stratification, ongoing follow-up with annual liver bloodwork, and monitoring.[29,33]

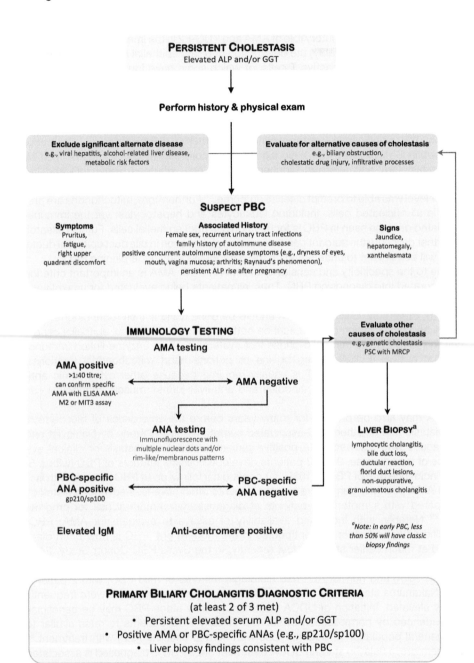

Fig. 1. Approach to persistent cholestasis and diagnosis of primary biliary cholangitis. ALP, alkaline phosphatase; AMA, antimitochondrial antibody; ANA, antinuclear antibody; GGT, gammaglutamyltransferase; IgM, immunoglobulin M; MRCP, magnetic resonance cholangiopancreatography; PBC, primary biliary cholangitis; PSC, primary sclerosing cholangitis.

Although both sensitive and specific for PBC, AMA can be seen in other hepatic and nonhepatic conditions. AMA positivity has been reported in patients with acute liver failure of any cause,[13] as well as other liver conditions including autoimmune hepatitis (AIH), hepatitis C, and alcohol-related liver disease.[28,34] In one series examining sera in patients with acute liver failure from multiple causes, AMAs were detected in 33% of patients, with reactivity found against the same major antigens also seen in PBC.[13] The authors concluded that this finding provides support for the hypothesis that oxidative stress-induced liver injury can lead to the induction of AMAs. Interestingly, AMA positivity waned with time from the initial onset of injury with only one patient retaining AMA positivity at 24 months.[13] AMAs have also been found in other autoimmune conditions such as systemic lupus erythematosus (SLE), Sjogren syndrome, and chronic graft versus host disease after allogeneic stem cell transplantation.[28,35] It is unclear whether AMA serologies persisted in these patients due to sparse longitudinal data. Additionally for such studies, it must be recognized that different AMA assays are usually used making generalization difficult.

Antimitochondrial Antibody-Negative Primary Biliary Cholangitis and Primary Biliary Cholangitis-Specific Antinuclear Antibodies

Depending on the laboratory assays used, 5% to 17% of patients with PBC do not have AMA reactivity. Previously, several studies have demonstrated that this could be partially overcome by using recombinant proteins for 2-oxo-acid dehydrogenase complexes in ELISA or using IgG and IgA specific isotopes of AMA in an M2-enhanced performance ELISA (MIT3), which incorporates the 3 immunodominant epitopes recognized by AMA.[26,36–38] It is thought that AMA-negative PBC is a similar disease process to AMA-positive PBC involving abnormal expression of PDC-E2 and/or molecular mimicry of PDC-E2. Tsuneyama and colleagues demonstrated that sera from AMA-negative patients react similarly to sera from AMA-positive patients, with intense staining of the apical region of the bile duct epithelial cells for PDC-E2, suggesting similar disease processes.[39] It has been previously proposed that a worse prognosis exists for patients diagnosed with AMA-negative PBC compared with AMA-positive PBC, with reduced transplant-free survival[40] and worse bile duct damage around portal areas on histopathology with increased levels of B-cell infiltrates in early phases of bile duct damage.[41] It is unclear whether this reflects diagnostic delay or true pathogenic differences; as such, contemporary research is required to evaluate this further. In clinical practice, it is important to manage patients with PBC the same regardless of AMA serology.

Table 1
Prevalence, sensitivity, and specificity of primary biliary cholangitis autoantibodies

| | | | PBC Diagnosis | |
| | | | Sensitivity (%) | Specificity (%) |
Autoantibody	PBC Prevalence (%)			
AMA	95		73–100[10]	76–100[10]
ANA	50–56[42,105]		-	-
	AMA positive	AMA negative		
Anti-gp210	16–18[105]	15–45[42,105]	6–55[42,106]	62–100[42,50,106]
Anti-sp100	24–31[59,105]	13–54[42,105]	8–42[42,106]	64–100[42,50,106]
Anti-hexokinase-1	39–56[66,67]	12–40[66,67]	45[67]	95[67]
Anti-Kelch	19–26[66,67]	10–29[66,67]	25[67]	95[67]

In the search for identifying other autoantibodies associated with PBC, researchers have also documented ANA serology in PBC patients, with 50% to 56% of all PBC having ANA positivity, and up to 85% of AMA-negative PBC patients having ANA positivity.[42,43] Approximately half of AMA-negative PBC patients will have at least 1 of 3 PBC-specific ANA: namely sp100 (a transcription stimulating factor), promyelocytic leukemia (a transcription coactivator), or gp210 (a nuclear pore glycoprotein).[38,44,45] These antibodies carry high specificity for PBC (**Table 1**)[46] and are particularly useful in diagnosing suspected AMA-negative PBC because these patients may experience a delay in diagnosis, and thus, a delay in appropriate care and treatment (see **Fig. 1**). PBC-specific ANA can be detected by IFT on rodent tissue, followed by confirmation with Hep-2 cell staining in various staining patterns depending on the nuclear antigen target. Nuclear body antigens (eg, sp100) stain in a "multiple nuclear dots pattern", whereas nuclear envelope antigens (eg, gp210) stain with a "dotted or discontinuous rim-like/membranous pattern."[47–49] Previously, multiple nuclear dots and/or rim-like/membranous patterns were found in 31 of 101 (31%) AMA-positive patients and 17 of 22 (77%) AMA-negative patients.[50] Hep-2 cells are usually avoided as an initial test due to the presence of low-titer ANA antibodies in healthy subjects.[27] ELISA can also be used to confirm results of IFT.

The mechanisms behind development and production of ANA in PBC remains unknown but is thought to be related to molecular mimicry with environmental or pathogenic antigens similar to the development of AMA,[51] or to mimicry between the nuclear proteins gp210 and sp100 to the E2 subunit of the PDC.[52] Studies have demonstrated human leukocyte antigen (HLA) alleles (including DRB1*rs9277535, DRB1*03:01, DRB1*15:01, DRB1*01, and DPB1*03:01) with the presence of sp100 antibodies, suggesting a significant genetic predisposition with the sp100 autoantibody.[53] Moreover, a study in Japanese patients reported association between the HLA alleles DRB1*04:04 and DRB1*08:03 with the presence of anti-gp210 and anti-centromere antibodies, respectively.[54] These specific ANA in PBC carry clinical significance. An sp100 autoantibody level may have prognostic utility with respect to the development of fibrosis on liver biopsy,[25] and positivity is associated with worse disease severity and worse prognosis in European studies[55,56]; however, this has not been consistently seen in other populations, particularly in Japan.[57] Of note, with treatment with UDCA, anti-sp100 has been shown to decrease in some patients (similar to AMA titer on UDCA treatment), suggesting modulation by UDCA in the response to the sp100 antigen; however, the clinical significance of this decrease in titer with treatment is not yet known.[58] In patients with high gp210 antibodies, these patients have worse cholestasis and impaired liver function[59] and are associated with more severe interface hepatitis lobular inflammation.[57,60] In a study evaluating serial anti-gp210 levels at diagnosis and with UDCA therapy, patients who had sustained anti-gp210 levels despite treatment were at increased risk of progressing to liver failure.[61] In another study evaluating newly diagnosed PBC patients, those with reactivity to gp210 and/or p62 (a nucleoporin) exhibited an unfavorable disease course characterized by decreased time to death, transplantation, and complication-free survival.[62] More recently, a study evaluating clinical utility of specific ANA in PBC found that anti-gp210 autoantibodies were significantly associated with elevated serum aminotransferase activity, bilirubin, and liver stiffness at presentation, as well as being independently associated with death or liver transplantation, even when accounting for other baseline determinants and UDCA treatment response.[42]

Besides the ANA described, other specific ANA targets in PBC include other nuclear body proteins such as sp140 and small ubiquitin-like modifiers, and nuclear envelope antigens such as the nucleoporin autophagy receptor p62.[48,59,63–65] Of note, patients with PBC-specific ANA to nuclear body proteins often react to 2 to 3 proteins in the family, suggesting clustering of autoantigens. Their exact contribution to PBC pathophysiology remains to be elucidated in future studies.

Other Novel Autoantibodies in Primary Biliary Cholangitis

Although advances in IFT solid phase immunoassays can detect most patients with PBC, a small proportion of patients remain both AMA and ANA negative. More recently, anti-kelch-like 12 protein (anti-Kelch) and anti-hexokinase-1 antibodies have been identified as potential new biomarkers for PBC, with a pooled prevalence of 24.9% positive for anti-Kelch and 45.7% positive for anti-hexokinase-1 in AMA-positive PBC patients, and 19.2% positive for anti-Kelch and 24.7% positive for hexo-kinase-1 in AMA-negative PBC patients.[66,67] The Kelch protein family participate in numerous cellular processes, including cytoskeletal organization, ion channel gating, transcription suppression, and targeting of proteins for ubiquitination.[68] The higher prevalence of hexokinase-1 in PBC may be related to the fact that this enzyme is found on the outer membrane of mitochondria and is responsible for phosphorylating glucose, as well as being involved in the adaptive coupling of mitochondrial metabolism to cell survival and sensitivity to apoptosis.[69] Anti-hexokinase-1 status was associated with lower transplant-free survival and time to liver decompensation.[56] Other autoantibodies of interest include anti-p97/valosin containing protein antibodies that have been found in approximately 13% of PBC patients.; The presence of these autoantibodies seem to suggest a slower progressive disease course and decreased mortality; however, further studies are required as the data is very preliminary.[70]

Secondary Hepatitis in Patients with Primary Biliary Cholangitis (Overlap/Primary Biliary Cholangitis with Features of Autoimmune Hepatitis)

A common clinical scenario is one where a patient presents with features of both PBC and AIH, including elevated transaminase activity and cholestatic liver chemistry, who is found to have AMA positivity along with serology or histology with features of AIH. In a recent study by Haldar and colleagues, 32 of 499 PBC patients (6.4%) had features of PBC with clinically classified overlapping AIH.[42] Such patients have been reported to have suboptimal responses to UDCA therapy, higher rates of decompensated liver disease complications (including bleeding and ascites), and lower transplant-free survival.[71–73] Whether patients with features of both PBC and AIH represent a high-risk PBC phenotype versus the coexistence of 2 disease entities is debated, as some studies show these patients benefit from initiation of UDCA alone, whereas other studies show augmented results with the addition of immunosuppression.[74] It is key to recognize that bile acid metabolism can affect immune responses, raising the concept that hepatitis activity in cholestatic liver disease could be secondary to the underlying biliary process. Two relevant articles recently demonstrated how bile acids can impact the balance of Th17 and Treg cells through the production of mitochondrial reactive oxygen species and modulating expression of key transcription factors as well as function.[75,76] Future studies are required to further understand and characterize these patients in objective ways.

Currently hepatology societal guidance suggests concurrent AIH with PBC can be diagnosed if 2 of 3 criteria are present: (1) elevation of ALT levels greater than 5 times upper limit the normal (ULN), (2) elevation of serum IgG levels greater than 2 times ULN or positive anti-smooth muscle antibody (SMA), and (3) moderate-to-severe interface hepatitis on histology.[7,77] Of note, the presence of anti-double stranded DNA (dsDNA) or anti-p53 (an important tumor-suppressor protein) has been associated with PBC-AIH overlap. In particular, double positivity for AMA and anti-dsDNA are reported to be present in 38% to 50% of AIH-PBC overlap patients, compared with 4% to 10% of PBC only patients and 26% of AIH only patients,[78–80] whereas autoantibodies to p53 were found in 50% of AIH-PBC overlap patients compared with 2% of PBC only patients.[79] Neither of these autoantibodies are specific to PBC, as anti-dsDNA are characteristically seen in SLE,[81] and anti-p53 are seen in variety of solid organ cancers[82] as well as SLE, rheumatoid arthritis, dermatomyositis, autoimmune thyroiditis, and type 1 diabetes.[79] Evaluation of other PBC-specific autoantibodies including anti-Kelch and anti-hexokinase-1 are not significantly associated with PBC-AIH overlap.[80] Further investigation and larger scale studies are required to evaluate the role of autoantibodies and other serum biomarkers in so-called PBC-AIH overlap.

Other Nonspecific Autoantibodies in Primary Biliary Cholangitis and Disease Associations

Patients with PBC will frequently test positive for other autoantibodies that associate with other rheumatological conditions, some of which may occasionally be concurrently present with PBC.[83] PBC is commonly associated with autoimmune thyroid disease; however, the presence of thyroid disease does not influence the natural history or progression of PBC.[83,84] Patients with PBC often have concurrent reactivity to thyroid disease antibodies, with increased anti-thyroglobulin antibody in 55% of patients and anti-thyroid peroxidase antibody in 46% of PBC patients without any known thyroid disease seen in one study.[85]

PBC is also associated with celiac disease, with variable prevalence of celiac disease diagnosis among PBC patients ranging from 1% to 12%.[86–88] However, the question as to whether to screen PBC patients for celiac disease is debated.[89] Some studies have demonstrated that not all PBC patients who screen positive for autoantibodies for celiac disease (such as anti-endomysium antibodies and transglutaminase antibodies) with have truly elevated titers of celiac autoantibodies, nor histologic patterns suggestive of celiac disease.[90,91] Bizzaro and colleagues concluded that a true association was present in only 2% of patients, and in most cases, false positives were due to substrate variability in the assay.

Commonly, patients with PBC also have autoantibodies for non-PBC-specific ANA and thrombophilia-associated autoantibodies.[92] Among the ANA family of autoantibodies, patients with PBC may exhibit positivity for anti-centromere, anti-nuclear envelope, anti-Sjögren's-syndrome-related antigen A (SSA) (both ro-52 and ro-60), anti-Sjögren's-syndrome-related antigen B (SSB) (La), anti-double stranded DNA (dsDNA), anti-single strand DNA (ssDNA), anti-histone, anti-topoisomerase I (aka. scl-70), anti-Smith, anti-Jo-1, and anti-U1RNP antibodies.[85,92,93] Anti-nuclear envelope antibodies target proteins of the nuclear lamina, the innermost layer of the nuclear envelope. These anti-lamin and anti-lamin receptor antibodies present with a smooth membrane fluorescence pattern on IFT in 6% to 9% of PBC patients[94]; however, their role is unclear, and anti-lamin antibodies are often also found in other autoimmune conditions such as SLE and chronic fatigue syndrome.[95] Anti-centromere antibodies present with a discrete speckled centromere pattern with IFT staining and are seen targeting the centromere–kinetochore macrocomplex in up to 30% of patients with PBC, while also being seen in a third of patients with systemic sclerosis (SSc) and 10% of those with Sjogren's syndrome.[47,57,96] In patients with both PBC and SSc, 9% to 30% have anti-centromere antibodies.[97–99] The importance of anti-centromere antibodies in PBC disease course is debated, with some data suggesting no difference, whereas others point to a higher risk for ductular reaction, progression to portal hypertension and cirrhosis.[57,100,101] It is also seen in practice that sometimes patients with AMA-negative PBC are anti-centromere positive with consistent PBC histology, and in this scenario, anti-centromere reactivity helps reach the PBC diagnosis.

Thrombophilia-associated autoantibodies (such as those reacting to cardiolipin, beta2-glycoprotein 1, phosphatidylserine, and prothrombin) also have notable presence in sera of PBC patients, with a range of 2% to 70% positivity reported depending on the specific antigen target.[102–104] The presence of these thrombophilia-associated autoantibodies have been reported (but not validated) with later PBC stage, with anti-prothrombin IgM associated with worse prognosis. The underlying mechanisms have yet to be elucidated[92], and additional studies are required to validate these findings and evaluate this association further.

SUMMARY

Testing for autoantibodies is essential to the diagnosis of PBC, as well as evaluation of related disease processes and potential prognostic factors. Future efforts to further characterize autoantibody profiles in PBC will be important in advancing our understanding of the pathophysiological mechanisms while providing new ways to risk stratify patients and possibly insights into therapeutic targets.

CLINICS CARE POINTS

- PBC is an archetypal autoimmune disease. Patients can be diagnosed accurately by appropriate use of immune serology. In particular upto 90-95% of patients are anti-mitochondrial antibody positive.
- Where patients are AMA negative, other serologic profiles based on anti-nuclear antibody patterns can be diagnostic. Some serologic findings, in particular gp210 reactivity, are associated with worse prognosis for patients.

DISCLOSURE

No relevant disclosures for all authors.

REFERENCES

1. Lleo A, Wang GQ, Gershwin ME, et al. Primary biliary cholangitis. Lancet 2020; 396(10266):1915–26.
2. Trivedi P, Hirschfield G. Recent advances in clinical practice: epidemiology of autoimmune liver diseases. Gut 2021;70(10):1989–2003.
3. Lv T, Chen S, Li M, et al. Regional variation and temporal trend of primary biliary cholangitis epidemiology: a systematic review and meta-analysis. J Gastroenterol Hepatol 2021;36(6):1423–34.
4. Gulamhusein AF, Hirschfield GM. Primary biliary cholangitis: pathogenesis and therapeutic opportunities. Nat Rev Gastroenterol Hepatol 2020;17(2):93–110.
5. Hirschfield GM, Dyson JK, Alexander GJM, et al. The British Society of Gastroenterology/UK-PBC primary biliary cholangitis treatment and management guidelines. Gut 2018;67(9):1568–94.
6. Harms MH, van Buuren HR, Corpechot C, et al. Ursodeoxycholic acid therapy and liver transplant-free survival in patients with primary biliary cholangitis. J Hepatol 2019;71(2):357–65.

7. Hirschfield GM, Corpechot C, Invernizzi P, et al. EASL Clinical Practice Guidelines: the diagnosis and management of patients with primary biliary cholangitis. J Hepatol 2017;67(1):145–72.

8. Weinberg SE, Sena LA, Chandel NS. Mitochondria in the regulation of innate and adaptive immunity. Immunity 2015;42(3):406–17.

9. Zhang Q, Raoof M, Chen Y, et al. Circulating mitochondrial DAMPs cause inflammatory responses to injury. Nature 2010;464(7285):104–7.

10. Hu S, Zhao F, Wang Q, et al. The accuracy of the anti-mitochondrial antibody and the M2 subtype test for diagnosis of primary biliary cirrhosis: a meta-analysis. Clin Chem Lab Med 2014;52(11):1533–42.

11. Zamfir O, Briaud I, Dubel L, et al. Anti-pyruvate dehydrogenase autoantibodies in extrahepatic disorders. J Hepatol 1999;31(5):964–5.

12. Mattalia A, Quaranta S, Leung PS, et al. Characterization of antimitochondrial antibodies in health adults. Hepatology 1998;27(3):656–61.

13. Leung PS, Rossaro L, Davis PA, et al. Antimitochondrial antibodies in acute liver failure: implications for primary biliary cirrhosis. Hepatology 2007;46(5): 1436–42.

14. Walker JG, Doniach D, Roitt IM, et al. Serological tests in diagnosis of primary biliary cirrhosis. Lancet 1965;1(7390):827–31.

15. Gershwin ME, Ansari AA, Mackay IR, et al. Primary biliary cirrhosis: an orchestrated immune response against epithelial cells. Immunol Rev 2000;174(1): 210–25.

16. Fregeau DR, Prindiville T, Coppel RL, et al. Inhibition of alpha-ketoglutarate dehydrogenase activity by a distinct population of autoantibodies recognizing dihydrolipoamide succinyltransferase in primary biliary cirrhosis. Hepatology 1990;11(6):975–81.

17. Fussey SP, Ali ST, Guest JR, et al. Reactivity of primary biliary cirrhosis sera with Escherichia coli dihydrolipoamide acetyltransferase (E2p): characterization of the main immunogenic region. Proc Natl Acad Sci U S A 1990;87(10):3987–91.

18. Gershwin ME, Selmi C, Worman HJ, et al. Risk factors and comorbidities in primary biliary cirrhosis: a controlled interview-based study of 1032 patients. Hepatology 2005;42(5):1194–202.

19. Tanaka A, Leung PSC, Gershwin ME. Pathogen infections and primary biliary cholangitis. Clin Exp Immunol 2019;195(1):25–34.

20. Yang Y, Choi J, Chen Y, et al. E. coli and the etiology of human PBC: antimitochondrial antibodies and spreading determinants. Hepatology 2022;75(2): 266–79.

21. Kita H, Matsumura S, He XS, et al. Quantitative and functional analysis of PDC-E2-specific autoreactive cytotoxic T lymphocytes in primary biliary cirrhosis. J Clin Invest 2002;109(9):1231–40.

22. Tsuneyama K, Van de Water J, Leung PS, et al. Abnormal expression of the E2 component of the pyruvate dehydrogenase complex on the luminal surface of biliary epithelium occurs before major histocompatibility complex class II and BB1/B7 expression. Hepatology 1995;21(4):1031–7.

23. Doniach D, Roitt IM, Walker JG, et al. Tissue antibodies in primary biliary cirrhosis, active chronic (lupoid) hepatitis, cryptogenic cirrhosis and other liver diseases and their clinical implications. Clin Exp Immunol 1966;1(3):237–62.

24. Van Norstrand MD, Malinchoc M, Lindor KD, et al. Quantitative measurement of autoantibodies to recombinant mitochondrial antigens in patients with primary biliary cirrhosis: relationship of levels of autoantibodies to disease progression. Hepatology 1997;25(1):6–11.

25. Tana MM, Shums Z, Milo J, et al. The significance of autoantibody changes over time in primary biliary cirrhosis. Am J Clin Pathol 2015;144(4):601–6.

26. Gabeta S, Norman GL, Liaskos C, et al. Diagnostic relevance and clinical significance of the new enhanced performance M2 (MIT3) ELISA for the detection of IgA and IgG antimitochondrial antibodies in primary biliary cirrhosis. J Clin Immunol 2007;27(4):378–87.

27. Sebode M, Weiler-Normann C, Liwinski T, et al. Autoantibodies in autoimmune liver disease—clinical and diagnostic relevance. Review. Front Immunol 2018; 9(609). https://doi.org/10.3389/fimmu.2018.00609.

28. Dahlqvist G, Gaouar F, Carrat F, et al. Large-scale characterization study of patients with antimitochondrial antibodies but nonestablished primary biliary cholangitis. Hepatology 2017;65(1):152–63.

29. Prince MI, Chetwynd A, Craig WL, et al. Asymptomatic primary biliary cirrhosis: clinical features, prognosis, and symptom progression in a large population based cohort. Gut 2004;53(6):865–70.

30. Terziroli Beretta-Piccoli B, Stirnimann G, Mertens J, et al. Primary biliary cholangitis with normal alkaline phosphatase: a neglected clinical entity challenging current guidelines. J Autoimmun 2021;116:102578.

31. Corpechot C, Carrat F, Bahr A, et al. The effect of ursodeoxycholic acid therapy on the natural course of primary biliary cirrhosis. Gastroenterology 2005;128(2): 297–303.

32. Carbone M, Nardi A, Flack S, et al. Pretreatment prediction of response to ursodeoxycholic acid in primary biliary cholangitis: development and validation of the UDCA Response Score. Lancet Gastroenterol Hepatol 2018;3(9):626–34.

33. Mitchison HC, Bassendine MF, Hendrick A, et al. Positive antimitochondrial antibody but normal alkaline phosphatase: is this primary biliary cirrhosis? Hepatology 1986;6(6):1279–84.

34. Tomizawa M, Shinozaki F, Fugo K, et al. Anti-mitochondrial M2 antibody-positive autoimmune hepatitis. Exp Ther Med 2015;10(4):1419–22.

35. Patriarca F, Skert C, Sperotto A, et al. The development of autoantibodies after allogeneic stem cell transplantation is related with chronic graft-vs-host disease and immune recovery. Exp Hematol 2006;34(3):389–96.

36. Miyakawa H, Tanaka A, Kikuchi K, et al. Detection of antimitochondrial autoantibodies in immunofluorescent AMA-negative patients with primary biliary cirrhosis using recombinant autoantigens. Hepatology 2001;34(2):243–8.

37. Nakanuma Y, Harada K, Kaji K, et al. Clinicopathological study of primary biliary cirrhosis negative for antimitochondrial antibodies. Liver 1997;17(6):281–7.

38. Bizzaro N, Covini G, Rosina F, et al. Overcoming a "probable" diagnosis in antimitochondrial antibody negative primary biliary cirrhosis: study of 100 sera and review of the literature. Clin Rev Allergy Immunol 2012;42(3):288–97.

39. Tsuneyama K, Van De Water J, Van Thiel D, et al. Abnormal expression of PDC-E2 on the apical surface of biliary epithelial cells in patients with antimitochondrial antibody—negative primary biliary cirrhosis. Hepatology 1995;22(5): 1440–6.

40. Juliusson G, Imam M, Björnsson ES, et al. Long-term outcomes in antimitochondrial antibody negative primary biliary cirrhosis. Scand J Gastroenterol 2016; 51(6):745–52.

41. Jin Q, Moritoki Y, Lleo A, et al. Comparative analysis of portal cell infiltrates in antimitochondrial autoantibody-positive versus antimitochondrial autoantibody-negative primary biliary cirrhosis. Hepatology 2012;55(5):1495–506.

42. Haldar D, Janmohamed A, Plant T, et al. Antibodies to gp210 and understanding risk in patients with primary biliary cholangitis. Liver Int 2021;41(3):535–44.

43. Muratori L, Parola M, Ripalti A, et al. Liver/kidney microsomal antibody type 1 targets CYP2D6 on hepatocyte plasma membrane. Gut 2000;46(4):553–61.

44. Saito H, Takahashi A, Abe K, et al. Autoantibodies by line immunoassay in patients with primary biliary cirrhosis. Fukushima J Med Sci 2012;58(2):107–16.

45. Liu H, Norman GL, Shums Z, et al. PBC screen: an IgG/IgA dual isotype ELISA detecting multiple mitochondrial and nuclear autoantibodies specific for primary biliary cirrhosis. J Autoimmun 2010;35(4):436–42.

46. Bandin O, Courvalin JC, Poupon R, et al. Specificity and sensitivity of gp210 autoantibodies detected using an enzyme-linked immunosorbent assay and a synthetic polypeptide in the diagnosis of primary biliary cirrhosis. Hepatology 1996; 23(5):1020–4.

47. Granito A, Muratori P, Quarneti C, et al. Antinuclear antibodies as ancillary markers in primary biliary cirrhosis. Expert Rev Mol Diagn 2012;12(1):65–74.

48. Granito A, Muratori L, Tovoli F, et al. Autoantibodies to speckled protein family in primary biliary cholangitis. Allergy Asthma Clin Immunol 2021;17(1):35.

49. von Mühlen CA, Garcia-De La Torre I, Infantino M, et al. How to report the antinuclear antibodies (anti-cell antibodies) test on HEp-2 cells: guidelines from the ICAP initiative. Immunol Res 2021;69(6):594–608.

50. Granito A, Muratori P, Muratori L, et al. Antinuclear antibodies giving the 'multiple nuclear dots' or the 'rim-like/membranous' patterns: diagnostic accuracy for primary biliary cirrhosis. Aliment Pharmacol Ther 2006;24(11–12):1575–83.

51. Bogdanos DP, Baum H, Butler P, et al. Association between the primary biliary cirrhosis specific anti-sp100 antibodies and recurrent urinary tract infection. Dig Liver Dis 2003;35(11):801–5.

52. Shimoda S, Nakamura M, Ishibashi H, et al. Molecular mimicry of mitochondrial and nuclear autoantigens in primary biliary cirrhosis. Gastroenterology 2003; 124(7):1915–25.

53. Wang C, Zheng X, Jiang P, et al. Genome-wide association studies of specific antinuclear autoantibody subphenotypes in primary biliary cholangitis. Hepatology (Baltimore, Md) 2019;70(1):294–307.

54. Umemura T, Joshita S, Ichijo T, et al. Human leukocyte antigen class II molecules confer both susceptibility and progression in Japanese patients with primary biliary cirrhosis. Hepatology 2012;55(2):506–11.

55. Rigopoulou EI, Davies ET, Pares A, et al. Prevalence and clinical significance of isotype specific antinuclear antibodies in primary biliary cirrhosis. Gut 2005; 54(4):528–32.

56. Reig A, Norman GL, Garcia M, et al. Novel anti-hexokinase 1 antibodies are associated with poor prognosis in patients with primary biliary cholangitis. Am J Gastroenterol 2020;115(10):1634–41.

57. Nakamura M, Kondo H, Mori T, et al. Anti-gp210 and anti-centromere antibodies are different risk factors for the progression of primary biliary cirrhosis. Hepatology 2007;45(1):118–27.

58. Züchner D, Sternsdorf T, Szostecki C, et al. Prevalence, kinetics, and therapeutic modulation of autoantibodies against Sp100 and promyelocytic leukemia protein in a large cohort of patients with primary biliary cirrhosis. Hepatology 1997;26(5):1123–30.

59. Muratori P, Muratori L, Ferrari R, et al. Characterization and clinical impact of antinuclear antibodies in primary biliary cirrhosis. Am J Gastroenterol 2003; 98(2):431–7.

60. Huang C, Han W, Wang C, et al. Early prognostic utility of gp210 antibody-positive rate in primary biliary cholangitis: a meta-analysis. Dis Markers 2019; 2019:9121207.

61. Nakamura M, Shimizu-Yoshida Y, Takii Y, et al. Antibody titer to gp210-C terminal peptide as a clinical parameter for monitoring primary biliary cirrhosis. J Hepatol 2005;42(3):386–92.

62. Wesierska-Gadek J, Penner E, Battezzati PM, et al. Correlation of initial autoantibody profile and clinical outcome in primary biliary cirrhosis. Hepatology 2006; 43(5):1135–44.

63. Szostecki C, Guldner HH, Will H. Autoantibodies against "nuclear dots" in primary biliary cirrhosis. Semin Liver Dis 1997;17(1):71–8.

64. Janka C, Selmi C, Gershwin ME, et al. Small ubiquitin-related modifiers: a novel and independent class of autoantigens in primary biliary cirrhosis. *Hepatology.* Mar 2005;41(3):609–16.

65. Bauer A, Habior A, Wieszczy P, et al. Analysis of Autoantibodies against promyelocytic leukemia nuclear body components and biochemical parameters in sera of patients with primary biliary cholangitis. Diagnostics (Basel) 2021; 11(4). https://doi.org/10.3390/diagnostics11040587.

66. Norman GL, Yang CY, Ostendorff HP, et al. Anti-kelch-like 12 and anti-hexokinase 1: novel autoantibodies in primary biliary cirrhosis. Liver Int 2015; 35(2):642–51.

67. Norman GL, Reig A, Viñas O, et al. The prevalence of anti-hexokinase-1 and anti-kelch-like 12 peptide antibodies in patients with primary biliary cholangitis is similar in Europe and North America: a large international, multi-center study. Front Immunol 2019;10:662.

68. Dhanoa BS, Cogliati T, Satish AG, et al. Update on the Kelch-like (KLHL) gene family. Hum Genomics 2013;7(1):13.

69. Robey RB, Hay N. Mitochondrial hexokinases: guardians of the mitochondria. Cell Cycle 2005;4(5):654–8.

70. Miyachi K, Hosaka H, Nakamura N, et al. Anti-p97/VCP antibodies: an autoantibody marker for a subset of primary biliary cirrhosis patients with milder disease? Scand J Immunol 2006;63(5):376–82.

71. Silveira MG, Talwalkar JA, Angulo P, et al. Overlap of autoimmune hepatitis and primary biliary cirrhosis: long-term outcomes. Am J Gastroenterol 2007;102(6): 1244–50.

72. Yang F, Wang Q, Wang Z, et al. The natural history and prognosis of primary biliary cirrhosis with clinical features of autoimmune hepatitis. Clin Rev Allergy Immunol 2016;50(1):114–23.

73. Chazouillères O, Wendum D, Serfaty L, et al. Long term outcome and response to therapy of primary biliary cirrhosis-autoimmune hepatitis overlap syndrome. J Hepatol 2006;44(2):400–6.

74. Freedman BL, Danford CJ, Patwardhan V, et al. Treatment of overlap syndromes in autoimmune liver disease: a systematic review and meta-analysis. J Clin Med 2020;9(5):1449.

75. Hang S, Paik D, Yao L, et al. Bile acid metabolites control TH17 and Treg cell differentiation. Nature 2019;576(7785):143–8.

76. Paik D, Yao L, Zhang Y, et al. Human gut bacteria produce TH17-modulating bile acid metabolites. Nature 2022;603(7903):907–12.

77. Chazouillères O, Wendum D, Serfaty L, et al. Primary biliary cirrhosis-autoimmune hepatitis overlap syndrome: clinical features and response to therapy. Hepatology 1998;28(2):296–301.

78. Muratori P, Granito A, Pappas G, et al. The serological profile of the autoimmune hepatitis/primary biliary cirrhosis overlap syndrome. Am J Gastroenterol 2009; 104(6):1420–5.

79. Himoto T, Yoneyama H, Kurokohchi K, et al. Clinical significance of autoantibodies to p53 protein in patients with autoimmune liver diseases. Can J Gastroenterol 2012;26(3):125–9.

80. Nguyen HH, Shaheen AA, Baeza N, et al. Evaluation of classical and novel autoantibodies for the diagnosis of primary biliary cholangitis-autoimmune hepatitis overlap syndrome (PBC-AIH OS). PLoS One 2018;13(3):e0193960.

81. Wang X, Xia Y. Anti-double stranded DNA antibodies: origin, pathogenicity, and targeted therapies. Review. Front Immunol 2019;10. https://doi.org/10.3389/fimmu.2019.01667.

82. Soussi T. p53 Antibodies in the sera of patients with various types of cancer: a review. Cancer Res 2000;60(7):1777–88.

83. Floreani A, Cazzagon N. PBC and related extrahepatic diseases. Best Pract Res Clin Gastroenterol 2018;34-35:49–54.

84. Floreani A, Mangini C, Reig A, et al. Thyroid dysfunction in primary biliary cholangitis: a comparative study at two european centers. Am J Gastroenterol 2017; 112(1):114–9.

85. Nakamura H, Usa T, Motomura M, et al. Prevalence of interrelated autoantibodies in thyroid diseases and autoimmune disorders. J Endocrinol Invest 2008;31(10):861–5.

86. Kingham JG, Parker DR. The association between primary biliary cirrhosis and coeliac disease: a study of relative prevalences. Gut 1998;42(1):120–2.

87. Lawson A, West J, Aithal GP, et al. Autoimmune cholestatic liver disease in people with coeliac disease: a population-based study of their association. Aliment Pharmacol Ther 2005;21(4):401–5.

88. Callichurn K, Cvetkovic L, Therrien A, et al. Prevalence of celiac disease in patients with primary biliary cholangitis. J Can Assoc Gastroenterol 2021; 4(1):44–7.

89. Narciso-Schiavon JL, Schiavon LL. To screen or not to screen? Celiac antibodies in liver diseases. World J Gastroenterol 2017;23(5):776–91.

90. Bizzaro N, Tampoia M, Villalta D, et al. Low specificity of anti-tissue transglutaminase antibodies in patients with primary biliary cirrhosis. J Clin Lab Anal 2006; 20(5):184–9.

91. Floreani A, Betterle C, Baragiotta A, et al. Prevalence of coeliac disease in primary biliary cirrhosis and of antimitochondrial antibodies in adult coeliac disease patients in Italy. Dig Liver Dis 2002;34(4):258–61.

92. Agmon-Levin N, Shapira Y, Selmi C, et al. A comprehensive evaluation of serum autoantibodies in primary biliary cirrhosis. J Autoimmun 2010;34(1):55–8.

93. Hu C-J, Zhang F-C, Li Y-Z, et al. Primary biliary cirrhosis: what do autoantibodies tell us? World J Gastroenterol 2010;16(29):3616–29.

94. Miyachi K, Hankins RW, Matsushima H, et al. Profile and clinical significance of anti-nuclear envelope antibodies found in patients with primary biliary cirrhosis: a multicenter study. J Autoimmun 2003;20(3):247–54.

95. Nesher G, Margalit R, Ashkenazi YJ. Anti-nuclear envelope antibodies: clinical associations. Semin Arthritis Rheum 2001;30(5):313–20.

96. Kajio N, Takeshita M, Suzuki K, et al. Anti-centromere antibodies target centromere–kinetochore macrocomplex: a comprehensive autoantigen profiling. Ann Rheum Dis 2021;80(5):651–9.

97. Bernstein RM, Callender ME, Neuberger JM, et al. Anticentromere antibody in primary biliary cirrhosis. Ann Rheum Dis 1982;41(6):612–4.

98. Chan HL, Lee YS, Hong HS, et al. Anticentromere antibodies (ACA): clinical distribution and disease specificity. Clin Exp Dermatol 1994;19(4):298–302.

99. Hansen BU, Eriksson S, Lindgren S. High prevalence of autoimmune liver disease in patients with multiple nuclear dot, anti-centromere, and mitotic spindle antibodies. Scand J Gastroenterol 1991;26(7):707–13.

100. Rigamonti C, Shand LM, Feudjo M. Clinical features and prognosis of primary biliary cirrhosis associated with systemic sclerosis. Gut 2006;55(3):388–94.

101. Shi TY, Zhang LN, Chen H, et al. Risk factors for hepatic decompensation in patients with primary biliary cirrhosis. World J Gastroenterol 2013;19(7):1111–8.

102. Zachou K, Liaskos C, Rigopoulou E, et al. Presence of high avidity anticardiolipin antibodies in patients with autoimmune cholestatic liver diseases. Clin Immunol 2006;119(2):203–12.

103. Mankaï A, Manoubi W, Ghozzi M, et al. High frequency of antiphospholipid antibodies in primary biliary cirrhosis. J Clin Lab Anal 2015;29(1):32–6.

104. Gabeta S, Norman GL, Gatselis N, et al. IgA anti-b2GPI antibodies in patients with autoimmune liver diseases. J Clin Immunol 2008;28(5):501.

105. Muratori L, Granito A, Muratori P, et al. Antimitochondrial antibodies and other antibodies in primary biliary cirrhosis: diagnostic and prognostic value. Clin Liver Dis 2008;12(2):261–76.

106. Hu S-L, Zhao F-R, Hu Q, et al. Meta-analysis assessment of gp210 and sp100 for the diagnosis of primary biliary cirrhosis. PLoS One 2014;9(7):e101916.

Prognostic Scoring Systems in Primary Biliary Cholangitis: An Update

Miki Scaravaglio, MD, Marco Carbone, MD, PhD*

KEYWORDS

- Primary biliary cholangitis • Autoimmune liver disease • Risk-stratification
- Prognostic models • Prediction

KEY POINTS

- The increasing availability of novel therapeutic molecules has prompted the need to improve our ability to predict primary biliary cholangitis (PBC) disease trajectory and thus to redefine the current standard of care.
- Validated prognostic systems based on the assessment of biochemical response to ursodeoxycholic acid (UDCA) accurately identify patients who might benefit from combination therapy with second-line drugs or clinical trials and have been the paradigm of risk stratification of PBC patients so far.
- Recent evidence highlighting the limits of a step-up approach waiting up to 12 months for first-line treatment failure to offer therapy escalation have shed lights on the urgent need of prediction models that enable us to define each patient's risk profile at disease onset and thus offer the best therapeutic option as early as possible.
- The integration of omics-technologies and artificial intelligence might offer a unique platform to develop personalized medicine in PBC.

NEED FOR PROGNOSTIC SCORING SYSTEMS IN PRIMARY BILIARY CHOLANGITIS

Prognostic modeling plays a fundamental role in modern medicine because it enables to predict the course of the disease with accuracy by using, ideally simple, available medical investigations. The availability of prognostic scoring systems is useful for supporting decision-making but also to provide potential surrogate markers of hard endpoints for clinical trials, particularly in slowly progressive diseases, such as primary biliary cholangitis (PBC). Furthermore, the process of biomarker discovery and model development might improve our comprehension of complex phenomena underlying disease progression.

The authors have no conflicts of interest to declare.

Division of Gastroenterology and Hepatology, Department of Medicine and Surgery, University of Milano-Bicocca, Via Cadore 48, 20900 Monza (MB), Italy

* Corresponding author.

E-mail addresses: m.scaravaglio@campus.unimib.it (M.S.); marco.carbone@unimib.it (M.C.)

Clin Liver Dis 26 (2022) 629–642

https://doi.org/10.1016/j.cld.2022.06.005

liver.theclinics.com

Abbreviations	
INR	International Normalized Ratio
AMA	Anti-mithocondrial antibody
ALP	Alkaline phosphatase
EASL	European Association for the Study of the Liver
NADPH	Nicotinamide adenine dinucleotide phosphate
NOX	oxidase
PPAR	Peroxisome Proliferator-activated Receptor
HCC	Hepatocellular carcinoma
SNP	Single-nucleotide polymorphism
BEC	Biliary epithelial cells
EU	European Union
AI	Artificial Intelligence

PBC is a chronic cholestatic liver disease characterized by an autoimmune-mediated destruction of small intrahepatic bile duct. Although the course of the disease is slowly progressive in most cases, a significant subgroup of patients experiences a more aggressive disease. This is generally characterized by a limited or lack of response to therapies that can lead to cirrhosis and the need for liver transplantation (LT).

Current standard of care of PBC patients is based on 3 pillars: (1) continuous management of patients' symptoms, (2) treatment and evaluation of therapeutic response, and (3) staging and surveillance.[1]

For at least 3 decades, in which UDCA has been the only drug available, criteria of response to UDCA have been the backbone of prognostic modeling in PBC because of the well-established relationship between serum liver tests that is, alkaline phosphatase, bilirubin, transaminases, and biliary injury and liver inflammation, which are the main drivers of disease progression. Patients who failed to control the disease had an invariable progress to end-stage liver disease (ESLD) in the absence of other treatment options.

The recent development of new drugs targeting different pathogenetic pathways has given us the chance to further reduce the group of patients who do not benefit from a disease-modifying treatment,[2] that is, the nonresponders to UDCA. Nonetheless, the current standard of care, by introducing a delay of 6 to 12 months in the definition of the patient's risk profile, might hamper the potential impact of these novel drugs on more aggressive disease phenotypes. Therefore, it has become crucial to change our paradigm of disease management and refine our ability to stratify patients early into different risk categories, ideally at the onset of the disease. Indeed, by predicting the patient's individual disease trajectory at diagnosis, we would be able to offer tailored follow-up and timely access to novel therapeutic strategy, ideally reversing the progression of the disease with a foreseeable significant impact on long-term outcomes.

Several prediction tools have been already validated to be used in clinical trials and in clinical practice providing a reliable support in medical decision-making throughout the disease course. They are mainly based on easy-to-collect serologic and clinical variables. Recently, the role of liver fibrosis assessment, ideally by noninvasive means using transient elastography, and thus the definition of baseline disease stage has gained prognostic significance because it provides insights on the risk of future liver-related event beyond response to treatment.[3]

In this review, we will focus on the main aspects associated with prognostication in PBC with particular interest on established and new emerging prediction tools highlighting their key role for clinical trial design and for progress toward a more personalized care in PBC.

HISTORICAL PROGNOSTIC SCORING SYSTEMS

Albumin, bilirubin, INR are well-recognized predictors of liver-related outcomes. As such, they have been included in the first models developed for PBC prognostication, that is, Mayo risk score (MRS), as well as they are part of the most widely used scores for ESLD, that is, albumin-bilirubin score, Child-Turcotte-Pugh score, and the model for ESLD.[4]

MRS was first developed in 1989 with the aim to aid clinicians in the selection of patients for and timing of LT in PBC patients. The current revised version of MRS includes the evaluation of both biochemical (serum albumin, total bilirubin, and prothrombin time) and clinical variables (patient's age, peripheral edema, and the use of diuretic treatments) from diagnosis throughout the disease course and give an estimation of survival at 6, 12, till 24 months.[5]

Before MRS, other 2 survival prediction models were validated, namely the Yale[6] and the European[7] models that include not only clinical and biochemical variables similar to MRS but also histologic parameters.

However, in the period when these models were developed, PBC was usually diagnosed at a late stage and there was no therapy available. The widespread availability of AMA testing, which improved of our ability to detect the disease at an earlier stage; and the introduction of UDCA therapy, which dramatically improved the disease course, made obsolete prognostic scores that included surrogate markers of ESLD.

THE BIOCHEMICAL RESPONSE TO TREATMENT

UDCA has been proved beneficial, at the optimized dose of 13 to 15 mg/kg/d, on liver function tests (LFTs) and histology. Moreover, LFTs improvement or normalization (particularly ALP and bilirubin) after UDCA treatment, the "UDCA response," has shown impact on long-term outcomes.[1,8] Efforts of the scientific community during the last decade have been focused on the development and validation of prognostic tools based on different criteria to define UDCA response by variably combining variables and testing different biochemical thresholds. The evaluation of UDCA response is nowadays the cornerstone of prognostication in PBC; indeed, an inadequate response to UDCA treatment is one of the most robust predictor of long-term prognosis[9] and thus widely used by health-care providers and in clinical trials.

Most of these prognostic models have been validated at 12 months after UDCA initiation. However, there is mounting evidence that the evaluation at 6 months might be more effective because it couples an equivalent prediction reliability with a shorter delay in stratifying patient's treatment response.[10]

Binary Prognostic Systems

Early definitions of UDCA response were based on specific thresholds of ALP, bilirubin, transaminases, and serum albumin with the aim to dichotomize the treatment response (ie, response vs nonresponse) and therefore prognosis (good vs poor). The currently recommended dichotomous definitions of UDCA response with their characteristics are listed in **Table 1**.[11–15] They have been developed from single-center longitudinal cohorts of PBC patients to predict death and LT, except for Toronto criteria, which predict histologic progression. Among them, Paris I criteria has been reported to be the more accurate in different large validation cohorts.[16,17]

Table 1
Characteristics of binary and continuous scoring systems for risk stratification in ursodeoxycholic acid-treated primary biliary cholangitis patients

Binary Prognostic Systems	Definitions	Evaluation Time Point (year)	No Patients	Centers	C statistical[a]
Barcelona, 2006[11]	Decrease in ALP >40% or normalization	1	192	Single	0.56, 0.61, 0.61
Paris I, 2008[12]	ALP<3xULN, AST<2xULN and bilirubin ≤ 1 mg/dl	1	292	Single	0.81, 0.81, 0.80
Rotterdam, 2009[13]	Normalization of bilirubin and/or albumin	1	375	Single	NA
Toronto, 2010[14]	ALP≤ 1.67xULN	2	69	Single	0.65, 0.70, 0.70
Paris II, 2011[15]	ALP≤1.5xULN, AST≤1.5xULN, bilirubin≤1 mg/dl	1	165	Single	0.75, 0.75, 0.74

Continuous Prognostic Systems	Scoring Variables	Evaluation Time Point (Year)	No Patients	Centers	C Statistical[b]
GLOBE score, 2015[17]	Bilirubin, albumin, ALP, platelet, baseline age	1	2488	15	0.82
UK-PBC score, 2016[16]	Bilirubin, AST/ALT, ALP, baseline platelet and albumin	1	1916	155	0.96, 0.95, 0.94 (5, 10, 15-y risk scores)

Abbreviations: ALP, alkaline phosphatase; ALT, alanine aminotransferase; AST, aspartate aminotransferase; ULN upper limit of normal.
[a] C statistics at 5, 10, 15 y calculated in the UK-PBC research cohort.
[b] C statistics calculated in the validation cohort.

The industry's preferred scoring system is a revised version of the Toronto criteria, namely the POISE (PBC OCA International Study of Efficacy) definition of UDCA response (ALP <1.67 × the upper limit of normal (ULN), ≥15% reduction in ALP, and normalization of total bilirubin), the most used dichotomous prognostic system in the setting of clinical trials given is higher sensibility compared with Paris I criteria.[18]

The great advantage of dichotomous definitions is that they are easy-to-use (and to remember) in clinical practice, including the primary care setting.

However, they also have methodological flaws in their development that limit their predictive accuracy potentially compromising a proper disease management. The stratification of patients in only 2 levels of risk is a simplification of the continuous relationship between the individual trend of LFTs and the risk of death or LT.[16] Moreover, dichotomous prognostic systems do not set in the time frame the probability of adverse event, thus classifying in the same risk category patients in actual need of LT and those who will need it in years.

Another important concern is that they neglect the influence of the stage of the disease on biochemical response to UDCA and on survival. Of note, although our diagnostic performance has improved over years and most of patients are detected at an early stage of the disease, still some patients may receive the diagnosis when the liver disease has already evolved to cirrhosis.

Furthermore, a neglected factor is the delta reduction in LFTs that has emerged in the definition of treatment benefit, which is only included in the Barcelona criteria.[11] Indeed, patients with highly elevated ALP and/or bilirubin at baseline may experience a significant biochemical improvement after UDCA introduction without meeting the thresholds defined for UDCA response. This is a key factor to evaluate the net benefit of a novel therapy.

More recently, although the EASL recommendations[1] advocate ALP less than 1.5×ULN and bilirubin less than 1×ULN as thresholds at which long-term risk becomes equally to a control healthy population, there is mounting evidence that the use of more restrictive goals of treatment might optimize PBC patients survival. Particularly, a threshold of 0.6×ULN for bilirubin and normalization for ALP has been proposed to refine previous definition criteria with the aim to identify a potential group of PBC patients that might benefit from second-line treatment.[19]

Continuous Prognostic Scores

In the attempt to overcome limitations of the binary stratification, the UK-PBC Research Group and the Global PBC Study Group independently proposed 2 continuous prognostic systems by analyzing large, multicenter PBC cohorts.[16,17] Both continuous risk scores, namely the UK-PBC risk score and the GLOBE score, respectively, were externally validated and outperformed previous binary models.[20]

These include LFTs after 12 months of UDCA treatment, with biochemical variables treated as continuous. Moreover, in contrast to binary criteria, they both include surrogate markers of disease stage (ie, albumin and platelet count). Particularly, age at diagnosis proved to correlate with the probability of response to UDCA with an approximately linear relationship with rates of response to UDCA ranging from 90% in patients aged more than 70 years to 50% in those younger than age 30.[21]

Instead of dichotomizing patients into responders or nonresponders, the UK-PBC risk score estimates the risk of LT or liver-related death within 5, 10, and 15 years; whereas the GLOBE score estimates the overall (cause of deaths) survival within 3, 5, 10, and 15 years.

Initially, both the UK-PBC and the GLOBE scores, similarly to the binary models, provided a snapshot at baseline of the patient's risk profile, whereas risk is dynamic throughout the disease course. Thereafter, they were both shown to work even when applied on follow-up data ignoring, although, the impact of second-line therapies.

Although continuous prognostic scoring systems have refined our ability to stratify PBC patients' risk profile, there are still some challenges that need to be addressed. Notably, there are no specific thresholds that identify patients at high risk in need of second-line therapies and those at low risk who can be de-escalated in intensity of management. Although health-economics, cost-effectiveness studies are needed to identify the threshold/s that define treatment benefit, such scores are nowadays limited to counseling of patients and families on long-term prognosis and to the clinical trial setting to explore the estimated survival benefit of new drugs targeting LFT's improvement.

In addition, no specific criterion to define response to second-line treatment has been developed, so far. Indeed, continuous prognostic systems have been mutualized to assess response to obeticholic acid (OCA)[22] and bezafibrate[23] ignoring potential biases given to different therapeutic mechanisms compared with UDCA.

Finally, scoring systems do not include gamma-glutamyl transferase (GGT), another serum marker of cholestasis that has been largely overlooked in predicting long-term outcomes in clinical practice and in clinical trials. The need for an alternative to ALP has emerged in specific clinical context characterized by a reduced reliability of

ALP levels as surrogate marker of disease activity (pregnancy, childhood, severe osteoporosis) and in clinical trials setting, as farnesoid X receptor (FXR) agonists, may induce the expression of bone-derived ALP gene.[24] Within the Global PBC study group, Gerussi and colleagues have recently provided the evidence of the independent, prognostic value of GGT toward LT-free survival in PBC patients,[25] thus supporting its use in clinical decision-making and in clinical trials when considered more appropriate by the investigators. Indeed, recent clinical trials in PBC such as anti-NOX agents (ie, setanaxib[26]) and nonsteroidal FXR agonists (ie, tropifexor[27]) have defined GGT as primary endpoint.

BRINGING FORWARD RISK-STRATIFICATION AT DISEASE ONSET

With the current PBC management, patients with aggressive disease who do not respond to UDCA, end up waiting for more than 12 months to receive treatment escalation, whereas the biliary injury and fibrosis potentially progress. Indeed, PBC has the potential to be an aggressive and rapidly progressive condition, especially in younger patients who are more likely to fail with UDCA and to develop debilitating symptoms.[21,28]

Given the current and forthcoming availability of several disease-modifying treatments such as PPAR-agonists, combinations of PPAR-OCA, anti-CD80,[18,29–31] this "wait-to-fail" approach might not be optimal. Efforts have been focused to bringing forward risk stratification at diagnosis by developing a novel prognostic tool, which enables pretreatment identification of patients who are unlikely to respond to UDCA and might therefore benefit from early introduction of add-on therapies (**Fig. 1**).

The Ursodeoxycholic Acid Response Score

The combined effort of the *UK-PBC Research Group* and the *Italian PBC study group* has recently brought to the identification of key clinical pretreatment parameters associated with inadequate response to UDCA. A novel predictive model based on these clinical parameters, the *UDCA response score* (URS), has been developed and externally validated demonstrating a high accuracy (area under the receiver operating characteristic [AUROC] curve = 0.83) to discriminated PBC patients who are unlikely to response to UDCA monotherapy before treatment initiation.[32] The online URS calculator is available at http://www.mat.uniroma2.it/~alenardi/URS.html.

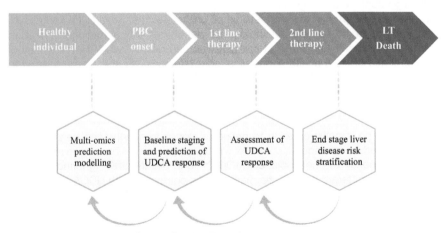

Fig. 1. Bringing forward risk stratification in PBC.

The following 6 pretreatment variables were included in the URS: ALP, total bilirubin, transaminases and age at diagnosis, interval from PBC diagnosis to UDCA initiation (in years), and the delta change of ALP from diagnosis to treatment initiation. Particularly, higher ALP at diagnosis and a further increase of ALP before UDCA start, together with higher total bilirubin, younger age and longer delay in treatment start were associated with a lower probability of response to UDCA. However, higher transaminases correlated with a higher probability of response, probably expressing parenchymal inflammation at an early hepatitic stage of the disease, more susceptible to the beneficial effect of UDCA. Of note, the delta ALP and the treatment delay possibly reflected the progression of biliary injury due to undertreatment, emphasizing the prognostic impact of delaying effective second-line therapy.

Importantly, the model received a "biological" validation by showing a significant correlation between treatment failure estimate and histologic features of disease severity, namely ductular reaction, biliary metaplasia, and the extent of fibrosis, thus highlighting the role of biliary damage severity—and ALP and bilirubin as its surrogate markers—as predictor of responsiveness to choleretic treatment.[32]

Although the application of URS in clinical practice is still to be implemented, this novel prediction model has been used to select high-risk patients at diagnosis for a UK ongoing trial investigating the feasibility and appropriateness of a novel top–down PBC treatment paradigm, characterized by a first-line treatment regimen of UDCA combined with OCA for those patients who were predicted to have a poor response to UDCA alone (for details, refer to https://fundingawards.nihr.ac.uk/award/NIHR131359).

Staging of the Disease

Paradoxically, although the historical scores (eg, MRS) were based on signs of end-stage disease, the recent ones overlooked markers of disease stage, such as the fibrosis stage, focusing only on markers of cholestasis and inflammation. This is likely due to the abandon of liver biopsy (LB) in clinical practice in PBC for diagnostic purposes, as per international guidelines.[1] Although LB is still the gold standard to assess the fibrosis extent in liver disease, its invasiveness and high rate of sampling error coupled with the availability of noninvasive tools for PBC diagnosis (AMA and cholestasis) made LB obsolete in PBC. It is nowadays performed only in specific scenario, that is, diagnosis of seronegative PBC, in patients with inadequate response to UDCA to identify mechanisms underlying treatment resistance, to exclude coexistence of autoimmune hepatitis (AIH), nonalcoholic steato-hepatitis, or other comorbidities when suspected. Lately, the evidence that adding liver fibrosis extent at diagnosis improved prediction accuracy of the *UK-PBC risk score* and the *GLOBE score* has marked a turning point, highlighting the need to incorporate liver fibrosis markers into paradigms of risk stratification of PBC patients because it is an independent predictor of outcomes during treatment response.

In recent years, we assisted to the development and validation of several noninvasive tests as surrogate markers of liver fibrosis that are now widely used for PBC staging and thus easy-to-use for prognostication purposes. Liver stiffness measure (LSM) by vibration-controlled transient elastography (VCTE), aspartate aminotransferase-to-platelet-ratio index (APRI) and enhanced liver fibrosis (ELF) are recommended by EASL as complementary approaches to assess PBC stage and prognosis.[4]

Serologic markers

In a large multicenter cohort of 3335 well-characterized PBC patients, an APRI greater than 0.54 after 12 months of UDCA treatment accurately predicted the risk of major nonneoplastic cirrhosis-related complications within 10 and 15 years beyond biochemical response to UDCA assessed by GLOBE score, thus improving thereof prognostic performance.[33] For its characteristics, easy-to-use and inexpensive, APRI score is widely applied in clinical practice.

Similarly, in a cohort of 161 PBC patients the ELF score[34] evaluated at baseline and prospectively has been proved to correlate with disease severity and the risk of long-term outcomes since the earlier stage of the disease. This algorithm is based on 3 proteomic markers of fibrosis, that is, hyaluronic acid, tissue inhibitor of metalloproteinase 1, and procollagen type III N-terminal propeptide, which are expressed during early stages of collagen deposition in liver parenchyma. Although it is widely adopted in clinical, the high cost of the equipment, the lack of study investigating its fluctuations over time and the possible existence of influence factors (gender, age, and ethnicity) might explain its limited application in clinical practice.

Elastography markers

There is large body of evidence on the accuracy of LSM in ruling in severe fibrosis or cirrhosis in several chronic liver diseases, including PBC. The historical study investigating the role of LSM by TE in PBC was a single-center study including 103 patients on UDCA treatment, at different times from diagnosis, including patients with overlap PBC/AIH syndrome under immunosuppressive therapy.[35] In this study, LSM by VCTE succeeded in discriminating advanced fibrosis (AF) with specificity and sensitivity greater than 90%. Moreover, an LSM greater than 9.6 kPa at baseline and a progression of ≥ 2.1 kPa/y in the overall cohort were associated with a 5-fold and 8-fold increased risk of liver-related adverse outcomes, respectively. However, the heterogeneity of the cohort limited the strength of these conclusions.

Recently, Cristoferi and colleagues have conducted a study on a multicenter cohort of 167 treatment naïve PBC patients at the disease onset from the *Italian PBC Registry*.[36] Authors have developed a "dual cut-off" approach characterized by a lower threshold of 6.5 kPa ruling out AF and a higher threshold of 11 kPa ruling in AF, with a sensitivity and specificity greater than 90%. Both values were externally validated with an AUROC of 0.89. A novel algorithm (**Fig. 2**) for early risk stratification of PBC patients has been proposed, which combines the prediction accuracy of URS with the dual cut-off approach to assess PBC stage by VCTE. This stratifies PBC patients in 3 categories at diagnosis based on the risk of future liver-related adverse outcomes (1) "*low risk patients*" without AF and high probability of UDCA response who can be deescalated in the intensity of care; (2) "*high risk patients*" with AF and low probability of UDCA response who can be offered early treatment escalation and HCC surveillance; (3) "*intermediate risk patients*" with "frozen" advanced disease or patients with active disease at an early stage, who should be offered HCC surveillance and cofactor management, and second-line drugs, respectively. Future studies are needed to establish whether timely repeated VCTE examination would improve the prediction accuracy of this model, in particular for intermediate risk patients.

POSSIBILITIES FROM INTEGRATING MULTIOMICS DATA THROUGH ARTIFICIAL INTELLIGENCE FOR PHENOTYPE DEFINITION AND DISEASE TRAJECTORIES

PBC pathogenesis is characterized by a high degree of complexity that involves the interaction between genes and environment. Most of the pathways underlying disease onset and progression are still not entirely clear, and this hinders the development of effective, disease-specific therapies. Patients have been observed to have different response to therapy and different disease trajectories. The biomarker discovery to support risk stratification has been mainly focused on available investigations (laboratory

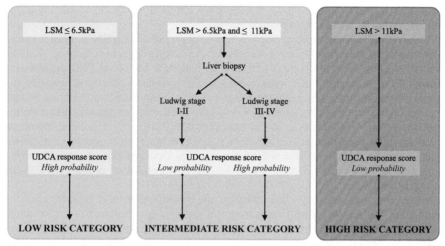

Fig. 2. A new algorithm combining disease stage and pretreatment likelihood of UDCA response for baseline risk stratification in PBC. (*Adapted from* Cristoferi L, Calvaruso V, Overi D, et al. Accuracy of Transient Elastography in Assessing Fibrosis at Diagnosis in Naïve Patients With Primary Biliary Cholangitis: A Dual Cut-Off Approach. *Hepatology* 2021; 74: 1496–1508.)

and radiological). The evolving landscape of high-throughput technologies might come in support to unravel the biological complexity of PBC by integrating and interpreting a large amount of clinical and biological data. The multiomics assessment of an individual—including genomic, epigenomic, transcriptomic, proteomic, metabolomic, microbiomic, and many others emerging[37]—combined with AI computational, provides the opportunity to deeply characterize the disease and accelerate the discovery of novel biomarkers, ideally more directly linked to the pathogenetic mechanisms.

Within the breadth of AI applications, machine learning (ML) is a computing process with the capability to recognize patterns within data and leverage them to make prediction on the behavior of upcoming instances. Given the foreseeable large amount of data, from standard laboratory and clinical variables to omics-derived biomarkers of disease, ML has the role to infer potential predictive disease models based on the interpretation of these data.

A recent promising application of ML, applied to an international, large cohort (N >10,000 patients) of well characterized PBC patients, identified clusters of patients with PBC having different biochemical phenotypes that correlated with different long-term prognosis providing a novel way of risk stratifying PBC patients. Particularly the cluster analysis process highlighted the prognostic impact of minimal variations of serum albumin within the normal range among different clusters of patients, leading to the finding that an improvement of serum albumin level above 1.2×ULN after 1 year of UDCA treatment is associated with survival.[38]

Genomics, in the form of genome wide association study (GWAS), has offered more insights in PBC susceptibility, as in other complex diseases[39] and the identification of new targetable drug pathways.[40] In comparison with other complex diseases, such as type 2 diabetes mellitus, no great attempts have been performed to explore risk prediction modeling from polygenic risk score (PRS). In a preliminary, post-GWAS attempt to explore outcome prediction based on genetic variants, we have identified a specific SNP, selected from GWAS in PBC[41] which when associated with tacrolimus-based regimen, was correlated with a higher risk of posttransplant recurrence of PBC.[42] International collaborative efforts are ongoing to identify a genetic signature of disease progression in PBC.[43,44]

Transcriptomic analysis, including both coding and noncoding RNAs, of liver tissue might identify transcriptional biomarkers that can then be sought in circulation. A study evaluating gene expression profile of a small historical cohort of PBC patients by means of the Nanostring nCounter applied to formalin-fixed paraffin-embedded biopsies from diagnosis, provided important insights on the association between high expression of inflammation-related gene and poor prognosis, suggesting also a signature of treatment response to immunosuppressive therapy.[45] In parallel, because blood sample-based biomarkers are more suitable, it has been suggested that differential expression profile of microRNAs in peripheral blood mononuclear cells correlates with disease progression, in particular the downregulation of hsa-miR-223-3p and hsa-miR-21-5p.[46]

Proteomics and metabolomics, through the identification and quantification of small-sized molecules, might offer support in generating hypothesis and biomarker discovery. Notably, the UK PBC consortium[47] has recently conducted a study investigating the serum proteome of PBC patients with the attempt to clarify molecular mechanisms underlying nonresponse to UDCA. They found differences in serum chemokines in patients with distinct UDCA response profile. Of note, they reported a reduction of chemokines production from baseline but not a complete thereof normalization in UDCA responder suggesting that UDCA attenuate without resolve disease associated inflammatory processes in PBC. In nonresponders, levels of chemokines were significant higher compared with UDCA responder, particularly CCL20 and CXCL11, the first being associated with the process of BEC senescence, a well-known key pathogenetic driver of PBC progression.[48] Importantly, these chemokines have been selected to be used as mechanistic disease biomarkers in an ongoing clinical trial evaluating the efficacy of a first-line combined therapy for UDCA plus OCA in inducing disease remission by the reversing of the BEC senescence process (https://fundingawards.nihr.ac.uk/award/NIHR131359).

Integrative Multiomics—Future Perspectives

Integrative multiomics represent the next field of research to be implemented. One of the first study aiming at integrating information derived from a multiomics approach was that of Wainberg and colleagues.[49] They combined whole genome sequencing with longitudinal multiomics collection in a wide cohort of healthy individual, generated PRS for 54 disease and complex traits previously investigated through GWAS and found correlations between PRS and alterations in proteomics, metabolomics, and standard clinical laboratory measurements. As a result, they demonstrated the presence of disease-specific omics-derived analytes alterations already in healthy individual at high genetic risks for that specific disease, providing insights on the possibilities of prognostic models able to predict the patient's risk profile before the disease onset.

Furthermore, recent advances in single-cell omics technologies, and in the development of personalized disease models, such as organoids, set the premises for the EU supported, LifeTimeInitiative,[50] which aims to identify molecular mechanisms of disease onset, create predictive computational models of disease progression and reveal new drug targets at a single-cell resolution thus achieving the concept of interceptive medicine, which is the ability to predict future disease phenotype at a cellular and molecular level. The derived amount of molecular mechanistic data collected will completely change our paradigm of clinical trial design and possibly our clinical decision-making processes.

Although multiomics technologies are growing rapidly, the implementation of omics-based prediction modeling is still difficult due to several hurdles related to the complexity of the cohort development and phenotyping, data acquisition and storage, and the computational component. Prognostic models in PBC should be developed on sufficiently large, databases of consecutive patients followed-up for sufficiently long periods of time, with appropriate quality control systems. Laboratory investigations from a centralized laboratory, information about treatment and intermediate events should be recorded at regular intervals,[51] in a longitudinal fashion.

A major challenge is to annotate, organize, and store these data so that they are suitable for downstream analysis. A well-designed, bespoke database (or data warehouse) may be required. Large sample collections should ideally be archived in well-equipped biorepositories, preferably with replicate collections in 2 or more locations. Use of Laboratory Information Management Systems, bar-coding, and robotics greatly facilitates management and maintenance of the collection, for example, rear-raying aliquots of selected samples for specific analyses or sharing with other researchers. With such massive volume of medical data, data-intensive computing is needed to increase efficiency and reduce costs.

SUMMARY

Recent advances in the understanding of the pathobiological mechanisms that drive the progression of biliary damage in PBC and the increasing availability of new drugs with different molecular targets has made the role of risk prediction modeling in PBC increasingly important. Driven by the evidence of early determinants of disease aggressiveness, during the last years, efforts have been made to bring forward risk stratification from evaluation of UDCA response after 1 year of treatment, to disease onset, thus enabling us to potentially individualize care, in terms of timely surveillance and treatment modulation, since the time of disease diagnosis. A further improvement of prognostic models will be possible by integrating novel biomarkers providing multiple layers of information including genetics, epigenetics, molecular, and metabolic alterations more directly linked to the pathogenetic mechanisms of the disease process. Indeed, the evolving landscape of omics technologies and AI applications, coupled with the current availability of large-scale patient cohorts in PBC, is creating a unique opportunity to reach a turning point in the paradigm of PBC treatment and management.

CLINICS CARE POINTS

- The potential role of early risk stratification in PBC and its cost-effectiveness should be tested in clinical practice
- Patients should have transient elastography and ultrasound within 3 to 6 months of diagnosis in order to assess stage of the disease
- Treatment response to UDCA and the need for a second-line treatment should be evaluated as early as 6 months, but no later than 12 months
- Effort should be focus to identify a omic-based disease signature to enhance prognostic modelling, ideally directly linked to the pathogenetic mechanisms.

REFERENCES

1. Hirschfield GM, Beuers U, Corpechot C, et al. EASL Clinical Practice Guidelines: the diagnosis and management of patients with primary biliary cholangitis. J Hepatol 2017;67:145–72.

2. Gerussi A, Lucà M, Cristoferi L, et al. New therapeutic targets in autoimmune cholangiopathies. Front Med 2020;7:117.
3. Murillo Perez CF, Hirschfield GM, Corpechot C, et al. Fibrosis stage is an independent predictor of outcome in primary biliary cholangitis despite biochemical treatment response. Aliment Pharmacol Ther 2019;50:1127–36.
4. Berzigotti A, Tsochatzis E, Boursier J, et al. EASL Clinical Practice Guidelines on non-invasive tests for evaluation of liver disease severity and prognosis – 2021 update. J Hepatol 2021;75:659–89.
5. Dickson ER, Grambsch PM, Fleming TR, et al. Prognosis in primary biliary cirrhosis: model for decision making. Hepatology 1989;10:1–7.
6. Roll J, Boyer JL, Barry D, et al. The prognostic importance of clinical and histologic features in asymptomatic and symptomatic primary biliary cirrhosis. N Engl J Med 1983;308:1–7.
7. Christensen E, Neuberger J, Crowe J, et al. Beneficial effect of azathioprine and prediction of prognosis in primary biliary cirrhosis. Gastroenterology 1985;89: 1084–91.
8. Leuschner U, Fischer H, Kurtz W, et al. Ursodeoxycholic acid in primary biliary cirrhosis: results of a controlled double-blind trial. Gastroenterology 1989;97: 1268–74.
9. Lammert C, Juran BD, Schlicht E, et al. Biochemical response to ursodeoxycholic acid predicts survival in a North American cohort of primary biliary cirrhosis patients. J Gastroenterol 2014;49:1414–20.
10. Zhang L-N, Shi T-Y, Shi X-H, et al. Early biochemical response to ursodeoxycholic acid and long-term prognosis of primary biliary cirrhosis: results of a 14-year cohort study. Hepatology 2013;58:264–72.
11. Parés A, Caballería L, Rodés J. Excellent long-term survival in patients with primary biliary cirrhosis and biochemical response to ursodeoxycholic acid. Gastroenterology 2006;130:715–20.
12. Corpechot C, Abenavoli L, Rabahi N, et al. Biochemical response to ursodeoxycholic acid and long-term prognosis in primary biliary cirrhosis. Hepatology 2008; 48:871–7.
13. Kuiper EMM, Hansen BE, de Vries RA, et al. Improved prognosis of patients with primary biliary cirrhosis that have a biochemical response to ursodeoxycholic acid. Gastroenterology 2009;136:1281–7.
14. Kumagi T, Guindi M, Fischer SE, et al. Baseline ductopenia and treatment response predict long-term histological progression in primary biliary cirrhosis. Am J Gastroenterol 2010;105:2186–94.
15. Corpechot C, Chazouillères O, Poupon R. Early primary biliary cirrhosis: biochemical response to treatment and prediction of long-term outcome. J Hepatol 2011;55:1361–7.
16. Carbone M, Sharp SJ, Flack S, et al. The UK-PBC risk scores: derivation and validation of a scoring system for long-term prediction of end-stage liver disease in primary biliary cholangitis: HEPATOLOGY, Vol. XX, NO. X, 2015. Hepatology 2016;63:930–50.
17. Lammers WJ, Hirschfield GM, Corpechot C, et al. Development and validation of a scoring system to predict outcomes of patients with primary biliary cirrhosis receiving ursodeoxycholic acid therapy. Gastroenterology 2015;149:1804–12.e4.
18. Nevens F, Andreone P, Mazzella G, et al. A placebo-controlled trial of obeticholic acid in primary biliary cholangitis. N Engl J Med 2016;375:631–43.
19. Murillo Perez CF, Harms MH, Lindor KD, et al. Goals of treatment for improved survival in primary biliary cholangitis: treatment target should Be bilirubin within

the normal range and normalization of alkaline phosphatase. Am J Gastroenterol 2020;115:1066–74.

20. Yang F, Yang Y, Wang Q, et al. The risk predictive values of UK-PBC and GLOBE scoring system in Chinese patients with primary biliary cholangitis: the additional effect of anti-gp210. Aliment Pharmacol Ther 2017;45:733–43.

21. Carbone M, Mells GF, Pells G, et al. Sex and age are determinants of the clinical phenotype of primary biliary cirrhosis and response to ursodeoxycholic acid. Gastroenterology 2013;144:560–9.e7.

22. Carbone M, Harms MH, Lammers WJ, et al. Clinical application of the GLOBE and United Kingdom-primary biliary cholangitis risk scores in a trial cohort of patients with primary biliary cholangitis. Hepatol Commun 2018; 2: 683–692.

23. Honda A, Tanaka A, Kaneko T, et al. Bezafibrate improves GLOBE and UK-PBC scores and long-term outcomes in patients with primary biliary cholangitis. Hepatology 2019; 70: 2035–2046.

24. Fujimori K, Iguchi Y, Yamashita Y, et al. Synthesis of novel farnesoid X receptor agonists and validation of their efficacy in activating differentiation of mouse bone marrow-derived mesenchymal stem cells into osteoblasts. Molecules 2019;24:E4155.

25. Gerussi A, Bernasconi DP, O'Donnell SE, et al. Measurement of gamma glutamyl transferase to determine risk of liver transplantation or death in patients with primary biliary cholangitis. Clin Gastroenterol Hepatol 2021;19:1688–97.e14.

26. Dalekos G, Invernizzi P, Nevens F, et al. GS-02-Efficacy of GKT831 in patients with primary biliary cholangitis and inadequate response to ursodeoxycholic acid: interim efficacy results of a phase 2 clinical trial. J Hepatol 2019;70:e1–2.

27. Schramm C, Hirschfield G, Mason AL, et al. Early assessment of safety and efficacy of tropifexor, a potent non bile-acid FXR agonist, in patients with primary biliary cholangitis: an interim analysis of an ongoing phase 2 study. J Hepatol 2018;68:S103.

28. Mells GF, Jones DE. Editorial: scoring systems in primary biliary cholangitis - time to make a move. Aliment Pharmacol Ther 2017;45:1163–4.

29. Corpechot C, Chazouillères O, Rousseau A, et al. A placebo-controlled trial of bezafibrate in primary biliary cholangitis. N Engl J Med 2018;378:2171–81.

30. Soret P-A, Lam L, Carrat F, et al. Combination of fibrates with obeticholic acid is able to normalise biochemical liver tests in patients with difficult-to-treat primary biliary cholangitis. Aliment Pharmacol Ther 2021;53:1138–46.

31. D'Amato D, Vincentis AD, Malinverno F, et al. Real-world experience with obeticholic acid in patients with primary biliary cholangitis. JHEPReport 2021;3. https://doi.org/10.1016/j.jhepr.2021.100248.

32. Carbone M, Nardi A, Flack S, et al. Pretreatment prediction of response to ursodeoxycholic acid in primary biliary cholangitis: development and validation of the UDCA Response Score. Lancet Gastroenterol Hepatol 2018;3:626–34.

33. Harms MH, Lammers WJ, Thorburn D, et al. Major hepatic complications in ursodeoxycholic acid-treated patients with primary biliary cholangitis: risk factors and time trends in incidence and outcome. Am J Gastroenterol 2018;113:254–64.

34. Mayo MJ, Parkes J, Adams-Huet B, et al. Prediction of clinical outcomes in primary biliary cirrhosis by serum enhanced liver fibrosis assay. Hepatology 2008; 48:1549–57.

35. Corpechot C, Carrat F, Poujol-Robert A, et al. Noninvasive elastography-based assessment of liver fibrosis progression and prognosis in primary biliary cirrhosis. Hepatology 2012;56:198–208.

36. Cristoferi L, Calvaruso V, Overi D, et al. Accuracy of transient elastography in assessing fibrosis at diagnosis in naïve patients with primary biliary cholangitis: a dual cut-off approach. Hepatology 2021; 74: 1496–1508.

37. Karczewski KJ, Snyder MP. Integrative omics for health and disease. Nat Rev Genet 2018;19:299–310.

38. Gerussi A, Verda D, Bernasconi DP, et al. Machine learning in primary biliary cholangitis: a novel approach for risk stratification. Liver Int 2022;liv:15141.

39. Gerussi A, Carbone M, Corpechot C, et al. The genetic architecture of primary biliary cholangitis. Eur J Med Genet 2021;64:104292.

40. Cordell HJ, Fryett JJ, Ueno K, et al. An international genome-wide meta-analysis of primary biliary cholangitis: novel risk loci and candidate drugs. J Hepatol 2021;75:572–81.

41. The UK PBC Consortium. The Wellcome Trust Case Control Consortium 3, Mells GF, et al. Genome-wide association study identifies 12 new susceptibility loci for primary biliary cirrhosis. Nat Genet 2011;43:329–32.

42. Carbone M, Mells GF, Alexander GJ, et al. Calcineurin inhibitors and the IL12A locus influence risk of recurrent primary biliary cirrhosis after liver transplantation. Am J Transplant 2013;13:1110–1.

43. Torkamani A, Wineinger NE, Topol EJ. The personal and clinical utility of polygenic risk scores. Nat Rev Genet 2018;19:581–90.

44. Tam V, Patel N, Turcotte M, et al. Benefits and limitations of genome-wide association studies. Nat Rev Genet 2019;20:467–84.

45. Hardie C, Green K, Jopson L, et al. Early molecular stratification of high-risk primary biliary cholangitis. EBioMedicine 2016;14:65–73.

46. Wang X, Wen X, Zhou J, et al. MicroRNA-223 and microRNA-21 in peripheral blood B cells associated with progression of primary biliary cholangitis patients. PLoS One 2017;12:e0184292.

47. Barron-Millar B, Ogle L, Mells G, et al. The serum proteome and ursodeoxycholic acid response in primary biliary cholangitis. Hepatology 2021;74:3269–83.

48. Meadows V, Baiocchi L, Kundu D, et al. Biliary Epithelial senescence in liver disease: there will Be SASP. Front Mol Biosci 2021;8:803098.

49. Wainberg M, Magis AT, Earls JC, et al. Multiomic blood correlates of genetic risk identify presymptomatic disease alterations. Proc Natl Acad Sci U S A 2020;117:21813–20.

50. Rajewsky N, Almouzni G, Gorski SA, et al. LifeTime and improving European healthcare through cell-based interceptive medicine. Nature 2020;587:377–86.

51. Cristoferi L, Nardi A, Ronca V, et al. Prognostic models in primary biliary cholangitis. J Autoimmun 2018;95:171–8.

Primary Biliary Cholangitis in Males

Pathogenesis, Clinical Presentation, and Prognosis

Mina Shaker, MD, MSc[a],*, Natalie Mansour, MD[a],
Binu V. John, MD, MPH[a,b]

KEYWORDS

- Primary biliary cholangitis ● Autoimmune hepatitis ● Men ● Epidemiology
- Clinical presentation ● Prognosis

Abbreviations	
HCC	hepatocellular carcinoma mRNA
mRNA	messenger ribonucleic acid SLE
SLE	Systemic lupus erythematosus MZ
MZ	monozygotic NK
NK	Natural killer cells CD
CD	cluster of differentiation dsDNA
dsDNA	double-standed deoxyribonucleic acid IgG
IgG	Immunoglobulin G igM
IgM	Immunoglobulin M

INTRODUCTION

Primary biliary cholangitis (PBC) is a chronic cholestatic liver disease characterized by an immune-mediated inflammatory destruction of small intrahepatic bile ducts, with progressive fibrosis that may lead to cirrhosis and subsequent liver failure.[1–3]

Studies from the United Kingdom suggest that PBC is the most frequent form of autoimmune liver diseases.[4]

The incidence and prevalence of PBC seem to be rising in several countries.[5,6] Differences in the clinical course have been noticed between Caucasian, African

[a] Division of Hepatology, Miami VA Medical Center 1201 NW 16th Street, Miami, FL 33125 USA;
[b] Department of Medicine, University of Miami Miller School of Medicine, Miami, FL, USA
* Corresponding author.
E-mail address: Mina.Shaker@va.gov

Clin Liver Dis 26 (2022) 643–655
https://doi.org/10.1016/j.cld.2022.06.008
1089-3261/22/Published by Elsevier Inc.

American, and Hispanic patients in the United States with cirrhosis presenting more frequently in non-Caucasians.[7] Migration studies indicated that the risk for PBC changes in accordance with local population which points to the significant role played by environmental factors in development of the disease.[6–8]

The typical patient with this disease is believed to be middle-aged woman; however, it is widely recognized now that men are affected in higher numbers than once believed with female-to-male ratio estimated to be 4–6:1.[9] There is limited data on the clinical presentation and natural history of PBC in males because most cohorts that have studied long-term outcomes in PBC have a small number of male participants. Recently, data from the United States Veterans Health Administration, which have greater number of males with PBC, have shed light on the outcomes of these patients.[10–13]

PATHOGENESIS

Exact etiology and mechanism by which PBC develops remain unclear. The disease seems to be initiated by variety of genetic susceptibility and environmental triggers. Thus, the prevalence varies geographically, with the highest incidence reported in northern Europe and North America.[1]

Autoantibodies

Antimitochondrial antibody (AMA) is a highly disease-specific autoantibody that targets the lipoic acid on the 2-oxoacid dehydrogenase complexes located on the inner mitochondrial membrane. In addition to a loss in humoral tolerance, there is an increase of autoreactive cluster of differentiation CD4+ CD8+ pyruvate dehydrogenase complex (PDC-E2)-specific T cells in the liver.[13–15]

A key feature of pathogenesis is the specific targeting of the biliary epithelial cells. AMA is produced by plasmablasts, undergo transcytosis through the biliary epithelium, and disrupt mitochondrial function. Incomplete proteolysis of PDC-E2 and other mitochondrial enzymes during apoptosis of biliary epithelial cells is another suspected mechanism.[16,17]

The inflammatory destruction of small intrahepatic bile ducts results in spectrum of cholangitis, varying degrees of fibrosis, and cirrhosis. This contributes significantly to disease-related morbidity and mortality. However, even in the absence of cirrhosis, PBC can severely impair the quality of life.[18]

Although AMAs are highly specific (95%) and sensitive (85%) for PBC, other autoantibodies such as antinuclear antibodies (ANAs) against glycoprotein 210 and sp100 are highly specific, excellent predictors of nonresponse to ursodeoxycholic acid (UDCA), and of death or transplantation. In a male predominant cohort of patients with PBC and cirrhosis, there was no difference in overall mortality, liver-related mortality, hepatic decompensation, or HCC between AMA-positive and AMA-negative patients.[12,17]

Genetic Predisposition/Familial Primary Biliary Cholangitis in Males

There are very few studies examining PBC in males from both pathogenesis and genetic predisposition viewpoint. Literature is limited to case reports and small retrospective studies.

The only twin study conducted in PBC consisted only of female pairs.[19] Brown and colleagues reported PBC in a set of brothers.[20] Tanaka and colleagues[21] noted two sets of brothers with PBC, one set in Britain and another in France, in addition to several father-daughter and two brother-sister pairs. Unfortunately, the AMA status and clinical course of these patients are unknown.[21] Lazaridis and colleagues examined AMA status in 306 first-degree relatives of 350 patients with PBC and found that AMA was present in 7.8% of brothers, 3.7% of fathers, and 0% of sons of patients with PBC.[22]

Familial studies of PBC in Europe and North America have suggested that genetic factors play a role in disease susceptibility. In Europe, the prevalence of PBC among people with family history of the disease is estimated to be 1% to 4.5%, which is about 1000-fold higher than in the general population.[22] One Japanese study cited a familial prevalence of PBC of 5.1%, which is like that in Europe, and noted that the second-generation family members frequently showed earlier onset of the disease.[23] A study from Mayo Clinic found that the first-degree relatives of patients with PBC were more likely than the general population to be AMA positive.[24] However, after 8 years of follow-up, only AMA-positive relatives with elevated alkaline phosphatase (ALP) levels showed an increased risk of developing PBC.

Environmental Triggers

Significant differences between and within geographic regions suggest that environmental agents may lead to PBC.

Prince and colleagues[25] found an evidence of disease clustering in Northeast England. The study involved two groups of patients with PBC: one consisting of 318 patients from an epidemiologic study and the other group consisted of 2258 patients from a PBC support group. The control group consisted of 2438 controls. Among patients with PBC from the epidemiologic study group, 8% were male, compared with 7% in the support group. No specific risk factors were identified for males, although it was noted in the study that less than 1% of males had a history of hair dye use, compared with over 50% of females, which is of interest given that hair dyes have been implicated as a possible risk factor for PBC development.

Similarly, Triger and colleagues[26] found clustering of cases in Sheffield, England, independently of family history. Specific water reservoirs were suspected to be associated with higher prevalence, although water analysis was inconclusive.

Corpechot and colleagues[27] involved a French cohort of 222 patients with PBC and 509 controls; all administered a questionnaire regarding demographic, lifestyle, and health factors, and 11% of the patients with PBC were male, as were 15% of the control groups. Several risk factors indicated the history of recurrent urinary tract infection (rUTI), smoking, and family history of PBC. No risk factors indicated which were related to male sex.

Several studies have linked PBC to smoking, use of certain cosmetics, and exposure to hair dyes, suggesting the possible involvement of xenobiotics. Similarly, UTI has been implicated in the development of PBC, with bacterial and viral proteins serving as the suspected culprits. It is unclear what proportion of men had a significant history of smoking or rUTI in those studies.[25–31]

Some clusters of patients with PBC have higher rates of affected men compared with the general population. Most of those clusters are centered on coal mines and steel working industries, which are primarily used by men.[29] Such observations warrant further studying of occupational exposures of men with PBC.

In the United States,[32] an increased incidence of PBC was noted among people living adjacent to toxic waste sites, further supporting a role for environmental toxins in disease pathogenesis. Finally, Ohba and colleagues showed increased incidence of PBC in atomic bomb survivors in Japan.[33]

X Chromosome

The role of the X chromosome has been investigated heavily, clinical data suggested links between X chromosome and immunity. X chromosome defects are also more frequent in women with late-onset autoimmune diseases.[34,35]

Epigenetic factors,[19] such as X chromosome inactivation, may also be involved in the development of PBC, giving variable rates of PBC among twins. These theories are of interest, given the increased X chromosome monosomy rate in the peripheral lymphocytes of female patients with PBC.[34–36] Mitchell and colleagues[37] analyzed 125 variable X chromosome inactivation status genes in peripheral blood mRNA and DNA from MZ discordant and concordant pairs. Consistently downregulated genes included CLIC2 and PIN4 in twins with PBC, which was not found in the healthy twin or in control subjects. Variable methylation was found in both genes and did not predict transcript levels or X inactivation status. This demonstrates the complexity of epigenetic factors which should be considered not only in twin studies but also in the comparison of men and women with PBC.[37]

Immunologic Differences

Immunologic differences may also explain the variable rates of PBC between men and women. For example, women demonstrate increased antibody production and cell-mediated responses following immunization, in addition to having an increased CD4 T-cell count.[38]

Men show increased inflammatory responses to infectious organisms,[39] and sex hormones seem to affect cytokine production, B-cell maturation, and antigen presentation, which is of interest given the association between hormone replacement therapy and PBC.[38] Sex hormones also can affect immune cell functioning by binding to steroid receptors. Estrogen and androgen receptors are expressed on B cells, whereas CD8 T cells, monocytes, neutrophils, and NK cells express estrogen but not androgen receptors.[39] One study has demonstrated that estrogen treatment of peripheral blood mononuclear cells from patients with SLE increased IgG production as well as anti-dsDNA autoantibody levels.[40]

Testosterone was found to decrease IgG and IgM production by peripheral blood mononuclear cells in healthy males and females.[41] It remains unclear what role sex hormones play in the pathogenesis of PBC as well as the preponderance of PBC in females versus males.

DIAGNOSIS

The diagnosis of PBC should be suspected in the setting of chronic cholestasis and a positive AMA. A liver biopsy can be used to further substantiate the diagnosis but is rarely needed.[42]

- Elevation of ALP of liver origin greater than 6 months
- Elevation of serum AMAs with high titer greater than 40

Liver biopsy is not necessary to establish a diagnosis if the above two criteria are already met but is occasionally needed for activity staging or to diagnose overlap syndrome: PBC with features of AIH.[3]

Characteristic histologic features on the liver biopsy include:[1–3]

- Destruction of biliary epithelial cells
- Loss of small bile ducts
- Portal inflammatory cell infiltrate primarily plasma cells and lymphocytes
- Noncaseating granuloma formation

Characteristic serologic markers include:[1–3,18–33,42]

- Increased levels of ALP
- Increased levels of gamma-glutamyl transferase

- IgM may be raised at times
- High titer of AMA
- Disease-specific ANA

AMAs and their titers do not affect the clinical outcome of the disease. However, a disease-specific ANA can identify a subgroup of patients with PBC with more severe histologic disease or may develop aggressive course compared with patients who test negative for those antibodies.[18,19,27,43,44]

Although a diagnosis of PBC in men and women is similar, the clinical picture and concomitant diseases are usually different between both. Trivial difference is noted regarding histologic, biochemical features or AMA reactivity.[1]

Nalbandian and colleagues[45] looked at serologic differences between men and women. That study involved 46 men and 42 women, all with high titer AMA. Reactivity patterns were similar in both groups. Testing of the optical densities did not reveal significant differences, which concluded that there was no difference of AMA reactivity between males and females.

EPIDEMIOLOGY

Most epidemiologic data on PBC have come from Europe, which report incidence and prevalence rates of 0.3 to 5.8 and 1.9 to 40 per 100,000 inhabitants, respectively.[4,6,8]

Northern Europe and North America have the highest prevalence of PBC, but this may be due to disparities in geographic populations.[30] The incidence and prevalence of PBC are increasing due to improved surveillance and increased reporting from Asia-Pacific region.[46]

PBC commonly develops in middle age (40–60 years of age) and is uncommon under 25 years of age.[4,5] It is now increasingly recognized that the female-to-male ratio is closer to 4–6:1, rather than the 10:1 ratio that was previously believed and widely cited.[6,8,9,47]

Fan and colleagues,[48] in the largest study from China to date, found significant increase in the number of patients with PBC between 2001 and 2016 with a female-to-male ratio of 6.1:1, a ratio that is remarkably similar to studies from South Korea 6.2:1 and Japan 7:1.[49,50] This suggests that the sex distribution of individuals with PBC in Asia is mirroring that observed in Europe and United States.[43]

It was Podda and colleagues who proposed initially the underestimation of male prevalence of PBC.[44] This was followed by two geoepidemiology research from Europe reporting female-to-male ratio could be as low as 1.6:1 from Swedish administrative database.[9,51]

CLINICAL, BIOCHEMICAL, AND HISTOPATHOLOGICAL DIFFERENCES IN MALE VERSUS FEMALE PRIMARY BILIARY CHOLANGITIS

Those differences in men versus women with PBC have been investigated in few studies.[47,52–55]

One of these was conducted at the Armed Forces Institute of Pathology and involved 30 male and 30 age-matched female patients with PBC, all AMA positive. In addition to histologic studies, symptoms and biochemical indices were also compared in each group.[53]

- Females experienced pruritus as a single symptom more often than males, in addition to experiencing more abdominal pain/discomfort and constitutional symptoms, malaise, anorexia, weight loss, fatigue, and weight loss.
- Males experienced more jaundice and upper gastrointestinal bleeding.

- ALP was slightly higher in symptomatic males compared with asymptomatic males, with both being higher than females in general.
- Histologically, the only difference found was that symptomatic female patients had more piecemeal necrosis and symptomatic males had more copper storage than asymptomatic males.

The overall data[53] indicate that the biochemical and histologic differences between males and females with PBC are relatively minor.

Another study, conducted by The Liver Unit at King's College Hospital, compared the clinical and biochemical profiles of males and females with PBC, in addition to long-term outcome; 39 men and 191 women with PBC were enrolled, with the age of diagnosis and disease severity being similar in both groups.[54]

- Pruritus again was more common in females than males (68% vs 45%). It was suggested that female sex hormones could be linked with pruritus, as there was an increased frequency of pruritus with use of oral contraceptives and during pregnancy.
- Gastrointestinal bleeding was more common among male patients (23%) than female patients (15%).
- Females demonstrated skin pigmentation more often than males (55% vs 35%).
- Females were more likely to have other autoimmune diseases
  - Sicca symptoms were present in 33% of females and 15% males
  - Scleroderma in 13% of females and 8% of males
  - Raynaud's in 13% females and 3% of males
- Males were more frequent to have of type 2 diabetes
- Males had increased rates of hepatocellular carcinoma.

Overall, there were no statistically significant differences observed with respect to AMA positivity or histology.[54]

An Italian study[52] compared clinical and serologic data of 30 male and 165 female PBC patients. Histology was available in 83% of the males and 79% of females.

- Males presented at older age, with median age of 68.5 years compared with 54.5 years in females. This was statistically significant.
- Jaundice was more common among males (13%) than females (11%).
- Biochemically, males had higher levels of alanine aminotransferase (ALT) and ALP.
- Histologically:
  - Stage I was present in 35% of females compared with 12% of males,
  - 36% and 28% of males were in stages III and IV, respectively, compared with 19% of females in both stages. However, this was not found to be statistically significant.
- Immunologic profiles regarding AMA and ANA were not different between the two groups, although a higher frequency of anti-centromere activity was noted in females (21.4%) than in males (3%).

That study concluded that more advanced disease in males was likely due to delayed diagnosis, as PBC was not initially suspected.[52]

Zakharia and colleagues[55] from the University of Iowa, USA, examined 290 patients with biopsy-proven PBC. Males were 12% of this cohort.

- Mean age of presentation was 54 for men versus 50 for women
- Mean ALP values were similar between men and women 334 U/L versus 320 U/L

- At the time of diagnosis, 31% of males had advanced fibrosis F3–F4, compared with 16% of females ($P = .09$)
- Disease progression was higher in males:
  - Portal hypertension developed 42% of males versus 16% in females ($P < .001$)
  - Decompensated cirrhosis was reported in 33% of males versus 10% in females ($P < .001$)
  - Kaplan Meier time to hepatic decompensation showed increased risk of development of hepatic decompensation in males as compared with females ($P < .001$)
- AMA-negative PBC was noted in 16% of females versus 0% of males
- Bone disease was higher in females compared with males
  - Osteopenia 22.5% versus 12.5, respectively
  - Osteoporosis 6% versus 3%, respectively.

Table 1 shows the difference in histologic findings between men and women of this study.

In a study of 532 US Veterans (418 male) with PBC and cirrhosis with 3231 person-years of follow-up, John and colleagues[47] showed that men with PBC cirrhosis have higher adjusted risk of death or transplantation (adjusted hazard ratio [HR], 1.80; 95% confidence interval [CI], 1.01–3.19; $P = .046$), and liver-related death or transplantation (subhazard ratio [sHR], 2.17; 95% CI, 1.15–4.08; $P = .02$). Similarly, Sayiner and colleagues in older Medicare population review showed higher 1-year mortality in male population with PBC ($P < .0001$).[56]

Cheung and colleagues[57] showed that male population were older had higher bilirubin and lower platelet counts at baseline. They also noted lower UDCA response in men, as previous study they found no differences on multivariate analysis.

Lleo and colleagues, in a large study, demonstrated that male sex was an independent predictor of all-cause mortality in both Italian and Danish populations (95% CI).[9]

Natarajan and colleagues,[58] in a recent metanalysis of 29 studies that examined incidence of HCC in patients with PBC from inception through November 2019, they identified 292 patients who were followed for an average of 76 months. The incidence of HCC in patients with PBC cirrhosis was 15.7 per 1000 patient-years (95% CI 8.73–28.24). The HCC incidence rate was 9.82 per 1000 person-years (95% CI 5.92–16.28) in men and 3.82 per 1000 person-years (95% CI 2.85–5.11) in women. It was concluded that Cirrhosis is the strongest risk factor for HCC in patients with PBC. Male gender was also a risk factor (**Table 2**).[58]

Table 1 Histological staging as investigated in Zacharia et al[55]		
Degree of Fibrosis at Time of Diagnosis	Women (172)	Men (26)
F0–1	107 (62%)	10 (38%)
F2	38 (22%)	8 (31%)
F3	15 (9%)	2 (8%)
F4	12 (7%)	8 (23%)

Table 2
Summary of major differences between men and women with primary biliary cholangitis[9,47,52–58]

Features	Men	Women
Ratio	1	4–6
1-y survival	78%	96%
5-y survival	64%	87%
10-y survival	0%	80%
Clinical Picture		
• Age	Older	Younger
• Pruritis	Less common	More common
• Fatigue	Less common	More common
• Abdominal pain	Less common	More common
• Concomitant autoimmune disorders	Less common	More common (sicca, scleroderma, and Raynaud's)
• Jaundice	More often	Less common
• GI bleeding	More often	Less common
• HCC	More often	Less common
• Type 2 diabetes	More often	Less common
Serology		
• ALT	Higher levels	Lower levels
• ALP	Higher levels	Lower levels
• Bilirubin	Higher levels	Lower levels
• PLT counts	Lower counts	Higher counts
• AMA	Similar reactivity	Similar reactivity
• Anti-centromere	Less common	More prevalent
Histopathology	Overall similar picture. More often to be diagnosed with advanced fibrosis. One study showed more copper storage in symptomatic men	Overall similar picture. More often to be diagnosed in stages 0–I fibrosis. One study showed more piecemeal necrosis and pseudoxanthomatous transformation in symptomatic women
Response to treatment (UDCA)	Lower response rate noted in men. More likely to progress to cirrhosis. More likely to transplant	More common to respond well to UDCA. Less likely to progress to cirrhosis. Less likely to need transplant
Morbidity and mortality	Higher rates of liver-related morbidity and mortality	Higher rates of extrahepatic disease-related complications like bone fractures and hyperlipidemia

MANAGEMENT OF PRIMARY BILIARY CHOLANGITIS IN MALES

Cheung and colleagues[57] evaluated the effects of age and sex on response to UDCA treatment and transplant-free survival period. In longitudinal analysis of 4355 adults, they found that younger age at initiation of therapy is associated with increased risk of treatment failure, liver transplant, and death.

- Male patients were older at start of treatment (58 vs 54, $P < .0001$)
- Males had higher bilirubin levels and lower platelet counts
- Males had lower biochemical response compared with female patients (statistically significant on univariate analysis but not on multivariable analysis)
- Males had a significantly lower rate of 10-year transplant-free survival compared with female patients (67.7% vs 80.1%, $P < .0001$) but on multivariable analysis, it was not statistically significant.

John and colleagues,[10] in a study of 501 participants with PBC cirrhosis (77% males), noted that UDCA response was associated with a lower risk of hepatic decompensation (sHR 0.54, 95% CI 0.31 to 0.95, $P = .03$), death from any cause or transplantation (adjusted HR 0.49, 95% CI 0.33–0.72, $P = .0002$), and liver-related death or transplantation (sHR 0.40, 95% CI 0.24–0.67, $P = .0004$), but not HCC (sHR 0.39, 95% CI 0.60–2.55, $P = .32$). However, no differences in UDCA response were noted between males and females in this study.

Regular follow-ups are recommended for both males and females with no differences apart from HCC screening. It is recommended to complete HCC screening with cross-sectional imaging in men with PBC and all patients with PBC-related advanced liver fibrosis every 6 months.[59–61] Those are most at risk to develop HCC, which was found at a rate of 3.9 cases in 1000 per year of follow-up.[59,60] Suboptimal response to UDCA is considered an important risk factor. Surveillance with regular imaging was associated with better clinical outcome of patients with PBC who develop HCC.[61]

SUMMARY

PBC remains a female predominant disease, but the disease is more prevalent in males than previously believed, with contemporary studies showing a 4–6:1 female-to-male ratio. Men present later in disease process, as evidenced by older age, higher bilirubin, lower platelet count, higher model for end-stage liver disease -Na, and lower UDCA exposure-time in several studies. Although males present at a more advanced stage of disease at diagnosis than females, male sex has been shown to be associated with a higher death or transplantation, or liver-related death or transplantation in PBC cirrhosis, even after adjusting for age, comorbidities, UDCA response, and the stage of disease.

A diagnosis of PBC is often delayed among males because of the myth that PBC is extremely rare in males. Greater research and education are needed to raise awareness, so that PBC is suspected and diagnosed at an earlier stage among males.

CLINICS CARE POINTS

- PBC is an immune-mediated chronic liver disease characterized by progressive cholestasis, bile duct destruction, biliary fibrosis, and cirrhosis.

- Although it is primarily a disease of females, incidence in male is not as rare as it was once thought.

- Diagnosis is usually late in males, thus the disease course in male tend to be more aggressive with worse outcomes.

- Earlier diagnosis allows earlier treatment. Patients who respond to ursodeoxycholic acid have an expected survival similar to the general population

DISCLAIMER

The authors prepared this work in their personal capacity. The opinions expressed in this article are the author's own and do not reflect the view of the Department of Veterans Affairs or the United States government.

CONFLICTS OF INTERESTS

None of the authors have personal or financial conflicts of interests to declare concerning this publication.

REFERENCES

1. Kaplan MM, Gershwin ME. Primary biliary cirrhosis. New Engl J Med 2005; 353(12):1261–73.
2. Hohenester S, Oude-Elferink RPJ, Beuers U. Primary biliary cirrhosis. Semin Immunopathology 2009;31(3):283–307.
3. Neuberger J. Primary biliary cirrhosis. The Lancet 1997;350(9081):875–9.
4. Smyk DS, Rigopoulou EI, Lleo A, et al. Immunopathogenesis of primary biliary cirrhosis: an old wives' tale. Immun Ageing 2011;8(1):12.
5. Sood S, Gow PJ, Christie JM, et al. Epidemiology of primary biliary cirrhosis in Victoria, Australia: high prevalence in migrant populations. Gastroenterology 2004;127(2):470–5.
6. Kim WR, Lindor KD, Locke GR, et al. Epidemiology and natural history of primary biliary cirrhosis in a U.S. community. Gastroenterology 2000;119(6):1631–6.
7. Anand AC, Elias E, Neuberger JM. End-stage primary biliary cirrhosis in a first-generation migrant south Asian population. Eur J Gastroenterol Hepatol 1996; 8(7):663–6.
8. Watson RG, Angus PW, Dewar M, et al. Low prevalence of primary biliary cirrhosis in Victoria, Australia. Melbourne Liver Group. Gut 1995;36(6):927–30.
9. Lleo A, Jepsen P, Morenghi E, et al. Evolving Trends in female to male incidence and male mortality of primary biliary cholangitis. Sci Rep 2016;6:25906.
10. John BV, Khakoo NS, Schwartz KB, et al. Ursodeoxycholic acid response is associated with Reduced mortality in primary biliary cholangitis with Compensated cirrhosis. Am J Gastroenterol 2021;116(9):1913–23.
11. John BV, Schwartz K, Levy C, et al. Impact of Obeticholic acid exposure on decompensation and mortality in primary biliary cholangitis and cirrhosis. Hepatol Commun 2021;5(8):1426–36.
12. John BV, Dahman B, Deng Y, et al. Rates of decompensation, hepatocellular carcinoma, and mortality in AMA-negative primary biliary cholangitis cirrhosis. Liver Int 2022;42(2):384–93.
13. Gershwin ME, Mackay IR, Sturgess A, et al. Identification and specificity of a cDNA encoding the 70 kd mitochondrial antigen recognized in primary biliary cirrhosis. J Immunol 1987;138:3525–31.
14. Moteki S, Leung PS, Dickson ER, et al. Epitope mapping and reactivity of autoantibodies to the E2 component of 2-oxoglutarate dehydrogenase complex in primary biliary cirrhosis using recombinant 2-oxoglutarate dehydrogenase complex. Hepatology 1996;23:436–44.
15. Kita H, Matsumura S, He XS, et al. Quantitative and functional analysis of PDCE2-specific autoreactive cytotoxic T lymphocytes in primary biliary cirrhosis. J Clin Invest 2002;109:1231–40.

16. Courvalin JC, Worman HJ. Nuclear envelope protein autoantibodies in primary biliary cirrhosis. Semin Liver Dis 1997;17(1):79–90 [34.

17. Bogdanos DP, Vergani D, Muratori P, Muratori L, et al. Specificity of anti-sp100 antibody for primary biliary cirrhosis. Scand J Gastroenterol 2004;39(4):405–7.

18. Pandit S, Samant H. Primary biliary cholangitis. [Updated 2021 Jul 18]. In: StatPearls [Internet]. Treasure Island (FL): StatPearls Publishing; 2022. Available at: https://www.ncbi.nlm.nih.gov/books/NBK459209/.

19. Selmi C, Mayo MJ, Bach N, et al. Primary biliary cirrhosis in monozygotic and dizygotic twins: genetics, epigenetics, and environment. Gastroenterology 2004;127(2):485–92.

20. Bown R, Clark ML, Doniach D. Primary biliary cirrhosis in brothers. Postgrad Med J 1975;51(592):110–5.

21. Tanaka A, Borchers AT, Ishibashi H, et al. Genetic and familial considerations of primary biliary cirrhosis. Am J Gastroenterol 2001;96(1):8–15.

22. Lazaridis KN, Juran BD, Boe GM, et al. Increased prevalence of antimitochondrial antibodies in first-degree relatives of patients with primary biliary cirrhosis. Hepatology 2007;46(3):785–92.

23. Tsuji K, Watanabe Y, Van De Water J, et al. Familial primary biliary cirrhosis in Hiroshima. J Autoimmune 1999;13:171e178.

24. Gulamhusein AF, Juran BD, Atkinson EJ, et al. Low incidence of primary biliary cirrhosis (PBC) in the first-degree relatives of PBC probands after 8 years of follow-up. Liver Int 2016;36:1378e1382.

25. Prince MI, Ducker SJ, James OFW. Case-control studies of risk factors for primary biliary cirrhosis in two United Kingdom populations. Gut 2010;59(4):508–12.

26. Triger DR. Primary biliary cirrhosis: an epidemiological study. Br Med J 1980;281:772e775.

27. Corpechot C, Chretien Y, Chazouilleres O, et al. Demographic, lifestyle, medical and familial factors associated with primary biliary cirrhosis. J Hepatol 2010;53(1):162–9.

28. Gershwin ME, Selmi C, Worman HJ, et al. Risk factors and comorbidities in primary biliary cirrhosis: a controlled interview-based study of 1032 patients. Hepatology 2005;42(5):1194–202.

29. Smyk D, Mytilinaiou MG, Rigopoulou EI, et al. PBC triggers in water reservoirs, coal mining areas and waste disposal sites: from Newcastle to New York. Dis Markers 2010;29(6):337–44.

30. Selmi C, Invernizzi P, Keeffe EB, et al. Epidemiology and pathogenesis of primary biliary cirrhosis. J Clin Gastroenterol 2004;38:264e271.

31. Prince MI, Chetwynd A, Diggle P, et al. The geographical distribution of primary biliary cirrhosis in a well-defined cohort. Hepatology 2001;34:1083e1088.

32. Ala A, Stanca CM, Bu-Ghanim, et al. Increased prevalence of primary biliary cirrhosis near Superfund toxic waste sites. Hepatology 2006;43:525e531.

33. Ohba K, Omagari K, Kinoshita H, et al. Primary biliary cirrhosis among atomic bomb survivors in Nagasaki, Japan. J Clin Epidemiol 2001;54:845e850.

34. Selmi C. The X in sex: how autoimmune diseases revolve around sex chromosomes. Best Pract Res Clin Rheumatol 2008;22(5):913–22.

35. Bianchi I, Lleo A, Gershwin ME, et al. The X chromosome and immune associated genes. J Autoimmun 2012;38(2–3):187–92.

36. Invernizzi P, Miozzo M, Battezzati PM, et al. Frequency of monosomy X in women with primary biliary cirrhosis. Lancet 2004;363(9408):533–5.

37. Mitchell MM, Lleo A, Zammataro L, et al. Epigenetic investigation of variably X chromosome inactivated genes in monozygotic female twins discordant for primary biliary cirrhosis. Epigenetics 2011;6(1):95–102.

38. Lleo A, Battezzati PM, Selmi C, et al. Is autoimmunity a matter of sex? Autoimmun Rev 2008;7(8):626–30.

39. Bouman A, Jan Heineman M, Faas MM. Sex hormones and the immune response in humans. Hum Reprod Update 2005;11(4):411–23.

40. Kanda N, Tsuchida T, Tamaki K. Estrogen enhancement of anti-double-stranded DNA antibody and immunoglobulin G production in peripheral blood mononuclear cells from patients with systemic lupus erythematosus. Arthritis Rheum 1999;42(2):328–37.

41. Kanda N, Tsuchida T, Tamaki K. Testosterone inhibits immunoglobulin production by human peripheral blood mononuclear cells. Clin Exp Immunol 1996;106(2):410–5.

42. Zein CO, Angulo P, Lindor KD. When is liver biopsy needed in the diagnosis of primary biliary cirrhosis? Clin Gastroenterol Hepatol 2003;1:89–95.

43. Prince M, Chetwynd A, Newman W, et al. Survival and symptom progression in a geographically based cohort of patients with primary biliary cirrhosis: follow-up for up to 28 years. Gastroenterology 2002;123:1044–51.

44. Podda M, Selmi C, Lleo A, et al. The limitations and hidden gems of the epidemiology of primary biliary cirrhosis. J Autoimmun 2013;46:81–7.

45. Nalbandian G, Van De Water J, Gish R, et al. Is there a serological difference between men and women with primary biliary cirrhosis? Am J Gastroenterol 1999;94(9):2482–6.

46. Tanaka A, Ma X, Yokosuka O, et al. Autoimmune liver diseases in the Asia-Pacific region: Proceedings of APASL symposium on AIH and PBC 2016. Hepatol Int 2016;10:909e915.

47. John BV, Aitcheson G, Schwartz KB, et al. Male sex is associated with higher rates of liver-related mortality in primary biliary cholangitis and cirrhosis. Hepatology 2021;74(2):879–91. Epub 2021 May 26. PMID: 33636012.

48. Fan X, Wang T, Shen Y, et al. Underestimated male prevalence of primary biliary cholangitis in China: results of a 16-yr cohort study involving 769 patients. Sci Rep 2017;7(1):6560. PMID: 28747696; PMCID: PMC5529550.

49. Kim KA, Ki M, Choi HY, Kim BH, Jang ES, Jeong SH. Population-based epidemiology of primary biliary cirrhosis in South Korea. Aliment Pharmacol Ther. 2016 Jan;43(1):154–62. doi: 10.1111/apt.13448. Epub 2015 Nov 2. PMID: 26526639.

50. Harada K, Hirohara J, Ueno Y, Nakano T, Kakuda Y, Tsubouchi H, Ichida T, Nakanuma Y. Incidence of and risk factors for hepatocellular carcinoma in primary biliary cirrhosis: national data from Japan. Hepatology. 2013 May;57(5):1942–9. doi: 10.1002/hep.26176. PMID: 23197466.

51. Zoller B, Li X, Sundquist J, et al. Risk of pulmonary embolism in patients with autoimmune disorders: a nationwide follow-up study from Sweden. Lancet 2012;379:244–9.

52. Muratori P, Granito A, Pappas G, et al. Clinical and serological profile of primary biliary cirrhosis in men. QJM 2007;100(8):534–5.

53. Rubel LR, Rabin L, Seeff LB, et al. Does primary biliary cirrhosis in men differ from primary biliary cirrhosis in women? Hepatology 1984;4(4):671–7.

54. Lucey MR, Neuberger JM, Williams R. Primary biliary cirrhosis in men. Gut 1986;27(11):1373–6.

55. Zakharia K, Robles J, Rasor M, et al. Primary biliary cholangitis (PBC): any differences between males and females? The Am J Gastroenterol 2019;114:S1543.

56. Sayiner M, Golabi P, Stepanova M, et al. Primary biliary cholangitis in Medicare population: the Impact on mortality and Resource Use. Hepatology 2019;69(1): 237–44.
57. Cheung AC, Lammers WJ, et al, Global PBC Study Group. Effects of age and sex of response to Ursodeoxycholic acid and transplant-free survival in patients with primary biliary cholangitis. Clin Gastroenterol Hepatol 2019;17(10):2076–84.e2. Epub 2019 Jan 4. PMID: 30616022.
58. Natarajan Y, Tansel A, Patel P, et al. Incidence of hepatocellular carcinoma in primary biliary cholangitis: a Systematic review and Meta-analysis. Dig Dis Sci 2021; 66(7):2439–51.
59. Suzuki A, Lymp J, Donlinger J, et al. Clinical predictors for hepatocellular carcinoma in patients with primary biliary cirrhosis. Clin Gastroenterol Hepatol 2007; 5:259–2564.
60. Silveira MG, Suzuki A, Lindor KD. Surveillance for hepatocellular carcinoma in patients with primary biliary cirrhosis. Hepatology 2008;48:1149–56.
61. Bruix J, Sherman M. Practice guidelines committee AASLD. Management of hepatocellular carcinoma. Hepatology 2005;42:1208–36.

The Inconvenient Truth of Primary Biliary Cholangitis/ Autoimmune Hepatitis Overlap Syndrome

Nasir Hussain, BSc, MBBS, MRCP[a,b],
Palak J. Trivedi, BSc (hons), MBBS, MRCP, PhD[a,b,c,d],*

KEYWORDS

- Autoimmune liver disease • Ursodeoxycholic acid • Obeticholic acid • Fibrates
- Immunosuppression

KEY POINTS

- Phenotypic manifestations of autoimmune liver disease are not static and can evolve over time.
- The majority of patients with PBC and elevated transaminases respond to bile acid therapy alone.
- Liver biopsy assessment of disease activity is essential to diagnose overlap presentations.
- Whilst some patients experience reduction in liver biochemistry, there is no high-quality data that shows improved transplant-free survival using combination immunosuppression and bile acid therapy over bile acid therapy alone.

INTRODUCTION

Primary biliary cholangitis (PBC) and autoimmune hepatitis (AIH) are distinct diseases with their own characteristics. For most patients, distinguishing between the two entities is without issue (**Fig. 1**). However, given the absence of defined etiological drivers, the authors recognize that the autoimmune liver spectrum is broad and occasionally disease boundaries become distorted. Indeed, in a minority of individuals,

---

[a] NIHR Birmingham BRC, Institute of Immunology and Immunotherapy, Centre for Liver and Gastrointestinal Research, University of Birmingham, Birmingham B15 2TT, United Kingdom; [b] Liver Unit, University Hospitals Birmingham National Health Service Foundation Trust Queen Elizabeth, Birmingham, United Kingdom; [c] Institute of Immunology and Immunotherapy, University of Birmingham, Birmingham, United Kingdom; [d] Institute of Applied Health Research, University of Birmingham, Birmingham, United Kingdom
* Corresponding author.
E-mail address: p.j.trivedi@bham.ac.uk

Clin Liver Dis 26 (2022) 657–680
https://doi.org/10.1016/j.cld.2022.06.007
1089-3261/22/© 2022 Elsevier Inc. All rights reserved.

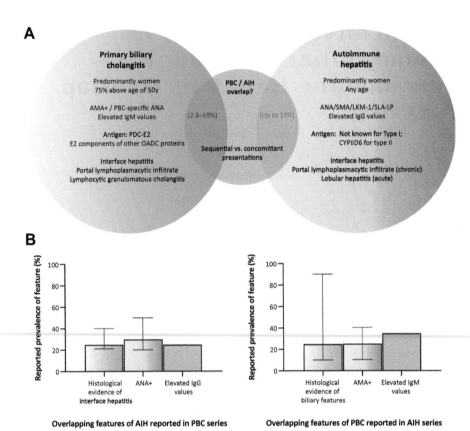

Fig. 1. Phenotypic features of PBC and AIH. An overview of the clinicopathological features of PBC and AIH are presented (*A*), with indicative percentages of overlap presentations provided in parenthesis. The proportion of patients who manifest histologic and immunoserological features of overlap are presented (*B*), as the median and range, derived from existing literature reports.

features of both diseases can present either concurrently or sequentially. The term "overlap syndrome" is often applied but can be misleading, as many interpret this to mean a separate disease. As a result, it is not infrequent for treatment paradigms to diverge from that of the predominant or original disease process, be that PBC or AIH, despite a lack of high-quality evidence to support this practice.

In this clinically focused review, the authors outline the definitions, presentation, and disease outcomes associated with PBC/AIH overlap syndromes, appraise the current evidence with regard to treatment strategy, and nominate areas for future research endeavor.

INCONVENIENT TRUTHS ABOUT DIAGNOSTIC CRITERIA FOR OVERLAP

The presentations in clinical practice that raise the question of overlap are variable but may include as follows:

1. A biochemical overlap: patients with PBC manifesting a "hepatitic" laboratory profile (aspartate aminotransferase [AST] or alanine aminotransferase [ALT] values

greater than 5x the upper limit of normal [ULN]); or patients with AIH who exhibit cholestatic liver biochemistry (alkaline phosphatase [ALP] greater than 3x ULN or gamma-glutamyltransferase [GGT] greater than 5x ULN)

2. An immunologic overlap: patients who test positive for anti-mitochondrial anti-bodies (AMAs), alongside elevated immunoglobulin G (IgG) values and/or positive antinuclear antibodies (ANAs)/anti-smooth muscle antibodies (ASMAs); or patients with otherwise classical AIH albeit testing positive for AMA.

3. A histologic overlap: florid bile duct lesions alongside a lymphoplasmacytic infiltrate with interface hepatitis.

Based on the above premise, definitions of overlap syndrome vary over time as our understandings of autoimmune liver disease continue to evolve. It is now generally accepted that the presence of a single phenotypic feature (eg, AMA positivity or bystander biliary inflammation in someone with otherwise typical AIH; or a patient with PBC having elevated aminotransferase activity or interface hepatitis) is not sufficient to claim an overlap diagnosis. Nevertheless, the rigor to which overlap definitions have been applied is likely biased by the interest and background viewpoint of reporting authors. Those with predominant interest in AIH are likely to claim greater prevalence of overlap in PBC cohorts, whereas individuals working in the biliary or cholestatic disease sphere tend to view overlap as an extreme presentation of PBC. As a result of these biases, quantifying the epidemiology of overlap presentations is difficult to do so accurately.[1]

Score-Based Criteria

Extensively validated, stringent criteria are lacking for PBC/AIH overlap, but the most commonly cited classifications are those proposed by the International Autoimmune Hepatitis Group (IAIHG),[2,3] and the Paris criteria developed by Chazouillères *and colleagues* (**Table 1**).[4] With regard to the former, it is important to recognize that neither the original nor revised IAIHG criteria were intended for this purpose, rather a means to ensure the homogeneity of patient populations entering AIH clinical trials. By assuming the character of a diagnostic index, IAIHG criteria risk weakening the legitimacy of other established diseases and drive clinicians toward AIH targets when treating patients with cholestasis.

To this effect, a position statement from the IAIHG categorically states that their scoring system should not be used to establish subgroups of patients with PBC.[5] By comparison, the Paris criteria are reported as having greater sensitivity and specificity for diagnosing overlap syndrome and in one study was claimed to reach greater than 90%.[3] However, it is important to recognize that the principled intent for defining overlap was not always a quantifiable metric in the index studies using Paris criteria (eg, the proportion of patients normalizing biochemistry, or a time-fixed event-free survival index). Instead, treatment superiority between UDCA monotherapy versus immunosuppression was determined based on the degree of improvement in laboratory values at different periods for different patients.[4]

Biochemical Criteria

Although biochemical thresholds for diagnosing overlap have been proposed, ALT and/or AST values greater than 5x ULN are common in >5% of patients with classical PBC. Preliminary data from the Global PBC Study Group (n = 3897) show that greater than 75% of patients manifest elevated ALT values at diagnosis, with 6.1% having readings >5x ULN.[6] However, the latter decreased to 1.1% after 1 year of ursodeoxycholic acid (UDCA) treatment, in the absence of immunosuppression. Phenotypic

Table 1
Caveats of primary biliary cholangitis and autoimmune hepatitis overlap scoring criteria

Parameter	Threshold	Comments
Original international AIH scoring criteria		
Sex	Male (0)	Criteria developed to
	Female (+2)	ensure homogeneity of
ALP:AST ratio	<1.5 (+2)	AIH patients entering
	1.5–3.0 (0)	into clinical trials and are
	>3.0 (−2)	not diagnostic of AIH
Serum globulin or IgG (× ULN)	>2.0 (+3)	Criteria never intended to
	1.5–2.0 (+2)	be applied to
	1.0–1.5 (+1)	discriminate specific
	<1.0 (0)	groups of patients with
ANA, SMA, and LKM1 antibodies	>1:80 (+3)	AILD
	1:80 (+2)	
	1:40 (+1)	
	<1:40 (0)	
Illicit drug use	Positive (−4)	
	Negative (+1)	
Average alcohol intake daily	<25 g/d (+2)	
	>60 g/d (−2)	
Histologic findings	Interface hepatitis (+3)	
	Lymphoplasmacytic infiltrate (+1)	
	Rosette formation (+1)	
	None of the above (−5)	
	Biliary changes (−3)	
	Other changes (+2)	
Other autoimmune disease	Yes (+2)	
AMA positivity	Yes (−4)	
Viral hepatitis markers	Positive (−3)	
	Negative (+3)	
Aggregate score (without treatment)	Definite AIH: >15	
	Probable AIH: 10–15	
Simplified AIH scoring criteria		
ANA or SMA	≥1:40 (+1)	Criteria developed to
	≥1:80 (+2)	ensure homogeneity of
	or LKM1 ≥1:40 (+2)	AIH patients entering
	or SLA positive (+2)	clinical trials and are not
Serum IgG	> ULN (+1)	diagnostic of AIH
	> 1.1 × ULN (+2)	Criteria never intended to
Histologic findings	Compatible with AIH (+1)	be applied to
	Typical of AIH (+2)	discriminate specific
Hepatitis viral markers	Negative (+2)	groups of patients with
Aggregate score (without treatment)	Definite AIH: ≥ 7	AILD
	Probable AIH: ≥ 6	

(continued on next page)

Table 1 (continued)		
Parameter	Threshold	Comments
Paris criteria for diagnosing AIH overlap in PBC		
ALT	5 × ULN	Criteria not validated at predicting response to treatments using contemporary response thresholds for either AIH or PBC
IgG	2 × ULN (or positive ASMA)	
Liver histology	Moderate or severe periportal or periseptal lymphocytic piecemeal necrosis	
		Transaminase elevations >5 × ULN detectable in >5% of patients with classical PBC, falling to 1% following UDCA monotherapy
		Up to 50% of patients treated with OCA second-line therapy normalize serum ALT values, in the absence of immunosuppression
		Validity of criteria in predicting response to immunosuppression in the absence of histologic confirmation of severe hepatitis activity has not been proven
Paris criteria for diagnosing PBC overlap in AIH		
ALP (or GGT)	2 × ULN	Poorly validated in non-White populations.
AMA	Positive 1:40	• Cholestatic biochemical presentations are evident in approximately 60% of AIH patients from the Middle East, Southern Africa, and those of Alaskan descent
Liver histology	Florid bile duct lesions	
		Isolated AMA positivity did not identify a separate clinical course in AIH for the vast majority
		Biliary features evident in up to 25% of AIH biopsies and do not associate with a distinct clinical course to AIH without biliary features

Abbreviations: AIH, autoimmune hepatitis; AILD, autoimmune liver disease; ALP, alkaline phosphatase; ALT, alanine aminotransferase; AMA, anti-mitochondrial antibody; ANA, antinuclear antibody; ASMA, anti-smooth muscle antibody; AST, aspartate aminotransferase; IgG, immunoglobulin G; LKM1, liver kidney microsomal antibody; OCA, obeticholic acid; PBC, primary biliary cholangitis; SLA, soluble liver antigen antibody; SMA, smooth muscle antibody; UDCA, ursodeoxycholic acid; ULN, upper limit of normal.

variation according to age is also apparent, with more than 50% of women diagnosed with PBC below 50 years of age being UDCA non-responders.[7,8]

Of interest, data from UK-PBC show that in young patients, biochemical non-response is most often on transaminase criteria.[7] Moreover, greater than 50% and ~30% of patients referred for the second-line therapy were found to normalize serum ALT and bilirubin values, respectively, when treated with obeticholic acid (OCA).[9] These studies emphasize the importance of gauging biochemical response to bile acid therapy before attributing overlap labels to patients with PBC.

Broader phenotypic variations are also evident geographically, with approximately 60% of Alaskan natives, alongside patients from the Middle East, Somalia, and Southern Africa, presenting with cholestatic biochemistry in the context of AIH.[1] Moreover, a single-center study from Miami found that Hispanic patients with PBC more often present with features of AIH than non-Hispanics (31% vs 13%), less commonly respond to UDCA monotherapy, and have a greater probability of experiencing hepatic decompensation.[10] For a more detailed epidemiology review of autoimmune liver disease, the authors refer the reader elsewhere.[1]

Immunologic Overlap

Up to 25% of patients reported as having PBC/AIH overlap are ASMA positive; despite the fact that this antibody is found in over 40% of the general adult population. Similarly, ANAs can be found in 46% to 47% and 68% to 100% of PBC patients who are AMA-positive and AMA-negative PBC, respectively. However, these include antigen-specific ANA subtypes (anti-gp210 and anti-sp100),[11] which are diagnostic of PBC rather than AIH, and stratify a group of patients at greater risk of liver disease progression.[12] However, true positivity for anti-liver kidney microsomal (LKM)-1 antibodies is seldom reported in cases of AIH/PBC overlap. This presumably exemplifies the antigen specificity of type-II AIH in terms of disease pathogenesis. Moreover, most patients with PBC tend to present above the age of 45 year old, whereas anti-LKM-1-positive AIH is most prevalent in childhood and adolescence.

By contrast, approximately 10% of AIH patients are AMA positive. One study from North America details 15 of 128 individuals with AIH who remained persistently AMA positive over a median of 8 years. The original report on this cohort found that no patient developed clinical or histologic evidence of PBC during this time.[13] However, a later series from the same group reported that 3 of 31 women with AMA-positive AIH went on to develop clinical, histologic, and serologic features of PBC, within 1 to 29 years following first presentation.[14] Clinical presentations are also seen with PBC manifesting first and features of AIH developing later.[14–16] An observational series from the Mayo clinic, capturing data from 1476 PBC patients, identified eight individuals (0.05%) who developed overt features of AIH over a period of 4 months to 9 years, despite UDCA.[15] The Paris group reports much greater prevalence, with 12 of 282 patients with PBC (4.2%) evolving disease phenotype into classical AIH between 6 months and 13 years from the first diagnosis.[16] These observations highlight that autoimmune phenotypes may not be static, have potential to change over the course of time, and the need for ongoing assessment of the predominant disease process in those with immunoserological crossover.

Histopathological Overlap

Liver biopsy is not necessary for a diagnosis of PBC but may be pursued in cases of diagnostic doubt. Conversely, histologic evidence of inflammatory activity is essential to diagnose AIH, fully assess treatment response, and identify those who may be able to wean immunosuppressive therapy. For all intents and purposes, histologic features of PBC and AIH are distinct (see **Fig. 1**), although some characteristics are common to both groups. As PBC is inherently an inflammatory disease, interface hepatitis can be detected in approximately 25% of patients[5] and in itself does not suggest a diagnosis of overlap. However, moderate-to-severe interface hepatitis is uncommon and an independent predictor of death or liver transplantation in UDCA-treated PBC patients (relative risk [RR]: 1.9), and alongside advanced histologic stage (RR 1.5), is risk factor for disease progression.[17] Disappointingly, a multicenter randomized control trial (RCT) of budesonide, in 62 PBC patients with confirmed hepatic inflammatory activity and persistently elevated ALP values despite UDCA, showed no significant improvement in liver histology over a median treatment duration of 32.3 months, questioning the added benefit of immunosuppression.[18] It is also notable that in a post hoc analysis of two RCTs, patients with PBC who were identified as having potential AIH overlap experienced the same clinical course on UDCA monotherapy as classical PBC patients.[19]

When comparing diseases, the magnitude of hepatocellular injury is often more severe in AIH than PBC, with more extensive lobular hepatitis, rosette formation, and emperipolesis.[20] In turn, biliary changes exist in >20% of patients with AIH alone. In one study of 84 AIH patients, 20 had evidence of biliary pathology, including nondestructive cholangitis ($n = 10$), ductopenia ($n = 4$), and destructive cholangitis ($n = 6$). Importantly, patients having such changes fared no different compared to those with no biliary changes, with regard to remission rates (90% vs 77%; $P = .3$) and incomplete response (5% vs 8%, $P>.9$). There were no significant differences in the rate of progression to cirrhosis (41% vs 34%, $P = .8$), requirement for liver transplantation (5% vs 11%, $P = .7$), or death from liver failure (5% vs 2%, $P = .4$).[21]

It has been proposed that hepatic inflammation in PBC (and in turn biliary damage in AIH) represents "bystander" injury resulting from the main mechanism of inflammation associated with the primary condition.[22] This is described by pathologists Tan and Goodman, where lymphoplasmacytic interface hepatitis in PBC resulted from the inflammation that accompanied bile duct destruction extending to adjacent and surrounding hepatocytes.[23] A retrospective review of liver biopsies from North America found that when immunostaining samples for IgG and IgM among patients with AIH ($n = 19$), PBC ($n = 22$), and PBC–AIH ($n = 13$), IgG levels were similar across all three groups. However, IgM levels were significantly lower in the AIH group, and similar among the PBC and PBC–AIH groups. This was mirrored when calculating the IgG/IgM plasma cell ratio; 5.2 (interquartile range (IQR), 2.6–13.3) in the AIH group, compared with 1.2 (IQR, 0.6–1.7) and 1.1 (IQR, 0.7–1.5) in the PBC and PBC–AIH group, respectively ($P<.01$), suggesting that PBC/AIH overlap is more similar to classical PBC than it is to AIH.[24] Additional evidence to support this claim stems from early studies of genetic risk, in which 17/20 patients with PBC/AIH overlap were found to be HLAB8, DR3, or DR6 positive (haplotypes more commonly associated with AIH), compared with 18 of 20 and 4 of 20 patients with AIH and PBC, respectively. The investigators concluded that overlap cases are in fact a form of PBC that develops a more "hepatitic" profile due to a predisposition in their genetic background.[25]

With these caveats in mind, overlap syndromes should be diagnosed conservatively and only considered in the differential when a patient deviates from the normal clinical course, when several (rather than singular) features of another disease are present and perhaps most importantly, when patients deviate from their expected response to therapy. Physicians must also be mindful of the varied presentation of non-autoimmune and drug-induced liver injury, for instance through vaccination, antibiotics, or the use of fibric acid derivatives, and the potential for clinical changes to be related to toxicity from prescribed and nonprescribed agents rather than concomitant AIH.[9,26,27]

EVIDENCE BEHIND EXISTING TREATMENT PARADIGMS

UDCA is well established as the first-line treatment of PBC. Long-term clinical outcome studies have shown attenuation in fibrosis progression, a reduction in liver cancer risk, and prolonged liver transplant-free survival, particularly among individuals attaining biochemical response after 1 to 2 years of therapy.[28–39] Second-line regimens vary but consist of licensed (OCA) and off-label bile acid therapies improve liver biochemistry and prolong transplant-free survival when combined with UDCA.[40–54] By contrast, induction regimens for AIH almost exclusively consist of corticosteroids (prednisolone or budesonide), followed by maintenance with steroid-sparing agents (azathioprine, mycophenolate mofetil, or calcineurin inhibitors).[55,56] Contemporary treatment targets also differ between diseases, and have evolved in recent years. For PBC, normalization in ALP values and a bilirubin $\leq$0.6x ULN are associated with the lowest risk of clinical events, and transplant-free survival rates akin to that of a control population.[57] For AIH, remission is defined as complete normalization in transaminases, bilirubin, and serum IgG values, ideally within 6 months of starting therapy.[56,58] Such treatment pathways have taken time to establish, with evidence being gathered over decades.[59] This reflects the chronic and slowly progressive nature of autoimmune liver diseases and highlights the need for robust slong-term observational cohort tudies.

Unfortunately, the low incidence and prevalence, as well as inconsistent definitions mean that there is lack of adequately powered prospective studies to support the implementation of a generic treatment pathway for overlap cases. Moreover, anecdotal experiences in the literature are largely derived from non-randomized, non-blinded studies. Early studies also do not use currently accepted definitions of biochemical remission (for AIH or PBC) when comparing treatment outcomes. Thus, it is unclear whether and/or which combination of therapies yields most benefit.

In a meta-analysis of eight RCTs, 214 patients were retrospectively identified as having features compatible with PBC/AIH overlap (using the Paris criteria), with 97 being treated with UDCA monotherapy and 117 a combination of UDCA and corticosteroids (mean follow-up ranging 10 to 90 months). Therein, combination therapy was found to be superior to UDCA monotherapy in lowering serum ALP, ALT, and other liver biochemical markers (odds ratio [OR]: 0.25, 95% CI: 0.13 to 0.48, P<.0001), However, death or liver transplantation occurred in one of 97 patients in the monotherapy groups and in 15 of 117 patients in the combination therapy group.[60] In one of the included studies, the outcomes of 17 patients over a median 7.5 year follow-up period was presented, in which four/six patients attained biochemical (transaminases $\leq$2x ULN) and immunologic (IgG <16 g/L) response alongside non-progression in fibrosis stage. This compared with overlap patients receiving UDCA alone, in whom biochemical response and stable/reduced fibrosis was observed in 3/11 patients, biochemical nonresponse in eight, and worsening of fibrosis in four.[61] Favorable responses to combination therapy are also reported in other cases series, although the overall frequency of nonresponders exceeds that in AIH alone (**Table 2**). In one evaluation of PBC/AIH overlap (identified by applying the IAIHG criteria to those with PBC), 40/52 patients attained biochemical remission within 12 months of treatment with corticosteroids, defined as complete normalization in ALT, AST, bilirubin, and IgG values, as well as reduction in ALP to $\leq$3x ULN at 12 months. Of note, severe interface hepatitis was a characteristic positively associate with treatment response, with an elevated serum

Table 2
Biochemical responses between treatment regimens in primary biliary cholangitis and autoimmune hepatitis overlap presentations

Author, Year	Location	Treatment Groups	Follow-up Period	Treatment Groups	Criteria to Determine Overlap	Biochemical Evaluation	Principal Results Reported
Chazouilleres et al,[4] 1998 *Retrospective cohort study*	France	UDCA monotherapy: 5 Combination: 9	23m (median)	UDCA 13–15 mg/kg/d Combination: UDCA 13–15 mg/kg/d + prednisolone 0.5 mg/kg/d +/– azathioprine 50–100 mg/d	Paris criteria	Biochemical improvement (not defined)	2/5 in UDCA group 6/6 in combination group
Chazouilleres et al,[61] 2006 *Retrospective cohort study*	France	UDCA monotherapy: 11 Combination: 6	90m (median)	UDCA 13–15 mg/kg/d Combination: UDCA 13–15 mg/kg/d + prednisolone 0.5 mg/kg/d +/– azathioprine 50–100 mg/d)	Paris criteria	Complete biochemical response (ALT < 2x ULN and IgG < 16 g/L) Absence of fibrosis progression (defined as no increase in 1 or more units on METAVIR five-point scale)	27% in UDCA group vs 67% in combo group (P = .11) 50% in the UDCA group 100% in the combination group (P = .08)
Saito et al,[84] 2006 *Retrospective cohort study*	Japan	UDCA monotherapy: 9 Combination: 6	84m (median)	UDCA 300–600 mg/d Combination: UDCA 300–600 mg/d + prednisolone 4–30 mg/d +/– azathioprine (dose not reported)	Paris criteria	The study aim was to characterize clinical laboratory characteristics of PBC–AIH overlap	Study reports normalization or near normalization in ALT and ALP after the addition of immunosuppression following initial treatment with UDCA monotherapy

(continued on next page)

Table 2
(continued)

Author, Year	Location	Treatment Groups	Follow-up Period	Treatment Groups	Criteria to Determine Overlap	Biochemical Evaluation	Principal Results Reported
Wu et al,[85] 2006 *Retrospective cohort study*	China	UDCA monotherapy: 3 Combination: 6	Not reported	UDCA 13–15 mg/kg/d Combination: UDCA 13–15 mg/kg/d + prednisolone 50 mg/d	Revised IAIHG scoring system	Biochemical remission achieved (not defined)	0/3 in the UDCA group (patients however achieved remission within 6 mo with the introduction of prednisolone) 6/6 in the combination group achieved remission within 6 mo.
Heurgue et al,[86] 2007 *Retrospective cohort study*	France	UDCA monotherapy: 6 Combination: 7	60m (median)	UDCA 11–14.7 mg/kg/d Combination: UDCA 11–14.7 mg/kg/d + corticosteroids 0.5-1 mg/kg/d +/– azathioprine 1.1–2.0 mg/kg/d	Paris criteria	Complete biochemical response (serum transaminase <2x ULN, and normalization of GGT and ALP)	3/6 in the UDCA group 7/7 in the combination group
Yokokawa et al,[87] 2010 *Retrospective cohort study*	Japan	UDCA monotherapy: 2 Combination: 13	119 (median)	UDCA 300–600 mg/d Combo UDCA 300–600 mg/d + prednisolone 20–40 mg d ± azathioprine 50 mg/d	Paris criteria	Mortality Normalization in ALT and ALP	2/2 in the UDCA group died of liver failure. 1/13 in the combination group died of a liver-unrelated cause Seen in all 13 patients in the combination group

Study	Country	Groups	Follow-up	Treatment	Criteria	Outcome	Results
Tanaka et al,[88] 2011 *Retrospective cohort study*	Japan	UDCA monotherapy: 15 Combination: 10	73m (mean)	UDCA (dose not reported) Combination: UDCA (dose not reported) + corticosteroids (dose not reported) +/– azathioprine (dose not reported)	Revised IAIHG scoring system	Improvement in liver biochemistry (not defined) Histologic disease progression (not defined)	8/15 in the UDCA group 10/10 in the combination group 7/15 in the UDCA group 0/10 in the combination group
Efe et al,[69] 2014 *Retrospective cohort study*	Multicenter (Turkey, France, Italy, Sweden, and USA)	UDCA monotherapy: 1 Combination: 18	50m (mean)	UDCA 12–15 mg/kg/d Combination UDCA 12–15 mg/kg/d + prednisolone 30–60 mg/d +/– azathioprine 50–150 mg/d	Paris criteria	Biochemical remission (defined as >40% decrease in ALP in 1 y and normalization of aminotransferases)	N = 1 pt in the UDCA monotherapy group entered remission N = 15/18 in the combination group went into remission
Levy et al,[10] 2014 *Retrospective cohort study*	USA	UDCA monotherapy: 18 Combination: 21	38m (median)	UDCA 14–15 mg/kg/d Combination: UDCA 14–15 mg/kg/d + azathioprine or prednisolone or MMF (doses not sated)	Paris criteria	Normalization of liver biochemistry	11/18 in the UDCA group 10/21 in the combination group
Liu et al,[89] 2014 *Retrospective cohort study*	China	UDCA monotherapy: 6 Combination: 5	9–48m (range)	UDCA 13–15 mg/kg/d Combination: UDCA 13–15 mg/kg + prednisolone (dose not reported) +/– azathioprine (dose not reported)	Simplified IAIHG scoring system	Complete biochemical response (defined as ALT < 2x ULN and IgG < 15.6 d/L or improvement in liver histology)	0/6 in the UDCA group 2/5 in the combination group

(continued on next page)

Table 2
(continued)

Author, Year	Location	Treatment Groups	Follow-up Period	Treatment Groups	Criteria to Determine Overlap	Biochemical Evaluation	Principal Results Reported
Ozaslan et al,[63] 2014 *Retrospective cohort study*	Turkey France Italy USA Sweden	UDCA monotherapy: 30 Combination: 67	66m (mean)	UDCA 13–15 mg/mg/d Combination: UDCA 13–15 mg/kg/d + prednisolone 30–60 mg/d +/– azathioprine 50–150 mg/d	Paris criteria	Biochemical remission (defined as >40% decrease in ALP in 1 y and normalization of aminotransferases)	21% in the UDCA group 56% in the combination group Severe interface hepatitis reported to be predictive of nonresponse to UDCA monotherapy (OR = 0.53, 95% CI: 0.004–0.68, P = .024)
Yoshioka et al,[90] 2014 *Retrospective cohort study*	Japan	UDCA monotherapy: 8 Combination: 20	94m (median)	UDCA (dose not reported) Combination: UDCA (dose not reported) and corticosteroids (30 mg/d)	Biochemical, serologic and histologic features of both diseases	Biochemical response (normalization of ALT)	Biochemical response not quantified for the UDCA monotherapy group Biochemical response in 15/20 of the combination group

Park et al,[66] 2015 South Korea *Retrospective cohort study*	UDCA monotherapy: 4 Combination: 5	70m (median)	UDCA (dose not stated) Combination: UDCA and corticosteroids (dose not stated)	Paris criteria	Response to UDCA (defined as ALP < 3x ULN, ALT < 2x ULN, bilirubin < 1x ULN) Clinical remission (defined as the disappearance of symptoms, normalisation of aminotransferases, bilirubin, and IgG levels)	50% in the UDCA monotherapy group (not assessed in the combination group) 20% in the of combination group (not assessed in the UDCA group)
Yang et al,[91] 2016 China *Retrospective cohort study*	UDCA monotherapy: 8 Combination: 27	38m (median)	UDCA 13–15 mg/kg/d Combination: UDCA 13–15 mg/kg/d + prednisolone 15–50 mg/d	Paris criteria	PBC response according to: Paris-I criteria (ALP < 3x ULN, AST < 2x ULN, bilirubin <1 mg/dL) Rotterdam criteria (normalization of albumin and/or bilirubin) Barcelona criteria (decrease in ALP by >40%, or ALP normalization) Toronto criteria (ALP ≤167 x ULN)	% in the UDCA group vs % in the combination group 0% vs 48% (*P* = .014) 13% vs 67% (*P* = .009) 38% vs 89% (*P* = .007) 25% vs 81% (*P* = .005)

(continued on next page)

Table 2
(continued)

Author, Year	Location	Treatment Groups	Follow-up Period	Treatment Groups	Criteria to Determine Overlap	Biochemical Evaluation	Principal Results Reported
Fan et al,[92] 2018 *Prospective cohort study*	China	UDCA monotherapy: 14 Combination: 14	18m (median)	UDCA 13–15 mg/kg/d Combination: UDCA 13–15 mg/kg/d + methylpredinosolone 12–40 mg/d +/− azathioprine 50–100 mg/d or MMF (dose not reported)	Paris criteria	Biochemical remission at 12 mo (normalization of transaminases and IgG) Liver related adverse events (worsening or new hepatic decompensation, liver failure, transplantation, or death attributable to decompensation)	9.1% in the UDCA group 60.0% in the combination group (*P* = .024) 64.3% in the UDCA group 14.3% in the combination group (*P* = .018)

Abbreviations: AIH, autoimmune hepatitis; ALP, alkaline phosphatase; ALT, alanine aminotransferase; AST, aspartate aminotransferase; CI, confidence intervals; GGT, gamma-glutamyl transferase; IAIHG, international autoimmune hepatitis group; IgG, immunoglobulin G; METAVIR, meta-analysis of histological data in viral hepatitis; MMF, mycophenolate mofetil; OR, odds ratio; PBC, primary biliary cholangitis; SLA, soluble liver antigen antibody; UDCA, ursodeoxycholic acid; ULN, upper limit of normal.

IgG value of greater than 1.3x ULN having a sensitivity and specificity of 60% and 97%, respectively, for defining steroid responsiveness.[62] This becomes important as the sensitivity reduced to 10% when applying the Paris criteria, which suggests IgG levels of greater than 2x ULN as its cutoff. This raises the possibility that potential patients who may benefit from steroids may be missed when the Paris criteria are applied. Regardless, Ozaslan and colleagues evaluated 88 patients with a diagnosis of PBC/AIH overlap (Paris criteria) from seven centers across five countries. In doing so, they found that severe interface hepatitis was independently associated with lack of biochemical response to UDCA alone, whereas advanced fibrosis was independently predictive of response to combination UDCA and immunosuppression.[63]

The benefit of corticosteroids is somewhat challenged in the study by Joshi and colleagues, who evaluated treatment with UDCA monotherapy ($n = 12$) in those with PBC/AIH overlap compared with classical PBC ($n = 171$). The investigators found similar percentage reductions in serum bilirubin, ALP, AST, cholesterol, and IgM values in both groups after 2 years of therapy with little change in histologic features.[19] Moreover, very little change in hepatic lobular inflammatory activity was observed during this period. A contemporary systematic review of 21 studies (17 of which compared UDCA monotherapy with UDCA and immunosuppression combination therapy) presented data from 402 patients in nine countries and showed no significant differences in the rate of symptomatic improvement, biochemical improvement, non-progression of liver fibrosis, or transplant-free survival between treatment regimens.[64] It is important to recognize that many studies are limited by the fact that the patients with PBC/AIH overlap were less likely to have received UDCA from the outset compared with those with PBC alone, and that delay in starting UDCA is a critical risk factor for primary biochemical nonresponse.[65] Furthermore, biochemical changes according to the total duration of UDCA therapy have not been rigorously evaluated.

Data from South Korea indicate that the rate to progression to liver cirrhosis may be greater among patients with PBC/AIH overlap group compared with those with AIH, but not significantly different when compared with PBC (**Table 3**).[66] These findings have been validated by single-center observations elsewhere, albeit with no differences in all-cause mortality between groups.[67] In turn, a small study from the Mayo clinic suggest that PBC/AIH overlap presentations ($n = 12$) experience worse clinical outcomes compared with PBC alone ($n = 123$), as evidenced by the development of portal hypertension, varices, gastrointestinal bleeding, ascites, need for liver transplantation, and death (see **Table 3**).[68] However, others report no significant difference in median transplant-free survival between PBC and PBC/AIH overlap presentations.[19] Limited data from historic observational cohorts suggest that PBC patients who develop AIH features sequentially experience more rapid progression to cirrhosis and chronic liver failure than those with classical PBC.[16] However, outcome data on sequential overlap presentations are conspicuous, with no baseline characteristics that predict which PBC patients are most likely to develop AIH (or vice versa),[15,69] nor any study which handles the development of an overlap syndrome as a time-dependent covariate.

PRACTICAL ADVICE AND FUTURE DIRECTIONS

It is the authors contention that in patients with PBC as the dominant disease entity, a label of AIH overlap should be attributed conservatively and robustly, following a "proper" trial of bile acid therapy (including for some, second-line treatments), with a good quality liver biopsy being the strongest means to diagnose and quantify the magnitude of overlap. Reciprocally, AMA positivity and biliary features are common in AIH, particularly among those of non-White race, and do not immediately qualify

Table 3
Clinical outcomes reported in primary biliary cholangitis and autoimmune hepatitis overlap presentations

Author and Year	Location	No of Patients	Groups Compared	Overlap Criteria	Outcomes Measured	Key Findings Against Outcomes
Silveira et al,[68] 2007	USA Mayo Clinic, Rochester, Minnesota	135 PBC/AIH overlap: 26 PBC: 109	PBC/AIH overlap vs PBC Follow up (mean): 6.1 y for overlap 5.4 y for PBC	Revised IAIHG criteria	Development of: 1. Portal hypertension 2. Esophageal varices 3. GI bleeding 4. Ascites 5. Adverse outcomes (death and or OLT)	Overlap vs PBC group 1. 54% vs 28% ($P = .01$) 2. 50% vs 23% ($P<.01$) 3. 35% vs 15% ($P = .03$) 4. 42% vs 15% ($P<.01$) 5. 38% vs 19% ($P<.05$)
Kuiper et al,[3] 2010	Holland Erasmus University Medical Center	134 PBC/AIH-overlap: 12 AIH: 65 PBC: 57	PBC/AIH overlap vs AIH vs PBC Follow-up (mean): 9.7 y	Paris criteria (Except one patient with: ALP > 2x ULN, ALT > 5x ULN, and florid bile duct lesions)	10-y transplant free survival	Overlap vs PBC vs AIH 92% vs 81% vs 88% (P values not provided
Neuhauser et al,[93] 2010	USA Mayo Clinic, Rochester, Minnesota	364 PBC/AIH overlap: 23 PBC: 341	PBC/AIH overlap vs PBC Follow-up (mean): 9.3 y overlap 9.8 y PBC	Simplified IAIHG scoring criteria	Frequency of: 1. Cirrhosis 2. Portal hypertension 3. GI bleeding 4. Ascites 5. Varices 6. Liver related death and/or liver transplantation	Overlap vs PBC group 1. 52% vs 42% ($P < .01$) 2. 74% vs 38% ($P < .01$) 3. 57% vs 14% ($P < .01$) 4. 43% vs22% ($P = .02$) 5. 74% vs 32% ($P<.01$) 6. 39% vs 21% ($P = .05$)
Kobayashi et al,[20] 2014	Japan Kanazawa University Hospital	84 liver biopsies PBC/AIH overlap				

Study	Country/Hospital	Patients	Comparison / Follow-up	Criteria	Outcomes	Results
Park et al,[66] 2015	Korea, *Seoul National university Hospital*	158, PBC/AIH-overlap: 9, AIH: 68, PBC: 81	PBC-AIH overlap vs AIH vs PBC, Follow-up (median): 5.8 y overlap, 5.3 y: AIH, 4.7 y: PBC	Revised and simplified IAIHG criteria	1. 5-y progression rate to cirrhosis 2. 5-y progression rate to hepatic decompensation	Overlap vs AIH vs PBC 1. 34.4% vs 9.8% vs 24.4% (P = .01, P = .16) 2. 0.0% vs 7.6% vs 11.4% (P = .996, P = .740)
Yang et al,[91] 2016	China, *Shanghai RenJi Hospital*	323, PBC/AIH-overlap: 46, PBC: 277	PBC-AIH overlap vs PBC, Follow-up (median): 38m overlap group, 41m PBC group	Paris criteria	5-y adverse outcome-free survival. Adverse outcomes defined as: complications of decompensation, OLT, and liver-related death	Overlap vs PBC -57% vs 81% (P = .38)
Casas et al,[67] 2018	Colombia	210, PBC/AIH-overlap: 32, AIH: 178	PBC-AIH overlap vs AIH, Follow-up (median): 52m overlap, 47.8m: AIH	Paris criteria	Progression to: 1. Cirrhosis 2. Liver transplantation	Overlap vs AIH 1. 22.2% vs 13.1% (P = .38) 2. 18% vs 5.6% (P = .009)

Abbreviations: AIH, autoimmune hepatitis; ALP, alkaline phosphatase; ALT, alanine transaminase; GI, gastrointestinal; HLA, human leukocyte antigens; IgG, immunoglobulin G; IgM, immunoglobulin M; OLT, orthotopic liver transplantation; PBC, primary biliary cholangitis (formerly primary biliary cirrhosis).

patients as having an overlap syndrome with PBC.[1,10] Although the vast majority of patients with AIH attain remission with immunosuppression alone, a very small proportion of patients evolve into PBC, emphasizing the need for long-term appraisal of diagnosis. This is perhaps most evident in transplant series of patients with AIH, wherein 14% to 31% of explant livers from patients with AIH are reclassified as either having PBC (12%) or 19% as primary sclerosing cholangitis (PSC).[70,71]

Clinicians must adopt a personalized approach when offering interventions to all patients, while being transparent about the strength (or lack) of evidence behind the treatment targets one hopes to achieve. Given the rare disease and heterogeneous nature of overlap presentations, RCTs are unlikely to be performed in this domain. However, the long-term national and international registries have greatly enhanced understandings of epidemiology and natural history in other autoimmune diseases.[72–80] Akin to studies in PSC,[73,81] multicenter data sets for PBC and AIH need to be interrogated and studied, to determine to what degree clinical outcomes differ among overlap presentations and whether treatment response criteria for PBC and AIH are valid for overlap presentations. The long-term goals may rest in the ability to reclassify patients based on the discovery of molecular signatures of disease (rather than by serology and biochemistry), particularly those that more accurately represent disease activity,[82] along with biomarkers that predict response to specific interventions.[82,83]

CLINICS CARE POINTS

- A high quality liver biopsy is essential before attributing a label of overlap
- Individualised and tailored management is required for all patients with autoimmune liver disease, including reglar appraisal of diagnosis
- PBC is an inflammatory disease. Elevated transaminases and interface hepatitis are common, and in themself do not quantify an ovrlap diagnosis.
- The majority of individuals with PBC and elevated transaminases show biochemical response to bile acid monotherapy

GRANT SUPPORT AND FUNDING

P.J. Trivedi receives institutional salary support from the National Institute for Health Research (NIHR) Birmingham Biomedical Research Centre (BRC). This article presents independent research supported by the Birmingham NIHR BRC based at the University Hospitals Birmingham National Health Service Foundation Trust and the University of Birmingham. The views expressed are those of the author(s) and not necessarily those of the National Health Service, the NIHR, or the Department of Health. Dr P.J. Trivedi has received grant support from the Wellcome Trust, the Medical Research Foundation, GSK, Guts UK, PSC Support, Intercept Pharma, Dr Falk Pharma, Gilead Sciences, and Bristol Myers Squibb. He has also received speaker fees from Intercept and Dr Falk, and advisory board / consultancy fees from Intercept, Dr Falk and GSK.

REFERENCES

1. Trivedi PJ, Hirschfield GM. Recent advances in clinical practice: epidemiology of autoimmune liver diseases. Gut 2021;70(10):1989–2003.

2. Alvarez F, Berg PA, Bianchi FB, et al. International Autoimmune Hepatitis Group Report: review of criteria for diagnosis of autoimmune hepatitis. J Hepatol 1999;31(5):929–38.

3. Kuiper EM, Zondervan PE, van Buuren HR. Paris criteria are effective in diagnosis of primary biliary cirrhosis and autoimmune hepatitis overlap syndrome. Clin Gastroenterol Hepatol 2010;8(6):530–4.

4. Chazouillères O, Wendum D, Serfaty L, et al. Primary biliary cirrhosis-autoimmune hepatitis overlap syndrome: clinical features and response to therapy. Hepatology 1998;28(2):296–301.

5. Boberg KM, Chapman RW, Hirschfield GM, et al. Overlap syndromes: the International Autoimmune Hepatitis Group (IAIHG) position statement on a controversial issue. J Hepatol 2011;54(2):374–85.

6. Sioufi A, Murillo Perez CF, Nevens F, et al. Characterising normal patterns of alanine aminotransferase elevations in ursodeoxycholic acid-treated patients with primary biliary cholangitis. Hepatology 2020;72(S1):739A–40A.

7. Carbone M, Mells GF, Pells G, et al. Sex and age are determinants of the clinical phenotype of primary biliary cirrhosis and response to ursodeoxycholic acid. Gastroenterology 2013;144(3):560–9.e7 [quiz: e13-4].

8. Cheung AC, Lammers WJ, Murillo Perez CF, et al. Effects of age and sex of response to ursodeoxycholic acid and transplant-free survival in patients with primary biliary cholangitis. Clin Gastroenterol Hepatol 2019;17(10):2076–84.e2.

9. Abbas N, Culver E, Thorburn D, et al. OWE-6 Multicentre evaluation of second line therapies in primary biliary cholangitis: UK experience. Gut 2021;70(Suppl 4):A10.

10. Levy C, Naik J, Giordano C, et al. Hispanics with primary biliary cirrhosis are more likely to have features of autoimmune hepatitis and reduced response to ursodeoxycholic acid than non-Hispanics. Clin Gastroenterol Hepatol 2014;12(8):1398–405.

11. Bogdanos DP, Komorowski L. Disease-specific autoantibodies in primary biliary cirrhosis. Clin Chim Acta 2011;412(7–8):502–12.

12. Haldar D, Janmohamed A, Plant T, et al. Antibodies to gp210 and understanding risk in patients with primary biliary cholangitis. Liver Int 2021;41(3):535–44.

13. O'Brien C, Joshi S, Feld JJ, et al. Long-term follow-up of antimitochondrial antibody-positive autoimmune hepatitis. Hepatology 2008;48(2):550–6.

14. Dinani AM, Fischer SE, Mosko J, et al. Patients with autoimmune hepatitis who have antimitochondrial antibodies need long-term follow-up to detect late development of primary biliary cirrhosis. Clin Gastroenterol Hepatol 2012;10(6):682–4.

15. Gossard AA, Lindor KD. Development of autoimmune hepatitis in primary biliary cirrhosis. Liver Int 2007;27(8):1086–90.

16. Poupon R, Chazouilleres O, Corpechot C, et al. Development of autoimmune hepatitis in patients with typical primary biliary cirrhosis. Hepatology 2006;44(1):85–90.

17. Corpechot C, Abenavoli L, Rabahi N, et al. Biochemical response to ursodeoxycholic acid and long-term prognosis in primary biliary cirrhosis. Hepatology 2008;48(3):871–7.

18. Hirschfield GM, Beuers U, Kupcinskas L, et al. A placebo-controlled randomised trial of budesonide for PBC following an insufficient response to UDCA. J Hepatol 2021;74(2):321–9.

19. Joshi S, Cauch-Dudek K, Wanless IR, et al. Primary biliary cirrhosis with additional features of autoimmune hepatitis: response to therapy with ursodeoxycholic acid. Hepatology 2002;35(2):409–13.

20. Kobayashi M, Kakuda Y, Harada K, et al. Clinicopathological study of primary biliary cirrhosis with interface hepatitis compared to autoimmune hepatitis. World J Gastroenterol 2014;20(13):3597–608.

21. Czaja AJ, Carpenter HA. Autoimmune hepatitis with incidental histologic features of bile duct injury. Hepatology 2001;34(4 Pt 1):659–65.

22. Trivedi PJ, Hirschfield GM. Review article: overlap syndromes and autoimmune liver disease. Aliment Pharmacol Ther 2012;36(6):517–33.

23. Tan D, Goodman ZD. Liver biopsy in primary biliary cholangitis: indications and interpretation. Clin Liver Dis 2018;22(3):579–88.

24. Lee BT, Wang Y, Yang A, et al. IgG:IgM ratios of liver plasma cells reveal similar phenotypes of primary biliary cholangitis with and without features of autoimmune hepatitis. Clin Gastroenterol Hepatol 2021;19(2):397–9.

25. Lohse AW, zum Büschenfelde KH, Franz B, et al. Characterization of the overlap syndrome of primary biliary cirrhosis (PBC) and autoimmune hepatitis: evidence for it being a hepatitic form of PBC in genetically susceptible individuals. Hepatology 1999;29(4):1078–84.

26. Boettler T, Csernalabics B, Salié H, et al. SARS-CoV-2 vaccination can elicit a CD8 T-cell dominant hepatitis. J Hepatol 2022. https://doi.org/10.1016/j.jhep.2022.03.040.

27. Lammert C, Zhu C, Lian Y, et al. Exploratory study of autoantibody profiling in drug-induced liver injury with an autoimmune phenotype. Hepatol Commun 2020;4(11):1651–63.

28. EASL Clinical Practice Guidelines: the diagnosis and management of patients with primary biliary cholangitis. J Hepatol 2017;67(1):145–72.

29. Hirschfield GM, Dyson JK, Alexander GJM, et al. The British Society of Gastroenterology/UK-PBC primary biliary cholangitis treatment and management guidelines. Gut 2018;67(9):1568–94.

30. Poupon RE, Poupon R, Balkau B. Ursodiol for the long-term treatment of primary biliary cirrhosis. The UDCA-PBC Study Group. N Engl J Med 1994;330(19):1342–7.

31. Lindor KD, Dickson ER, Baldus WP, et al. Ursodeoxycholic acid in the treatment of primary biliary cirrhosis. Gastroenterology 1994;106(5):1284–90.

32. Heathcote EJ, Cauch-Dudek K, Walker V, et al. The Canadian Multicenter Double-blind Randomized Controlled Trial of ursodeoxycholic acid in primary biliary cirrhosis. Hepatology 1994;19(5):1149–56.

33. Turner IB, Myszor M, Mitchison HC, et al. A two year controlled trial examining the effectiveness of ursodeoxycholic acid in primary biliary cirrhosis. J Gastroenterol Hepatol 1994;9(2):162–8.

34. Poupon RE, Lindor KD, Cauch-Dudek K, et al. Combined analysis of randomized controlled trials of ursodeoxycholic acid in primary biliary cirrhosis. Gastroenterology 1997;113(3):884–90.

35. Combes B, Carithers RL Jr, Maddrey WC, et al. A randomized, double-blind, placebo-controlled trial of ursodeoxycholic acid in primary biliary cirrhosis. Hepatology 1995;22(3):759–66.

36. Van Hoogstraten HJ, De Smet MB, Renooij W, et al. A randomized trial in primary biliary cirrhosis comparing ursodeoxycholic acid in daily doses of either 10 mg/kg or 20 mg/kg. Dutch Multicentre PBC Study Group. Aliment Pharmacol Ther 1998;12(10):965–71.

37. Goulis J, Leandro G, Burroughs AK. Randomised controlled trials of ursodeoxycholic-acid therapy for primary biliary cirrhosis: a meta-analysis. Lancet 1999;354(9184):1053–60.

38. Corpechot C, Carrat F, Bonnand AM, et al. The effect of ursodeoxycholic acid therapy on liver fibrosis progression in primary biliary cirrhosis. Hepatology 2000;32(6):1196–9.

39. Shi J, Wu C, Lin Y, et al. Long-term effects of mid-dose ursodeoxycholic acid in primary biliary cirrhosis: a meta-analysis of randomized controlled trials. Am J Gastroenterol 2006;101(7):1529–38.

40. Hirschfield GM, Mason A, Luketic V, et al. Efficacy of obeticholic acid in patients with primary biliary cirrhosis and inadequate response to ursodeoxycholic acid. Gastroenterology 2015;148(4):751–61.e8.

41. Nevens F, Andreone P, Mazzella G, et al. A placebo-controlled trial of obeticholic acid in primary biliary cholangitis. N Engl J Med 2016;375(7):631–43.

42. Yin Q, Li J, Xia Y, et al. Systematic review and meta-analysis: bezafibrate in patients with primary biliary cirrhosis. Drug Des Devel Ther 2015;9:5407–19.

43. Tanaka A, Hirohara J, Nakanuma Y, et al. Biochemical responses to bezafibrate improve long-term outcome in asymptomatic patients with primary biliary cirrhosis refractory to UDCA. J Gastroenterol 2015;50(6):675–82.

44. Kanda T, Yokosuka O, Imazeki F, et al. Bezafibrate treatment: a new medical approach for PBC patients? J Gastroenterol 2003;38(6):573–8.

45. Hosonuma K, Sato K, Yamazaki Y, et al. A prospective randomized controlled study of long-term combination therapy using ursodeoxycholic acid and bezafibrate in patients with primary biliary cirrhosis and dyslipidemia. Am J Gastroenterol 2015;110(3):423–31.

46. Lens S, Leoz M, Nazal L, et al. Bezafibrate normalizes alkaline phosphatase in primary biliary cirrhosis patients with incomplete response to ursodeoxycholic acid. Liver Int 2014;34(2):197–203.

47. Ohira H, Sato Y, Ueno T, et al. Fenofibrate treatment in patients with primary biliary cirrhosis. Am J Gastroenterol 2002;97(8):2147–9.

48. Levy C, Peter JA, Nelson DR, et al. Pilot study: fenofibrate for patients with primary biliary cirrhosis and an incomplete response to ursodeoxycholic acid. Aliment Pharmacol Ther 2011;33(2):235–42.

49. Grigorian AY, Mardini HE, Corpechot C, et al. Fenofibrate is effective adjunctive therapy in the treatment of primary biliary cirrhosis: a meta-analysis. Clin Res Hepatol Gastroenterol 2015;39(3):296–306.

50. Cheung AC, Lapointe-Shaw L, Kowgier M, et al. Combined ursodeoxycholic acid (UDCA) and fenofibrate in primary biliary cholangitis patients with incomplete UDCA response may improve outcomes. Aliment Pharmacol Ther 2016;43(2):283–93.

51. Yano K, Kato H, Morita S, et al. Is bezafibrate histologically effective for primary biliary cirrhosis? Am J Gastroenterol 2002;97(4):1075–7.

52. Kurihara T, Maeda A, Shigemoto M, et al. Investigation into the efficacy of bezafibrate against primary biliary cirrhosis, with histological references from cases receiving long term monotherapy. Am J Gastroenterol 2002;97(1):212–4.

53. Hegade VS, Khanna A, Walker LJ, et al. Long-term fenofibrate treatment in primary biliary cholangitis improves biochemistry but not the UK-PBC risk score. Dig Dis Sci 2016;61(10):3037–44.

54. Zhang Y, Li S, He L, et al. Combination therapy of fenofibrate and ursodeoxycholic acid in patients with primary biliary cirrhosis who respond incompletely to UDCA monotherapy: a meta-analysis. Drug Des Devel Ther 2015;9:2757–66.

55. Gleeson D, Heneghan MA. British Society of Gastroenterology (BSG) guidelines for management of autoimmune hepatitis. Gut 2011;60(12):1611–29.

56. EASL clinical practice guidelines: autoimmune hepatitis. J Hepatol 2015;63(4): 971–1004.

57. Murillo Perez CF, Harms MH, Lindor KD, et al. Goals of treatment for improved survival in primary biliary cholangitis: treatment target should Be bilirubin within the normal range and normalization of alkaline phosphatase. Am J Gastroenterol 2020;115(7):1066–74.

58. Pape S, Snijders R, Gevers TJG, et al. Systematic review of response criteria and endpoints in autoimmune hepatitis by the International Autoimmune Hepatitis Group. J Hepatol 2022;76(4):841–9.

59. Lammers WJ, van Buuren HR, Hirschfield GM, et al. Levels of alkaline phosphatase and bilirubin are surrogate end points of outcomes of patients with primary biliary cirrhosis: an international follow-up study. Gastroenterology 2014;147(6): 1338–49.e5 [quiz: e15].

60. Zhang H, Li S, Yang J, et al. A meta-analysis of ursodeoxycholic acid therapy versus combination therapy with corticosteroids for PBC-AIH-overlap syndrome: evidence from 97 monotherapy and 117 combinations. Prz Gastroenterol 2015; 10(3):148–55.

61. Chazouillères O, Wendum D, Serfaty L, et al. Long term outcome and response to therapy of primary biliary cirrhosis-autoimmune hepatitis overlap syndrome. J Hepatol 2006;44(2):400–6.

62. Wang Q, Selmi C, Zhou X, et al. Epigenetic considerations and the clinical reevaluation of the overlap syndrome between primary biliary cirrhosis and autoimmune hepatitis. J Autoimmun 2013;41:140–5.

63. Ozaslan E, Efe C, Heurgué-Berlot A, et al. Factors associated with response to therapy and outcome of patients with primary biliary cirrhosis with features of autoimmune hepatitis. Clin Gastroenterol Hepatol 2014;12(5):863–9.

64. Freedman BL, Danford CJ, Patwardhan V, et al. Treatment of overlap syndromes in autoimmune liver disease: a systematic review and meta-analysis. J Clin Med 2020;9(5). https://doi.org/10.3390/jcm9051449.

65. Carbone M, Nardi A, Flack S, et al. Pretreatment prediction of response to ursodeoxycholic acid in primary biliary cholangitis: development and validation of the UDCA Response Score. Lancet Gastroenterol Hepatol 2018;3(9):626–34.

66. Park Y, Cho Y, Cho EJ, et al. Retrospective analysis of autoimmune hepatitis-primary biliary cirrhosis overlap syndrome in Korea: characteristics, treatments, and outcomes. Clin Mol Hepatol 2015;21(2):150–7.

67. Martínez Casas OY, Díaz Ramírez GS, Marín Zuluaga JI, et al. Autoimmune hepatitis - primary biliary cholangitis overlap syndrome. Long-term outcomes of a retrospective cohort in a university hospital. Gastroenterol Hepatol 2018;41(9): 544–52. Síndrome de superposición: hepatitis autoinmune y colangitis biliar primaria. Resultados a largo plazo de una cohorte retrospectiva en un hospital universitario.

68. Silveira MG, Talwalkar JA, Angulo P, et al. Overlap of autoimmune hepatitis and primary biliary cirrhosis: long-term outcomes. Am J Gastroenterol 2007;102(6): 1244–50.

69. Efe C, Ozaslan E, Heurgué-Berlot A, et al. Sequential presentation of primary biliary cirrhosis and autoimmune hepatitis. Eur J Gastroenterol Hepatol 2014; 26(5):532–7.

70. Puustinen L, Boyd S, Arkkila P, et al. Histologic surveillance after liver transplantation due to autoimmune hepatitis. Clin Transplant 2017;31(5). https://doi.org/10.1111/ctr.12936.

71. Montano-Loza AJ, Ronca V, Ebadi M, et al. Risk factors and outcomes associated with recurrent autoimmune hepatitis following liver transplantation. J Hepatol 2022. https://doi.org/10.1016/j.jhep.2022.01.022.

72. Trivedi PJ, Crothers H, Mytton J, et al. Effects of primary sclerosing cholangitis on risks of cancer and death in people with inflammatory bowel disease, based on sex, race, and age. Gastroenterology 2020;159(3):915–28.

73. Weismüller TJ, Trivedi PJ, Bergquist A, et al. Patient Age, sex, and inflammatory bowel disease phenotype Associate with course of primary sclerosing cholangitis. Gastroenterology 2017;152(8):1975–84.e8.

74. Harms MH, van Buuren HR, Corpechot C, et al. Ursodeoxycholic acid therapy and liver transplant-free survival in patients with primary biliary cholangitis. J Hepatol 2019;71(2):357–65.

75. Murillo Perez CF, Goet JC, Lammers WJ, et al. Milder disease stage in patients with primary biliary cholangitis over a 44-year period: a changing natural history. Hepatology 2018;67(5):1920–30.

76. Gordon V, Adhikary R, Appleby V, et al. Treatment and outcome of autoimmune hepatitis (AIH): audit of 28 UK centres. Liver Int 2022. https://doi.org/10.1111/liv.15241.

77. Gordon VM, Adhikary R, Aithal GP, et al. Provision and standards of care for treatment and follow-up of patients with Autoimmune Hepatitis (AIH). Frontline Gastroenterol 2022;13(2):126–32.

78. Jensen MD, Jepsen P, Vilstrup H, et al. Increased cancer risk in autoimmune hepatitis: a Danish nationwide cohort study. Am J Gastroenterol 2022;117(1):129–37.

79. Grønbaek L, Otete H, Ban L, et al. Incidence, prevalence and mortality of autoimmune hepatitis in England 1997-2015. A population-based cohort study. Liver Int 2020;40(7):1634–44.

80. Trivedi PJ, Lammers WJ, van Buuren HR, et al. Stratification of hepatocellular carcinoma risk in primary biliary cirrhosis: a multicentre international study. Gut 2016;65(2):321–9.

81. Deneau MR, El-Matary W, Valentino PL, et al. The natural history of primary sclerosing cholangitis in 781 children: a multicenter, international collaboration. Hepatology 2017;66(2):518–27.

82. Laschtowitz A, Zachou K, Lygoura V, et al. Histological activity despite normal ALT and IgG serum levels in patients with autoimmune hepatitis and cirrhosis. JHEP Rep 2021;3(4):100321.

83. Günsar F, Akarca US, Ersöz G, et al. Clinical and biochemical features and therapy responses in primary biliary cirrhosis and primary biliary cirrhosis-autoimmune hepatitis overlap syndrome. Hepatogastroenterology 2002;49(47):1195–200.

84. Saito H, Rai T, Takahashi A, et al. Clinicolaboratory characteristics of Japanese patients with primary biliary cirrhosis-autoimmune hepatitis overlap. Fukushima J Med Sci 2006;52(2):71–7.

85. Wu CH, Wang QH, Tian GS, et al. Clinical features of the overlap syndrome of autoimmune hepatitis and primary biliary cirrhosis: retrospective study. Chin Med J (Engl) 2006;119(3):238–41.

86. Heurgué A, Vitry F, Diebold MD, et al. Overlap syndrome of primary biliary cirrhosis and autoimmune hepatitis: a retrospective study of 115 cases of autoimmune liver disease. Gastroenterol Clin Biol 2007;31(1):17–25.

87. Yokokawa J, Saito H, Kanno Y, et al. Overlap of primary biliary cirrhosis and autoimmune hepatitis: characteristics, therapy, and long term outcomes. J Gastroenterol Hepatol 2010;25(2):376–82.

88. Tanaka A, Harada K, Ebinuma H, et al. Primary biliary cirrhosis - autoimmune hepatitis overlap syndrome: a rationale for corticosteroids use based on a nation-wide retrospective study in Japan. Hepatol Res 2011;41(9):877–86.

89. Liu F, Pan ZG, Ye J, et al. Primary biliary cirrhosis-autoimmune hepatitis overlap syndrome: simplified criteria may be effective in the diagnosis in Chinese patients. J Dig Dis 2014;15(12):660–8.

90. Yoshioka Y, Taniai M, Hashimoto E, et al. Clinical profile of primary biliary cirrhosis with features of autoimmune hepatitis: importance of corticosteroid therapy. Hepatol Res 2014;44(9):947–55.

91. Yang F, Wang Q, Wang Z, et al. The natural history and prognosis of primary biliary cirrhosis with clinical features of autoimmune hepatitis. Clin Rev Allergy Immunol 2016;50(1):114–23.

92. Fan X, Zhu Y, Men R, et al. Efficacy and safety of immunosuppressive therapy for PBC-AIH overlap syndrome accompanied by decompensated cirrhosis: a real-world study. Can J Gastroenterol Hepatol 2018;2018:1965492.

93. Neuhauser M, Bjornsson E, Treeprasertsuk S, et al. Autoimmune hepatitis-PBC overlap syndrome: a simplified scoring system may assist in the diagnosis. Am J Gastroenterol 2010;105(2):345–53.

Noninvasive Evaluation of Fibrosis and Portal Hypertension in Primary Biliary Cholangitis

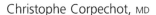

Christophe Corpechot, MD

KEYWORDS

• PBC • Elastography • VCTE • Serum fibrosis markers • Baveno criteria • Prognosis

KEY POINTS

- The extent of liver fibrosis and the degree of portal hypertension (PH) have a major prognostic role in PBC.
- In patients with PBC, the non-invasive evaluation of fibrosis and PH should be based on liver stiffness measurement (LSM) and platelet count.
- LSM, platelet count, and biochemical response to therapy are the 3 keys to PBC assessment in 2022.
- PBC patients with compensated advanced disease, clinically significant PH, or inadequate biochemcial response to therapy require optimized monitoring and treatment.

INTRODUCTION

Primary biliary cholangitis (PBC) is a chronic cholestatic autoimmune liver disease that, similar to most other chronic liver diseases, naturally progresses to cirrhosis and its complications, namely portal hypertension (PH), chronic liver failure, and hepatocellular carcinoma.[1] Chronic cholestasis is the main driver of disease progression, which is why, to date, only anticholestatic drugs, including ursodeoxycholic acid (UDCA), obeticholic acid, and fibrates, have shown signs of efficacy.[2–4]

Long-term oral administration of UDCA is currently the standard-of-care therapy for PBC.[5–7] UDCA has been shown to delay histologic progression and the development of PH and to prolong liver transplantation (LT)-free survival regardless of disease stage and biochemical response.[8–10] However, even treated with UDCA, PBC remains a progressive

Reference Center for Inflammatory Biliary Diseases and Autoimmune Hepatitis, French network for rare liver diseases FILFOIE, European Reference Network ERN RARE-LIVER, Saint-Antoine Hospital, Assistance Publique – Hôpitaux de Paris, Inserm UMR_S938, Saint-Antoine Research Center (CRSA), Sorbonne University, 184 rue du Faubourg Saint-Antoine, Paris 75571 Cedex 12, France
E-mail address: christophe.corpechot@aphp.fr

Clin Liver Dis 26 (2022) 681–689
https://doi.org/10.1016/j.cld.2022.06.010
1089-3261/22/© 2022 Elsevier Inc. All rights reserved.

liver.theclinics.com

disease associated with an increased risk of liver complication and related death, in particular in patients with a poor response to UDCA and/or advanced disease.[11,12]

The average incidence rate of major complications (ascites, variceal bleeding, hepatic encephalopathy) in PBC patients treated with UDCA is approximately 1% per year but this rate is 4 times higher in those with both inadequate biochemical response and indirect evidence for advanced liver fibrosis.[13] This shows that, in patients with PBC, disease prognosis depends on two key factors: biochemical response to UDCA and initial disease stage.

During the past 30 years, the concept of disease stage in PBC has gradually shifted from purely histologic to biochemical and/or biophysical (liver elastography) definitions.[5,14] The purpose of this article is to review the noninvasive tools that can be used in routine practice to accurately and robustly screen for advanced (ie, clinically significant) stages of PBC.

FROM HISTOLOGIC STAGE TO NONINVASIVE DIAGNOSIS OF COMPENSATED ADVANCED PRIMARY BILIARY CHOLANGITIS

As histologic examination of the liver is no longer mandatory for the diagnosis of PBC and surrogate markers for staging have been developed in parallel, the residual place of liver biopsy in the management of the disease is now limited. However, it is clear that, similar to other chronic liver diseases, the diagnosis of cirrhosis or advanced (ie, bridging) liver fibrosis in patients with PBC is associated with decreased long-term survival.[11,15] In addition, evidence of PH, which can precede cirrhosis in PBC, is known to be a major poor prognostic factor in this disease.[16,17] Therefore, any noninvasive evaluation of PBC should aim at screening for patients with clinically significant advanced disease and/or PH.

In the general trend associated with the development of noninvasive liver-assessment methods, and specifically liver stiffness measurement (LSM) by vibration-controlled transient elastography (VCTE), the Baveno VI consensus conference introduced in 2015 the concept of compensated advanced chronic liver disease (cACLD) to better reflect the continuous spectrum in terms of risk stratification between severe fibrosis and cirrhosis, the distinction of which is often not possible on clinical or even histologic grounds.[18] The initial aim of this concept was to avoid screening endoscopy in patients with low risk of clinically significant PH (CSPH) as diagnosed with VCTE and platelet count results. The Baveno VII consensus conference in 2021 extended this noninvasive approach based on elastography (irrespective of the technique used) and platelet count to the screening and early treatment with nonselective beta-blockers of patients with CSPH.[19] A rule of 5 for LSM by VCTE (10–15–20–25 kPa) was further proposed to denote progressively higher relative risks of decompensation and liver-related death independently of the cause of chronic liver disease (**Fig. 1**).

In this context, PBC should not be distinguished from other fibrosing chronic liver diseases. Most correlations made in PBC between LSM by VCTE and histologic fibrosis stage show that any value of LSM equal or greater to 10-11 kPa rules in severe fibrosis or advanced histologic stages.[20,21] In addition, an LSM threshold of approximately 10 kPa (exactly 9.6 kPa) has been shown to optimally discriminate PBC patients between low-risk and high-risk groups for liver-related complications or death, thus defining what is clinically significant advanced PBC according to VCTE.[20] The 2021 update of EASL (The European Association for the Study of the Liver) clinical practice guidelines on noninvasive test for the evaluation of liver disease severity and prognosis recently confirmed the relevance of using LSM by VCTE to diagnose or exclude

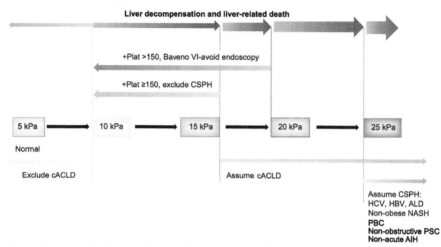

Fig. 1. Algorithm for the noninvasive determination of cACLD and CSPH. AIH, autoimmune hepatitis; ALD, alcohol-related liver disease; NASH, nonalcoholic steatohepatitis; PSC, primary sclerosing cholangitis. (*From* Roberto de Franchis, et al. Baveno VII - Renewing consensus in portal hypertension, Journal of Hepatology, 76 (4), 2022, 959-974, https://doi.org/10.1016/j.jhep.2021.12.022.)

advanced PBC with a threshold of 10 kPa (strong recommendation).[14] Furthermore, a large international cohort study including more than 3000 patients has recently validated the prognostic value of LSM by VCTE in PBC. In this study, the cutoffs of 8 and 15 kPa were found to distinguish PBC patients into low-risk, medium-risk, and high-risk groups regardless of biochemical response to UDCA, thus providing more accurate risk prediction for patients. Finally, the Baveno VI prediction criteria for CSPH have been validated in PBC and thus should be considered in PBC patients to avoid futile endoscopies.[23,24]

NONINVASIVE EVALUATION OF FIBROSIS IN PRIMARY BILIARY CHOLANGITIS
Serum Biomarkers

Several serum biomarkers and composite scores of fibrosis have been investigated in PBC, including in particular aspartate aminotransferase/platelet ratio index (APRI), FIB-4 (Fibrosis-4 index) score, Forns score, aspartate to alanine aminotransferases ratio (AAR), enhanced liver fibrosis (ELF) test, FibroTest, FibroMeter, hyaluronic acid, and procollagen III propeptide.[11,20,25–30] Among them, APRI, FIB-4, and AAR were by far the most extensively studied. The performance of these biomarkers for the diagnosis of severe fibrosis or cirrhosis varies from study to study, probably due to the small size of these studies and significant discrepancies in the populations studied and the histologic scoring systems used.[31] However, in most of these studies, including the largest and most recent, none of these blood markers have shown an adequate accuracy to differentiate mild from severe fibrosis or early from advanced histologic stage (AUROC (Area Under the Receiver Operating Characteristic curve) < 0.80). Consequently, their use for the evaluation of fibrosis in PBC is currently not recommended.[14]

However, it is noteworthy that, despite inadequate accuracy to properly quantify fibrosis in PBC, ELF and APRI indices were both associated with disease severity and able to provide meaningful long-term prognostic information.[26,32] These blood markers might therefore be useful as risk-stratification tools in clinical trials of second-line or third-line therapies for PBC.

Table 1
Performance of elastography-based techniques for the diagnosis of histologically proven severe fibrosis and cirrhosis in primary biliary cholangitis

Reference	Technique	Patients	Severe Fibrosis AUROC (Cutoff)	Cirrhosis AUROC (Cutoff)
Corpechot et al,[37] 2006	VCTE	73	0.95 (9.8 kPa)	0.96 (17.3 kPa)
Gomez et al,[38] 2008	VCTE	55	0.86 (14.7 kPa)	0.96 (15.6 kPa)
Friedrich et al,[27] 2010	VCTE	45	N/A (N/A)	0.95 (N/A)
Floreani et al,[25] 2011	VCTE	120	0.88 (7.6 kPa)	0.99 (11.4 kPa)
Corpechot et al,[20] 2012	VCTE	103	0.95 (10.7 kPa)	0.99 (16.9 kPa)
Koizumi et al,[44] 2017	VCTE	44	0.91 (N/A)	0.91 (N/A)
Wu et al,[47] 2018	VCTE	70	0.91 (10.5 kPa)	0.97 (14.5 kPa)
Joshita et al,[53] 2020	VCTE	69	0.76 (8.9 kPa)	0.91 (23.7 kPa)
Osman et al,[45] 2021	VCTE	63	0.73 (7.5 kPa)	0.94 (14.4 kPa)
Cristoferi et al,[21] 2021	VCTE	167	0.89 (11.0 kPa)	N/A (N/A)
Zachou et al,[29] 2021	VCTE	56	0.99 (11.9 kPa)	N/A (N/A)
Zhang et al,[39] 2014	ARFI	61	0.93 (1.79 m/s)	0.91 (2.01 m/s)
Goertz et al,[40] 2019	ARFI	26	N/A (N/A)	N/A (N/A)
Park et al,[41] 2019	SWE	41	0.91 (6.04 kPa)	N/A (N/A)
Manesis et al,[42] 2021	SWE	53	0.85 (10.0 kPa)	0.90 (11.9 kPa)
Schulz et al,[43] 2022	SWE	22	N/A (N/A)	N/A (N/A)
Koizumi et al,[44] 2017	RTE	44	0.95 (N/A)	0.97 (N/A)
Osman et al,[45] 2021	MRE	98	0.71 (3.7 kPa)	0.82 (4.6 kPa)

Abbreviations: ARFI, acoustic radiation force impulse elastography; AUROC, area under the ROC curve; MRE, magnetic resonance elastography; RTE, real-time tissue elastography; SWE, shear wave elastography; VCTE, vibration-controlled transient elastography.

Elastography Techniques

The use of LSM as a noninvasive marker of liver fibrosis in routine medical practice has developed considerably during the last 15 years.[33,34] Among the different techniques available, VCTE (Fibroscan) was the first to be marketed, has been the most extensively evaluated, in particular in PBC, and is today one of the most popular and commonly used, especially in hepatology units.[35,36] LSM by VCTE was previously shown to correlate with both liver fibrosis and histologic stage in PBC with high performance (AUROC ≥ 0.90) for the diagnosis of cirrhosis or advanced fibrosis (**Table 1**).[20,25,37,38] Although fibrosis thresholds differ between studies, it seems acceptable to consider from the compilation of these results that LSM values ≥7 to 8 kPa and ≥10 to 11 kPa are diagnostic of significant fibrosis and advanced fibrosis, respectively, whereas cirrhosis should be considered for values ≥ 14 to 17 kPa (**Fig. 2**). In a recent large Italian study of treatment-naïve patients with PBC, thresholds of 6.5 and 11 kPa enabled to exclude and confirm, respectively, advanced fibrosis with accuracy.[21] LSM by VCTE is therefore to date the best surrogate marker in PBC for ruling in severe fibrosis/cACLD and should be used for this purpose using a cutoff of 10 kPa in line with the Baveno VII conference consensus and last EASL clinical practice guidelines.[14,19]

Other techniques of liver elastography, including acoustic radiation force impulse (ARFI) elastography, shear wave elastography (SWE), real-time tissue elastography

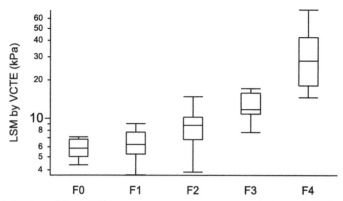

Fig. 2. Distribution of liver stiffness measurement across fibrosis stages in PBC. Box plot of liver stiffness measured by VCTE (logarithm scale) depending on biopsy METAVIR fibrosis stage. The bottom and top of the boxes are the first and third quartiles, and the band inside the boxes is the median. The ends of the whiskers are the minimum and maximum of the data. (*Adapted from* Corpechot C, Carrat F, Poujol-Robert A, Gaouar F, Wendum D, Chazouil-leres O, et al. Noninvasive elastography-based assessment of liver fibrosis progression and prognosis in primary biliary cirrhosis. Hepatology 2012;56:198-208, with permission.)

(RTE), and magnetic resonance elastography (MRE), have shown comparable performance with VCTE in assessing fibrosis in PBC, although current data are still limited to relatively small studies.[39–45] It should be noted that LSM units and thresholds can differ across elastography techniques and are therefore not always comparable.

There is little data on the time course of LSM in PBC. In 150 PBC patients treated with UDCA followed-up with VCTE for an average of 5 years in a French tertiary center, the overall progression rate of LSM was significant (0.48 ± 0.21 kPa/y; $P < .05$) but was mainly related to a faster progression in cirrhotic patients (4.06 ± 0.72 kPa/y; $P < .001$), whereas no significant change was observed in noncirrhotic patients in the same time frame.[20] In this study, a cutoff value of 2.1 kPa/y was associated with an 8.4-fold increased risk of liver decompensation, LT, or death, thus suggesting that LSM might be used as a relevant surrogate marker of clinical outcomes in PBC, an assumption recently confirmed in a large international longitudinal study.[22] Despite the lack of evidence regarding the optimal time frame between consecutive LSMs but considering that both advanced disease and response to UDCA are predictors of poor outcomes in PBC, it seems reasonable to repeat LSM every year in high-risk patients, that is, those with advanced disease (LSM $\geq$ 10 kPa) and/or inadequate biochemical response to UDCA, and every 2 to 3 years in those with nonadvanced disease (<10 kPa) and no resistance to UDCA.[14]

In liver disease, in particular autoimmune hepatitis (AIH), it has been shown that histologic inflammatory activity is able to increase LSM independently of fibrosis.[46] In pure PBC, where histologic activity grade is generally low, LSM by VCTE was not found to correlate with periportal necroinflammatory activity.[20] However, in a recent study, LSM by SWE was affected by portal inflammation grade.[42] Unfortunately, periportal and lobular inflammatory activity grade in this study was not assessed. Finally, in a relatively large series of patients with PBC-AIH overlap syndrome, LSM by VCTE closely correlated with histologic fibrosis stage, with diagnostic thresholds for severe fibrosis and cirrhosis of 10.5 and 14.5 kPa, respectively, thus suggesting that LSM remains a reliable measure of fibrosis even in this singular active form of the disease.[47]

Imaging Techniques

Ultrasound scan of the liver can help to detect signs of cACLD in PBC, including dysmorphic liver, nontumoral heterogeneous parenchyma, or features associated with compensated PH (enlarged spleen or portal vein, portosystemic shunts). However, these signs are usually present in very late stage of the disease when clinical and/or biological features associated with cirrhosis or PH are evident. Therefore, ultrasound imaging alone, that is, not coupled with elastography, is of very limited value in accurately assessing fibrosis in PBC. Contrast-enhanced ultrasound and diffusion-weighted MRI could provide more accurate diagnostic information, independently of the existence of typical morphologic signs of cirrhosis or PH.[48–52] The presence of periportal halo sign, in particular, could be indicative for significant fibrosis in PBC.

NONINVASIVE EVALUATION OF PORTAL HYPERTENSION IN PRIMARY BILIARY CHOLANGITIS

The factors associated with the presence of gastro-esophageal varices (GOV) in PBC have specifically been assessed in a large cross-sectional retrospective study.[17] These factors included platelets count, albumin, alkaline phosphatase, and the presence of splenomegaly. A continuous predictive score called the Newcastle Varices in PBC score has been developed and validated. This score was shown to have good performance (AUROC 0.86) and accuracy in discriminating between patients with or without GOV and was predicted to be cost-effective in reducing the number of screening endoscopies significantly. However, this score, which is calculated from a complex formula, is rarely used in clinical practice.

More recently, the Baveno VI guidelines, recommending that patients with chronic liver disease with LSM by VCTE less than 20 kPa and platelets count greater than 150,000 G/L do not need endoscopy to screen for GOV, have been validated in PBC in 2 independent studies with a false-negative rate of 0% and 5%, respectively, and an estimated rate of saved endoscopy of 39% and 74%, respectively, thus showing that these simple binary criteria based on VCTE and platelet cutoffs can be applied with confidence in patients with cACLD due to PBC.[23,24] In line with these results, LSM has been shown to correlate with spleen size and platelets counts in patients with PBC.[43] Currently, there is no data on the potential value of measuring spleen stiffness in PBCs.

SUMMARY

Liver fibrosis and PH are major prognostic factors of PBC. Their noninvasive evaluation is a crucial step in identifying patients with cACLD or CSPH, that is, PBC patients requiring optimized monitoring and treatment. For this purpose, LSM by VCTE or other techniques, used in conjunction with platelets count (Baveno criteria) and biochemical response to UDCA, has emerged as an essential measure for assessing the severity of PBC and anticipating the risk of poor long-term clinical outcomes. The combination of LSM with UDCA response should be considered as the key element of PBC evaluation in 2022.

CONFLICT OF INTEREST

None.

REFERENCES

1. Lleo A, Wang GQ, Gershwin ME, et al. Primary biliary cholangitis. Lancet 2020; 396:1915–26.
2. Poupon RE, Balkau B, Eschwege E, et al. A multicenter, controlled trial of ursodiol for the treatment of primary biliary cirrhosis. N Engl J Med 1991;324:1548–54.
3. Nevens F, Andreone P, Mazzella G, et al. A Placebo-controlled trial of obeticholic acid in primary biliary cholangitis. N Engl J Med 2016;375:631–43.
4. Corpechot C, Chazouilleres O, Rousseau A, et al. A Placebo-controlled trial of Bezafibrate in primary biliary cholangitis. N Engl J Med 2018;378:2171–81.
5. EASL Clinical Practice Guidelines. The diagnosis and management of patients with primary biliary cholangitis. J Hepatol 2017;67:145–72.
6. Lindor KD, Bowlus CL, Boyer J, et al. Primary biliary cholangitis: 2018 practice guidance from the American association for the study of liver diseases. Hepatology 2019;69:394–419.
7. Hirschfield GM, Dyson JK, Alexander GJM, et al. The British Society of Gastroenterology/UK-PBC primary biliary cholangitis treatment and management guidelines. Gut 2018;67:1568–94.
8. Poupon RE, Lindor KD, Pares A, et al. Combined analysis of the effect of treatment with ursodeoxycholic acid on histologic progression in primary biliary cirrhosis. J Hepatol 2003;39:12–6.
9. Lindor KD, Jorgensen RA, Therneau TM, et al. Ursodeoxycholic acid delays the onset of esophageal varices in primary biliary cirrhosis. Mayo Clin Proc 1997;72:1137–40.
10. Harms MH, van Buuren HR, Corpechot C, et al. Ursodeoxycholic acid therapy and liver transplant-free survival in patients with primary biliary cholangitis. J Hepatol 2019;71:357–65.
11. Murillo Perez CF, Hirschfield GM, Corpechot C, et al. Fibrosis stage is an independent predictor of outcome in primary biliary cholangitis despite biochemical treatment response. Aliment Pharmacol Ther 2019;50:1127–36.
12. Pares A, Caballeria L, Rodes J. Excellent long-term survival in patients with primary biliary cirrhosis and biochemical response to ursodeoxycholic Acid. Gastroenterology 2006;130:715–20.
13. Harms MH, Lammers WJ, Thorburn D, et al. Major hepatic complications in ursodeoxycholic acid-treated patients with primary biliary cholangitis: risk factors and time trends in incidence and outcome. Am J Gastroenterol 2018;113:254–64.
14. EASL Clinical Practice Guidelines on non-invasive tests for evaluation of liver disease severity and prognosis - 2021 update. J Hepatol 2021;75:659–89.
15. Poupon RE, Bonnand AM, Chretien Y, et al. Ten-year survival in ursodeoxycholic acid-treated patients with primary biliary cirrhosis. Hepatology 1999;29:1668–71.
16. Huet PM, Vincent C, Deslaurier J, et al. Portal hypertension and primary biliary cirrhosis: effect of long-term ursodeoxycholic acid treatment. Gastroenterology 2008;135:1552–60.
17. Patanwala I, McMeekin P, Walters R, et al. A validated clinical tool for the prediction of varices in PBC: the Newcastle Varices in PBC Score. J Hepatol 2013;59:327–35.
18. de Franchis R, Baveno VIF. Expanding consensus in portal hypertension: Report of the Baveno VI Consensus Workshop: Stratifying risk and individualizing care for portal hypertension. J Hepatol 2015;63:743–52.
19. de Franchis R, Bosch J, Garcia-Tsao G, et al. Baveno VII - Renewing consensus in portal hypertension. J Hepatol 2022;76:959–74.

20. Corpechot C, Carrat F, Poujol-Robert A, et al. Noninvasive elastography-based assessment of liver fibrosis progression and prognosis in primary biliary cirrhosis. Hepatology 2012;56:198–208.
21. Cristoferi L, Calvaruso V, Overi D, et al. Accuracy of Transient Elastography in assessing fibrosis at diagnosis in naive patients with Primary Biliary Cholangitis: a dual cut-off approach. Hepatology 2021;74:1496–508.
22. Corpechot C, Carrat F, Gaouar F, et al. Liver stiffness measurement by vibration-controlled transient elastography improves outcome prediction in primary biliary cholangitis. J Hepatol 2022;Jun 28;S0168-8278.
23. Moctezuma-Velazquez C, Saffioti F, Tasayco-Huaman S, et al. Non-invasive prediction of high-risk varices in patients with primary biliary cholangitis and primary sclerosing cholangitis. Am J Gastroenterol 2019;114:446–52.
24. Pariente A, Chazouilleres O, Causse X, et al. Baveno-VI-guided prediction of Eso-gastric varices in primary biliary cholangitis. Am J Gastroenterol 2019;114:361–2.
25. Floreani A, Cazzagon N, Martines D, et al. Performance and utility of transient elastography and noninvasive markers of liver fibrosis in primary biliary cirrhosis. Dig Liver Dis 2011;43:887–92.
26. Mayo MJ, Parkes J, Adams-Huet B, et al. Prediction of clinical outcomes in primary biliary cirrhosis by serum enhanced liver fibrosis assay. Hepatology 2008; 48:1549–57.
27. Friedrich-Rust M, Muller C, Winckler A, et al. Assessment of liver fibrosis and steatosis in PBC with FibroScan, MRI, MR-spectroscopy, and serum markers. J Clin Gastroenterol 2010;44:58–65.
28. Corpechot C, Rousseau A, Lefèvre G, et al. Bezafibrate Add-on therapy in high-risk primary biliary cholangitis is associated with an Improvement of FibroMeter and FibroMeter-VCTE, two high-accuracy non-invasive fibrosis tests extensively validated in Frequent chronic liver diseases. J Hepatol 2019;70:e387.
29. Zachou K, Lygoura V, Arvaniti P, et al. FibroMeter scores for the assessment of liver fibrosis in patients with autoimmune liver diseases. Ann Hepatol 2021;22: 100285.
30. Nyberg A, Lindqvist U, Engstrom-Laurent A. Serum hyaluronan and aminoterminal propeptide of type III procollagen in primary biliary cirrhosis: relation to clinical symptoms, liver histopathology and outcome. J Intern Med 1992;231:485–91.
31. Corpechot C. Utility of noninvasive markers of fibrosis in cholestatic liver diseases. Clin Liver Dis 2016;20:143–58.
32. Trivedi PJ, Bruns T, Cheung A, et al. Optimising risk stratification in primary biliary cirrhosis: AST/platelet ratio index predicts outcome independent of ursodeoxycholic acid response. J Hepatol 2014;60:1249–58.
33. Friedrich-Rust M, Poynard T, Castera L. Critical comparison of elastography methods to assess chronic liver disease. Nat Rev Gastroenterol Hepatol 2016; 13:402–11.
34. Mueller S. Liver elastography. In: Mueller S, editor. Clin Use InterpretationXIX. Cham: Springer; 2020. p. 737.
35. Sandrin L, Fourquet B, Hasquenoph JM, et al. Transient elastography: a new noninvasive method for assessment of hepatic fibrosis. Ultrasound Med Biol 2003;29:1705–13.
36. Friedrich-Rust M, Ong MF, Martens S, et al. Performance of transient elastography for the staging of liver fibrosis: a meta-analysis. Gastroenterology 2008; 134:960–74.

37. Corpechot C, El Naggar A, Poujol-Robert A, et al. Assessment of biliary fibrosis by transient elastography in patients with PBC and PSC. Hepatology 2006;43: 1118–24.
38. Gomez-Dominguez E, Mendoza J, Garcia-Buey L, et al. Transient elastography to assess hepatic fibrosis in primary biliary cirrhosis. Aliment Pharmacol Ther 2008; 27:441–7.
39. Zhang DK, Chen M, Liu Y, et al. Acoustic radiation force impulse elastography for non-invasive assessment of disease stage in patients with primary biliary cirrhosis: a preliminary study. Clin Radiol 2014;69:836–40.
40. Goertz RS, GaBmann L, Strobel D, et al. Acoustic radiation force impulse (ARFI) elastography in autoimmune and cholestatic liver diseases. Ann Hepatol 2019; 18:23–9.
41. Park DW, Lee YJ, Chang W, et al. Diagnostic performance of a point shear wave elastography (pSWE) for hepatic fibrosis in patients with autoimmune liver disease. PLoS One 2019;14:e0212771.
42. Manesis EK, Schina M, Vafiadis I, et al. Liver stiffness measurements by 2-dimensional shear wave elastography compared to histological and ultrasound parameters in primary biliary cholangitis. Scand J Gastroenterol 2021;56:1187–93.
43. Schulz M, Wilde AB, Demir M, et al. Shear wave elastography and shear wave dispersion imaging in primary biliary cholangitis-a pilot study. Quant Imaging Med Surg 2022;12:1235–42.
44. Koizumi Y, Hirooka M, Abe M, et al. Comparison between real-time tissue elastography and vibration-controlled transient elastography for the assessment of liver fibrosis and disease progression in patients with primary biliary cholangitis. Hepatol Res 2017;47:1252–9.
45. Osman KT, Maselli DB, Idilman IS, et al. Liver stiffness measured by Either magnetic resonance or transient elastography is associated with liver fibrosis and is an independent predictor of outcomes Among patients with primary biliary cholangitis. J Clin Gastroenterol 2021;55:449–57.
46. Hartl J, Denzer U, Ehlken H, et al. Transient elastography in autoimmune hepatitis: Timing determines the impact of inflammation and fibrosis. J Hepatol 2016;65: 769–75.
47. Wu HM, Sheng L, Wang Q, et al. Performance of transient elastography in assessing liver fibrosis in patients with autoimmune hepatitis-primary biliary cholangitis overlap syndrome. World J Gastroenterol 2018;24:737–43.
48. Yoshimine N, Wakui N, Nagai H, et al. Arrival-time Parametric imaging in Contrast-enhanced ultrasound for diagnosing fibrosis in primary biliary cholangitis. Ultrasound Q 2022;38:191–9.
49. Kovac JD, Jesic R, Stanisavljevic D, et al. Integrative role of MRI in the evaluation of primary biliary cirrhosis. Eur Radiol 2012;22:688–94.
50. Meng Y, Liang Y, Liu M. The value of MRI in the diagnosis of primary biliary cirrhosis and assessment of liver fibrosis. PLoS One 2015;10:e0120110.
51. Takeyama Y, Tsuchiya N, Kunimoto H, et al. Gadolinium-ethoxybenzyl-diethylene-triamine pentaacetic acid-enhanced magnetic resonance imaging as a useful detection method for advanced primary biliary cirrhosis. Hepatol Res 2015;45: E108–14.
52. Idilman IS, Venkatesh SH, Eaton JE, et al. Magnetic resonance imaging features in 283 patients with primary biliary cholangitis. Eur Radiol 2020;30:5139–48.
53. Joshita S, Yamashita Y, Sugiura A, et al. Clinical utility of FibroScan as a non-invasive diagnostic test for primary biliary cholangitis. J Gastroenterol Hepatol 2020;35:1208–14.

Hepatocellular Carcinoma in Primary Biliary Cholangitis

Alexander M. Sy, MD[a,b,*], Raphaella D. Ferreira, MD[a], Binu V. John, MD, MPH[a]

KEYWORDS

- Cirrhosis • Autoimmune liver disease • Epidemiology • Primary liver cancer

KEY POINTS

- Primary biliary cholangitis (PBC) with cirrhosis has the strongest association with hepatocellular carcinoma (HCC) development. Thus, surveillance for HCC is currently recommended in all patients with PBC and cirrhosis.
- PBC without cirrhosis confers a risk of developing HCC, although at a lower rate compared with other chronic liver diseases.
- Multiple factors have been implicated in the development of HCC in PBC: age, male sex, comorbid conditions such as diabetes, previous viral infections, and alcohol consumption. Currently, the American Association for the Study of Liver Diseases recommends screening for HCC in all patients with PBC and cirrhosis and in male patients with PBC even in the absence of cirrhosis. Further risk stratification is needed to update recommendations for surveillance in PBC patients with coexisting factors.
- There are conflicting studies regarding the biochemical response to ursodeoxycholic acid (UDCA) in reducing the risk of HCC in PBC patients.
- HCC in PBC has a poor prognosis: the 5-year survival rate in this population is 50% compared with 75% in other chronic liver diseases with HCC, and liver transplantation offers the best survival rate among available therapies.

INTRODUCTION

Primary biliary cholangitis (PBC), formerly known as primary biliary cirrhosis, is an autoimmune, T-cell-mediated condition affecting the biliary epithelial cells. It presents in a spectrum of disease severity ranging from asymptomatic, cholestasis to cirrhosis, portal hypertension, and ultimately resulting in end-stage liver disease requiring liver transplantation.

[a] Division of Hepatology, Miami VA Medical System, Department of Medicine, University of Miami Miller School of Medicine, 1201 Northwest 16th Street, Miami, FL 33125, USA; [b] Department of Translational Medicine, Florida International University, Herbert Wertheim College of Medicine, Miami, FL, USA
* Corresponding author:
E-mail address: alexander.sy3@va.gov

Clin Liver Dis 26 (2022) 691–704
https://doi.org/10.1016/j.cld.2022.06.011
1089-3261/22/© 2022 Elsevier Inc. All rights reserved.

liver.theclinics.com

Hepatocellular carcinoma (HCC) is one of the complications of PBC, particularly among patients with advanced fibrosis. Histopathological findings of granulomatous destruction and subsequent breakdown of cholangiocytes causing accumulation of inflammatory infiltrate results in cholestasis and fibrosis. Advanced fibrosis is the most important risk factor for the development of HCC, but there are other reports showing the development of HCC in PBC without an evidence of advanced disease. Without treatment, the overall survival is poor, with a median survival of 36 months following the diagnosis of HCC in PBC.[1] Animal studies have also provided hypothesized mechanism involving the nuclear Farnesoid X receptor (FXR) in the development of HCC in cholestatic liver disease as it acts regulating bile acid (BA) homeostasis and tumor suppressor genes.[2]

Hepatocellular Carcinoma

In 2020, primary liver cancer was the sixth most common cancer diagnosis worldwide and the third most common cause of death, with males having two to three times higher mortality rates.[3] Primary liver cancer includes HCC, intrahepatic cholangiocarcinoma, and other rare types of liver cancers; among these, HCC comprises 75% to 85% of all cases and is considered the most common primary liver malignancy globally.[3] The previous studies have shown that the incidence of HCC has doubled over the past 2 decades, becoming the fastest-rising cause of cancer-related deaths.

In the United States alone, HCC was the third most common diagnosis for liver transplantation from 2017 to 2019.[4,5] A 2016 study using the Surveillance Epidemiology End Result (SEER) registry demonstrated a decreasing or plateauing incidence of HCC in American Asian/Pacific Islanders and patients younger than 65 years, whereas the incidence of HCC in African Americans, Hispanics, and patients older than 65 years was predicted to rise steadily to 2030.[6]

Hepatocellular Carcinoma and Primary Biliary Cholangitis

Homeostasis of the gut-liver axis relies on tight control of BA levels to avoid BA overload associated with the development of cholestasis and consequently injury to liver cells, induction of chronic inflammation, cell proliferation, and liver tumors.[7] FXR is a ligand-activated transcription factor highly expressed in the liver and intestines. It is a major regulator of genes involved in BA synthesis, conjugation, transportation, and enterohepatic circulation.[8,9] In addition, regulating BA levels, lipid, and glucose metabolism, FXR also contributes to the regulation of liver regeneration, hepatic inflammation, tumor suppressor genes, and hepatic fibrosis.[9] FXR−/− mice models exhibit increased BA pool size and display cell hyperproliferation leading to spontaneous HCC at 12 months.[2,7] **Fig. 1** presents the effects of FXR suppression on HCC development. FXR inhibits BA synthesis by activating the V-maf avian musculoaponeurotic fibrosarcoma oncogene homolog G (MAFG). At least one animal study found that MAFG was induced in chronic cholestasis contributing to cholestatic liver injury and HCC.[10]

Growing evidence suggests that autoimmune liver diseases confer an increased risk of HCC, but at lower frequencies than is the case with other liver diseases. A study by McGee and colleagues using the SEER registry data found a wide range of increased risk for hepatobiliary cancer following a diagnosis of several autoimmune diseases,[11] among which PBC had the strongest association with HCC development (Odds Ratio (OR): 31.33 [95% Confidence Interval (CI): 23.63–41.56]) as compared with primary sclerosing cholangitis (OR: 4.42 [95% CI: 2.06, 9.45]).[11] Unfortunately, this study did not differentiate autoimmune hepatitis (AIH) from other hepatobiliary-related autoimmune conditions.

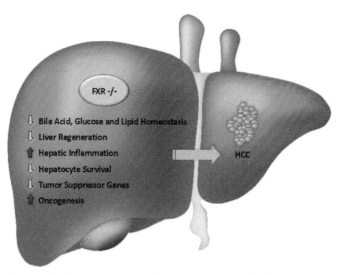

Fig. 1. The effects of FXR suppression on the development of HCC.

Table 1 lists the studies of the incidence of HCC in PBC without regard to fibrosis status. The range of incidences reported between the studies is noted, possibly due to varying methodologies.[1,12–16]

Table 2 lists the studies of the incidence of HCC in PBC, specifically in cases of advanced fibrosis in which there is a wide range of incidences ranging from 1.9% to 14%.[12,17–23] Natarajan and colleagues performed a systematic review using several databases where they found an incidence of 13.05 per 1000 person-years in PBC with cirrhosis (95% CI 7.17–23.75), although the HCC risk in PBC without cirrhosis was 2.68 per 1000 person-years (95% CI 1.78–4.05).[12] This compares to the HCC risk in AIH with cirrhosis which stands at 10.07 per 1000 person-years and without cirrhosis at only 3.06 per 1000 person-years.[24]

Risk Factors for the Development of Hepatocellular Carcinoma in Primary Biliary Cholangitis (Fig.2)

There is no cure for PBC. However, early treatment with ursodeoxycholic acid (UDCA) at a dose of 13 to 15 mg/kg/d with biochemical response has been shown to delay the progression to cirrhosis (13% in UDCA-treated vs 49% in placebo-treated patients, $P < .009$),[25] and reduction in hepatic decompensation and transplantation even in cases of cirrhosis.[26] Without treatment, the early stages of PBC can develop into biliary cirrhosis in 10 to 20 years.[27]

Reports of the biochemical response to UDCA affecting the development of HCC have been conflicting. Some studies found that biochemical nonresponse to UDCA is a risk for HCC development.[13,17] In another study of cirrhotic PBC patients, response to UDCA was not associated with HCC development after adjusting for potential confounders (sHR 0.39, 95% CI 0.06–2.55, $P = .33$).[26] This finding was also seen in a meta-analysis by Natarajan, where treatment with UDCA did not reduce the risk of HCC in PBC patients with or without cirrhosis.[12]

Cirrhosis is the final pathologic consequence of liver damage that can result from a number of chronic liver diseases, including PBC. Multiple studies found that progression to advanced stages of PBC is associated with an increased incidence of HCC.

Table 1
Incidence of hepatocellular carcinoma in primary biliary cholangitis

Study	Patients with HCC/ Total PBC	Cumulative Incidence	Follow-Up	Study Period	Study Design
Cavazza et al,[1] 2009	24/716	0.35 cases per 100 patient-years	Mean 9.3 y		Prospective
Harada et al,[16] 2013	71/2946	2.4%	Mean 6.7 y Median 4.8 y	1980–2009	Retrospective
Tomiyama et al,[14] 2013	11/210	5.2%	Median 8.5 y	May 1984–May 2010	Retrospective
Rong et al,[15] 2015	70/1865	2.6% (5 y) and 8.9% (10 y)	Median 5.5 y	Jan 1994–June 2014	Retrospective
Trivedi et al,[13] 2016	123/4565	3.4 per 1000 patient-years	Mean 8 y	1959–2012	Retrospective
Natarajan et al,[12] 2021	559/22,615	4.17 per 1000 person-years	Mean 6.3 y	Inception to November 30, 2019	Meta-analysis

Table 2
Incidence of hepatocellular carcinoma in primary biliary cholangitis with advanced fibrosis

Study	Patients with HCC/ Total PBC	Cumulative Incidence	Follow-Up	Study Period	Study Design
Jones et al,[23] 1997	16/667	5.9%	Mean 7.3 y	October 1975–October 1995	Retrospective
Caballería et al,[19] 2001	5/140	11.1%	Mean 5.6 y	January 1977–October 1996	Retrospective
Shibuya et al,[20] 2002	14/396	12.3% (10 y)	Median 3.6 y	1980–1998	Prospective
Findor et al,[22] 2002	4/292	3.4%	Mean 2.2 y	1978–1998	Prospective
Deutsch et al,[18] 2008	8/212	3% (1 y) 5% (5 y) and 14% (10 y)	Median 6 y	1987–2005	Prospective
Kuiper et al,[17] 2010	9/375	1.9%	Median 9.7 y	1990–2007	Prospective
Zhang et al,[21] 2015	52/1255	4.13%	Mean 3.6 y	Jan 2002–December 2013	Retrospective
Natarajan et al,[12] 2021	559/22,615	13.05 per 1000 person-years	Mean 6.3 y	Inception to November 30, 2019	Meta-analysis

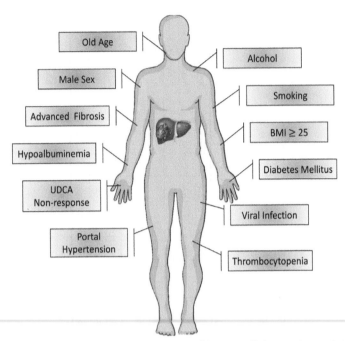

Fig. 2. Factors associated with the development of hepatocellular carcinoma in PBC.

However, only a minority of patients can progress to cirrhosis. For that reason, primary biliary cirrhosis was changed to PBC.[28] The true incidence of PBC with cirrhosis is difficult to determine due to wide variability and uneven distribution worldwide. It is well described in Western populations but scant information from Africa and parts of Asia.[29]

Table 2 shows the cumulative incidences of PBC with advanced fibrosis as reported in several studies. The difference in the incidences between these studies may be secondary to a relatively extended period of follow-up and dropout rates. Four studies show an increased risk of HCC development in PBC patients with advanced fibrosis.[13,14,18,19] A recent meta-analysis found that PBC with cirrhosis at baseline was the most substantial risk factor for HCC development.[12] In comparison to other liver diseases, PBC without cirrhosis has a lower incidence of HCC at 0.35 to 6.02 per 1000 person-years compared with chronic hepatitis B with 1 to 10 per 1000 person-years and 1 to 8 per 1000 person-years in chronic hepatitis C.[12] In the study by Caballeria, the high incidence of HCC in PBC with cirrhosis was comparable to the incidence of HCV with cirrhosis.[19]

PBC is a predominantly female disease. Studies show that females with PBC cirrhosis have a lower frequency of HCC than males. The possible protective effect of estrogen against hepatocellular cancer through inhibiting cytokine and interleukin-6 has been proposed.[30]

Five studies have found that being male with PBC confers an increased risk of HCC (see **Table 3**).[13,15,16,20,31] A study by Trivedi and colleagues involving 4565 patients with PBC from 15 centers in North America and Europe demonstrated that male sex was a risk factor for HCC development in PBC (adjusted HR 2.41 [95% CI 1.5–3.86] *P* < .0001) and men with advanced disease at baseline were found to have an increased HCC incidence.[13] In addition, a history of hepatitis B virus (HBV) infection, hepatitis C virus (HCV) infection, smoking, and alcohol consumption is significantly

Table 3
Risk factors of hepatocellular carcinoma in primary biliary cholangitis

Factors	Study	HCC/ Total Patients	Median Follow Up	Statistics
Demographics				
Age	Shibuya A (25) (>70 years and above)	14/396	43 months	HR: 1.0769 (95% CI 1.0190-1.1380)
	Suzuki A (26) (>70 years and above)	17 cases/ 56 control	-	OR: 1.6 (95% CI 1.2 -2.2) p value: .003
	Deutsch M (21) (Mean age 67 years)	8/212	6 years	HR: 1.16; 95% CI 1.02-1.32; p=0.027
	Rong G (27) (>54 years old)	70/1865	65.8 months	OR: 5.49, 95% CI 2.99-10.07 p=0.001
Male sex	Shibuya A (25)	14/396	43 months	HR: 6.7736 (95% CI 1.7795-25.7832)
	Suzuki A (26)	17 cases/ 56 control	-	OR: 4.2 (95% CI 1.2-14.3) p value: .021
	Harada K (28)	71/2946	58 months	OR: 3.09 (p value 0.0012)
	Rong G (27)	70/1865	65.8 months	OR= 2.19, 95% CI 1.23 – 3.93, p=0.001
	Trivedi PJ (18)	123/4565	96.1 months	(Adjusted HR 2.41, p<0.0001)
Clinical Features				
Advanced stage	Deutsch M (21)	8/212	6 years	HR: 31.50; 95% CI 1.59-625.30; p=0.024
	Cavazza A (1)	24/716	9.3 years	OR: 5.80, 95% CI 2.34-14.38, p<0.001
	Tomiyama Y (22)	11/210	8.5 years	(OR: 6.27, 95%CI: 1.80-21.83, p=0.004)
	Trivedi PJ (18)	123/4565	96.1 months	HR 2.72, p=0.022
Albumin	Hosonuma K (40)	13/179	97 months	OR: 0.205 (95% CI 0.091 – 0.459) p<0.001

(continued on next page)

Table 3
(continued)

Factors	Study	HCC/ Total Patients	Median Follow Up	Statistics
Non responder to UDCA	Kuiper EM (17)	9/375	9.7 years	(p<0.001)
	Trivedi PJ (18)	123/4565	36,577 patient-years	(HR 3.44, p<0.0001)
Presence of portal hypertension	Suzuki A (26)	17 cases/ 56 control	-	OR: 22.9; 95% CI: 3.4-155.3, p<0.01
Thrombocytopenia	Trivedi PJ (18)	123/4565	36,577 patient-years	HR: 1.41;95% CI: 1.25-1.58, p<0.0001
Co-existing factors				
Alcohol consumption	Zhang XX (36)	52/1255	43.4 months	(AOR = 10.294, 95% CI: 1.108 -95.680, p=0.040)
Blood transfusion	Shibuya A (25)	14/396	43 months	HR: 3.855 (95% CI 1.1515-12.9055)
	Suzuki A (26)	17 cases/ 56 control	-	OR: 3.3 (95% CI 1.1 -10.1) p value .038
BMI> = 25	Zhang XX (36)	52/1255	43.4 months	(AOR = 1.116, 95% CI: 1.002 - 1.244, p=0.045)
Diabetes mellitus	Rong G (27)	70/1865	65.8 months	(OR = 3.14, 95% CI 1.59-6.19, p=0.002)
HCV antibody +	Floreani A (35)	4/175	6.8 years/person	OR: 22.5 (p value .02)
	Watanabe T (34)	50 PBC with HCC/50 HCC	-	P<0.001
Previous HBV infection (HBc +)	Watanabe T (34)	50 PBC with HCC/50 HCC	-	P<0.001
	Rong G (27)	70/1865	65.8 months	(OR=6.60, 95% CI 3.69-11.89, p=0.001)
Smoking	Floreani A (35)	4/175	6.8 years/person	OR: 26.5 (p value .02)

higher in males than in females,[32–34] are also associated with a higher risk for HCC in PBC, and may contribute to the higher incidence of HCC in male PBC patients.[15,21,35,36] In multiple studies, older age at the time of diagnosis was associated with an increased risk of HCC in PBC patients.[18,20,31] In another study, a median of 54 years has an odds of 5.49 times of developing HCC (95% CI 2.99–10.07 P = .001).[15] PBC diagnosis in males is frequently delayed, often presenting in advanced disease with hepatic decompensation such as gastrointestinal bleeding, hepatoma, and jaundice,[37] which may play a role in the higher incidence of HCC in males due to age. Despite these proposed indicators of increased risk in males, there is an opposing large population-based study by Boonstra and colleagues, in which an association between male sex and an increased risk for HCC was not seen.[38]

Other predisposing factors associated with HCC in PBC were comorbid diabetes mellitus and increased body mass indices (BMIs).[15,21] Diabetes mellitus increases the risk of HCC among patients with HBV and HCV infections.[39,40] In nonalcoholic steatohepatitis patients, baseline diagnosis of diabetes was the strongest independent predictor of HCC and fibrosis progression.[41] Diabetes and obesity were associated with insulin resistance and hyperinsulinemia. Both are believed to be the key factors in HCC oncogenesis, primarily through multiple pathways of inflammatory processes and hepatocyte injury leading to cellular proliferation, increased angiogenesis, and decreased apoptosis.[39] These factors with underlying inflammation from PBC increase the risk for HCC development.

Hypoalbuminemia, thrombocytopenia, and evidence of portal hypertension have also been shown to be risk factors for the development of HCC with OR: 0.205 (95% CI 0.091–0.459), P < .001, HR: 1.41; 95% CI 1.25–1.58, P < .0001 and OR: 22.9; 95% CI: 3.4–155.3, P < .01, respectively.[13,31,42] Taken together, all these parameters are indicators of advanced PBC, supporting the recommendation to screen PBC with cirrhosis for HCC.

Surveillance for Hepatocellular Carcinoma in Primary Biliary Cholangitis

The current recommendation is to do surveillance for HCC when the risk of HCC is at least 1.5% per year in patients with cirrhosis and 0.2% per year in non-cirrhotic patients.[43] These patients are eligible to receive curative therapy for HCC, which is considered cost-effective surveillance for HCC. As a result, all major liver societies around the world currently recommend offering surveillance for HCC in PBC patients with cirrhosis,[43–45] except for patients with Child's Pugh Class C cirrhosis who are not on a transplant waiting list given the low-anticipated survival and are not eligible to receive therapy for HCC.[43–45]

As liver biopsy is not required in the diagnosis of PBC, it was recommended that PBC patients with low-platelet count, a Mayo risk score greater than 4.1 or a transient elastography value of 17 kPa and above should be screened for HCC as these patients are most likely to have cirrhosis.[43] Furthermore, the European Association for the Study of the Liver recommended that non-cirrhotic F3 patients, regardless of etiology, be considered for surveillance based on an individual risk assessment.[44]

The recommended screening modality for HCC in PBC is the same as for any chronic liver disease with HCC: ultrasound (US) with or without alpha–fetoprotein (AFP) testing every 6 months is the initial screening modality used as it is widely available, noninvasive, and relatively safe with a sensitivity of 84% at any stage (95% CI 76%–92%).[46] However, it is less effective in the early stages of HCC with a sensitivity of 47% (95% CI 33%–61%), but the sensitivity increases to 63% (95% CI 48%–75%) with the addition of AFP.[46] Small HCC will show a hypoechoic or isoechoic lesion in the US and progress with increased echogenicity as the tumor enlarges. Other modalities such as multidetector computed tomography (CT) or dynamic MRI are not effective for surveillance due to high cost, exposure to radiation, and the need for contrast agents in these imaging. If the US is inadequate, as it can be in obese patients, cross-sectional imaging using CT or MRI can be used as a screening tool. The current recommendation is to proceed to diagnostic cross-sectional imaging for lesions ≥ 10 mm found on a surveillance US or a serum AFP level of ≥ 20 ng/mL.[43] The cross-sectional imaging using a multidetector CT or dynamic MRI shows a typical vascular pattern of HCC lesions, characterized by hyper-enhancement in the arterial phase followed by contrast media washout in the venous phase corresponding to Liver Imaging Reporting and Data System (LIRADS) 5, which confirms the diagnosis of HCC. These imaging findings and LI-RADS categorization of liver lesions are the same for PBC with HCC as with any etiology of chronic liver disease with HCC.

Aside from the presence of cirrhosis, the American Association Study of Liver Disease (AASLD) guidelines for PBC recommends regular screening with cross-sectional imaging for males with PBC, same as for patients with cirrhosis[47] as multiple studies had found that the male gender confers increased risk of HCC development as discussed earlier. However, these recommendations are based on consensus opinion of experts, with limited data showing that the prevalence of HCC in males with PBC without cirrhosis is high enough to be cost-effective to warrant surveillance.

Treatment and Survival of Hepatocellular Carcinoma in Primary Biliary Cholangitis

Currently, the indications for liver transplantation for HCC in PBC are similar to any form of chronic liver disease with HCC. In terms of treatment, Imam and colleagues looked at 38 patients with PBC developing HCC: 23 patients had a single treatment modality and 12 had more than one treatment, 7 of which had a combination of arterial chemoembolization and transplant. Findings showed that only liver transplantation had better survival than locoregional treatment, surgical resection, or combined multiple modalities (OR: 0.06, $P < .0001$).[48] The survival was higher with a single nodule compared with multinodular HCC in PBC ($P < .05$).[1] The Barcelona-Clinic Liver Cancer staging system is also used to stratify PBC patients with HCC for prognostic staging and treatment strategy. Surgical resection is recommended for the non-cirrhotic liver with HCC. In the United States, patients with HCC meeting the Milan criteria (one lesion 2 to 5 cm or up to three lesions 1 to 3 cm) have been granted access to liver transplantation by Model for End-Stage Liver Disease (MELD) exception point allocation. Despite the study by Imam and colleagues, the AASLD suggests that patients within the Milan criteria be bridged with any form of locoregional therapy such as transarterial chemoembolization, Y90, ablative therapy, or combination to transplant in patients listed for a liver transplant to decrease the progression of the disease and subsequent dropout from the waiting list.[43]

The diagnosis of HCC in PBC carries a poor prognosis compared with other autoimmune liver diseases. HCC is a critical event in the clinical course of PBC and is associated with significantly poorer transplant-free survival. The interval from HCC diagnosis in PBC to death was shorter (8.4 ± 14 months) as compared with AIH with HCC (14 ± 12 months) ($P = .047$).[35] Median survival after diagnosis in the study of Cavazza and colleagues was 36 months.[1] Survival among PBC patients with HCC was almost 50% in 5 years[48] compared with general HCC, which is 74% in 5 years.[49]

SUMMARY

Several studies have shown PBC to confer increased risk to develop HCC. Parameters recognized as risk factors for the development of HCC in PBC include advanced age, male sex, and comorbidities. Advanced liver fibrosis is the most significant risk factor. Moreover, future studies should aim to clarify the role of treatment response as a risk factor for HCC development in PBC patients. To date, the only indication for HCC screening that is agreed on by all scientific societies is in patients with cirrhosis. HCC in PBC carries a poor prognosis compared with other chronic liver diseases with HCC, and liver transplantation offers the best survival rate among available therapies.

CLINICS CARE POINTS

- PBC patients and cirrhosis should undergo routine screening for hepatocellular carcinoma with a liver imaging every 6 months.

DISCLAIMER

The authors prepared this work in their personal capacity. The opinions expressed in this article are the author's own and do not reflect the view of the Department of Veterans Affairs or the United States government.

CONFLICTS OF INTERESTS

None of the authors have personal or financial conflicts of interests to declare concerning this publication.

REFERENCES

1. Cavazza A, Caballería L, Floreani A, et al. Incidence, risk factors, and survival of hepatocellular carcinoma in primary biliary cirrhosis: comparative analysis from two centers. Hepatology 2009;50(4):1162-8.
2. Yang F, Huang X, Yi T, et al. Spontaneous development of liver tumors in the absence of the bile acid receptor farnesoid X receptor. Cancer Res 2007;67(3): 863-70.
3. Sung H, Ferlay J, Siegel RL, et al. Global Cancer Statistics 2020: GLOBOCAN estimates of incidence and mortality worldwide for 36 cancers in 185 countries. CA Cancer J Clin 2021;71(3):209-49.
4. Kulik L, El-Serag HB. Epidemiology and management of hepatocellular carcinoma. Gastroenterology 2019;156(2):477-91.e1.
5. Health Resources and Services Administration. OPTN/SRTR 2019 Annual data report: liver. Available at: https://srtr.transplant.hrsa.gov/annual_reports/2019/Liver.aspx. Accessed February 17, 2022.
6. Petrick JL, Kelly SP, Altekruse SF, et al. Future of hepatocellular carcinoma incidence in the United States forecast through 2030. J Clin Oncol 2016;34(15): 1787-94.
7. Huang X-F, Zhao W-Y, Huang W-D. FXR and liver carcinogenesis. Nat Publ Gr 2015;36:37-43.
8. Gadaleta RM, Scialpi N, Peres C, et al. Suppression of hepatic bile acid synthesis by a non-tumorigenic FGF19 analogue protects mice from fibrosis and hepatocarcinogenesis. Scientific Rep 2018;8:17210.
9. Sun L, Cai J, Gonzalez FJ. The role of farnesoid X receptor in metabolic diseases, and gastrointestinal and liver cancer. Nat Rev Gastroenterol Hepatol 2021;18: 335-47.

10. Liu T, Yang H, Fan W, et al. Mechanisms of MAFG dysregulation in cholestatic liver injury and development of liver cancer. Gastroenterology 2018;155(2): 557–71.e14.

11. McGee EE, Castro FA, Engels EA, et al. Associations between autoimmune conditions and hepatobiliary cancer risk among elderly US adults. Int J Cancer 2019; 144(4):707–17.

12. Natarajan Y, Tansel A, Patel P, et al. Incidence of hepatocellular carcinoma in primary biliary cholangitis: a systematic review and meta-Analysis. Dig Dis Sci 2021; 66(7):2439–51.

13. Trivedi PJ, Lammers WJ, van Buuren HR, et al, Global PBC Study Group. Stratification of hepatocellular carcinoma risk in primary biliary cirrhosis: a multicentre international study. Gut 2016;65(2):321–9.

14. Tomiyama Y, Takenaka K, Kodama T, et al. Risk factors for survival and the development of hepatocellular carcinoma in patients with primary biliary cirrhosis. Intern Med 2013;52(14):1553–9.

15. Rong G, Wang H, Bowlus CL, et al. Incidence and risk factors for hepatocellular carcinoma in primary biliary cirrhosis. Clin Rev Allergy Immunol 2015;48(2–3): 132–41.

16. Harada K, Hirohara J, Ueno Y, et al. Incidence of and risk factors for hepatocellular carcinoma in primary biliary cirrhosis: national data from Japan. Hepatology 2013;57(5):1942–9.

17. Kuiper EM, Hansen BE, Adang RP, et al, Dutch PBC Study Group. Relatively high risk for hepatocellular carcinoma in patients with primary biliary cirrhosis not responding to ursodeoxycholic acid. Eur J Gastroenterol Hepatol 2010;22(12): 1495–502.

18. Deutsch M, Papatheodoridis GV, Tzakou A, et al. Risk of hepatocellular carcinoma and extrahepatic malignancies in primary biliary cirrhosis. Eur J Gastroenterol Hepatol 2008;20(1):5–9.

19. Caballería L, Parés A, Castells A, et al. Hepatocellular carcinoma in primary biliary cirrhosis: similar incidence to that in hepatitis C virus-related cirrhosis. Am J Gastroenterol 2001;96(4):1160–3.

20. Shibuya A, Tanaka K, Miyakawa H, et al. Hepatocellular carcinoma and survival in patients with primary biliary cirrhosis. Hepatology 2002;35(5):1172–8.

21. Zhang XX, Wang LF, Jin L, et al. Primary biliary cirrhosis-associated hepatocellular carcinoma in Chinese patients: incidence and risk factors. World J Gastroenterol 2015;21(12):3554–63.

22. Findor J, He XS, Sord J, et al. Primary biliary cirrhosis and hepatocellular carcinoma. Autoimmun Rev 2002;1(4):220–5.

23. Jones DE, Metcalf JV, Collier JD, et al. Hepatocellular carcinoma in primary biliary cirrhosis and its impact on outcomes. Hepatology 1997;26(5):1138–42.

24. Tansel A, Katz LH, El-Serag HB. Incidence and determinants of hepatocellular carcinoma in autoimmune hepatitis: a systematic review and meta-analysis. Clin Gastroenterol Hepatol 2017;15(8):1207–17.e4.

25. Angulo P, Batts KP, Therneau TM, et al. Long-term ursodeoxycholic acid delays histological progression in primary biliary cirrhosis. Hepatology 1999;29(3): 644–7.

26. John BV, Khakoo NS, Schwartz KB, et al. Ursodeoxycholic acid response is associated with reduced mortality in primary biliary cholangitis with compensated cirrhosis. Am J Gastroenterol 2021;116(9):1913–23.

27. Janmohamed A, Trivedi PJ. Patterns of disease progression and incidence of complications in primary biliary cholangitis. Best Pract Res Clin Gastroenterol 2018;34-35:71–83.

28. Beuers U, Gershwin ME, Gish RG, et al. Changing nomenclature for PBC: from 'cirrhosis' to 'cholangitis. J Hepatol 2015;63(5):1285–7.

29. Lleo A, Colapietro F. Changes in the epidemiology of primary biliary cholangitis. Clin Liver Dis 2018;22(3):429–41.

30. Yeh SH, Chen PJ. Gender disparity of hepatocellular carcinoma: the roles of sex hormones. Oncology 2010;78(Suppl 1):172–9.

31. Suzuki A, Lymp J, Donlinger J, et al. Clinical predictors for hepatocellular carcinoma in patients with primary biliary cirrhosis. Clin Gastroenterol Hepatol 2007; 5(2):259–64.

32. Baden R, Rockstroh JK, Buti M. Natural history and management of hepatitis C: does sex play a role? J Infect Dis 2014;209(Suppl 3):S81–5.

33. Higgins ST, Kurti AN, Redner R, et al. A literature review on prevalence of gender differences and intersections with other vulnerabilities to tobacco use in the United States, 2004-2014. Prev Med 2015;80:89–100.

34. Centers for Disease Control and Prevention. Behavioral risk factor surveillance system data. Available at: https://www.cdc.gov/brfss/index.html. Accessed February 17, 2022.

35. Watanabe T, Soga K, Hirono H, et al. Features of hepatocellular carcinoma in cases with autoimmune hepatitis and primary biliary cirrhosis. World J Gastroenterol 2009;15(2):231–9.

36. Floreani A, Baragiotta A, Baldo V, et al. Hepatic and extrahepatic malignancies in primary biliary cirrhosis. Hepatology 1999;29(5):1425–8.

37. Smyk DS, Rigopoulou EI, Pares A, et al. Sex differences associated with primary biliary cirrhosis. Clin Dev Immunol 2012;2012:610504.

38. Boonstra K, Bokelaar R, Stadhouders PH, et al. Increased cancer risk in a large population-based cohort of patients with primary biliary cirrhosis: follow-up for up to 36 years. Hepatol Int 2014;8(2):266–74.

39. Tan Y, Wei S, Zhang W, et al. Type 2 diabetes mellitus increases the risk of hepatocellular carcinoma in subjects with chronic hepatitis B virus infection: a meta-analysis and systematic review. Cancer Manag Res 2019;11:705–13.

40. Dyal HK, Aguilar M, Bartos G, et al. Diabetes Mellitus increases risk of hepatocellular carcinoma in chronic hepatitis C virus patients: a systematic review. Dig Dis Sci 2016;61(2):636–45.

41. Alexander M, Loomis AK, van der Lei J, et al. Risks and clinical predictors of cirrhosis and hepatocellular carcinoma diagnoses in adults with diagnosed NAFLD: real-world study of 18 million patients in four European cohorts. BMC Med 2019;17(1):95.

42. Hosonuma K, Sato K, Yanagisawa M, et al. Incidence, mortality, and predictive factors of hepatocellular carcinoma in primary biliary cirrhosis. Gastroenterol Res Pract 2013;2013:168012.

43. Marrero JA, Kulik LM, Sirlin CB, et al. Diagnosis, staging, and management of hepatocellular carcinoma: 2018 practice guidance by the American Association for the Study of Liver Diseases. Hepatology 2018;68(2):723–50.

44. European Association for the Study of the Liver. EASL Clinical Practice Guidelines: the diagnosis and management of patients with primary biliary cholangitis. J Hepatol 2017;67(1):145–72.

45. Omata M, Cheng AL, Kokudo N, et al. Asia-Pacific clinical practice guidelines on the management of hepatocellular carcinoma: a 2017 update. Hepatol Int 2017; 11(4):317–70.

46. Tzartzeva K, Obi J, Rich NE, et al. Surveillance imaging and alpha fetoprotein for early Detection of hepatocellular carcinoma in patients with cirrhosis: a meta-analysis. Gastroenterology 2018;154(6):1706–18.e1.

47. Lindor KD, Bowlus CL, Boyer J, et al. Primary biliary cholangitis: 2018 practice guidance from the American association for the study of liver diseases. Hepatology 2019;69(1):394–419.

48. Imam MH, Silveira MG, Sinakos E, et al. Long-term outcomes of patients with primary biliary cirrhosis and hepatocellular carcinoma. Clin Gastroenterol Hepatol 2012;10(2):182–5.

49. Singal AK, Guturu P, Hmoud B, et al. Evolving frequency and outcomes of liver transplantation based on etiology of liver disease. Transplantation 2013;95(5): 755–60.

Treatment of Primary Biliary Cholangitis

First-Line and Second-Line Therapies

Chung-Heng Liu, BS[a], Christopher L. Bowlus, MD[b],*

KEYWORDS

- Autoimmune liver disease • Therapy • Bile acids • Farnesoid X receptor

KEY POINTS

- Up to 40% of patients with PBC do not have an adequate response to the first-line treatment with ursodeoxycholic acid (UDCA) and remain at risk of disease progression.
- The farnesoid X receptor agonist obeticholic acid (OCA) improves liver biochemistries associated with better transplant-free survival but is contraindicated in patients with PBC and decompensated cirrhosis or portal hypertension.
- Real-world data supports the effectiveness of OCA in improving liver biochemistries but pruritus remains a limiting adverse effect in some patients.
- Peroxisome proliferator-activated receptor agonists, fenofibrate and bezafibrate, have potential benefit for patients with PBC and an incomplete response to UDCA but further study is needed to demonstrate their safety.
- Fatigue is a common symptom of PBC but current therapies do not affect fatigue.

INTRODUCTION

Primary biliary cholangitis (PBC) is a progressive, rare, autoimmune, inflammatory disease of the interlobular bile ducts, leading to cholestasis and secondary damage of hepatocytes that may ultimately progress to cirrhosis and liver failure (**Fig. 1**).[1] A prototypical autoimmune disease, PBC affects predominantly middle-aged women in whom loss of tolerance to specific epitopes on mitochondrial antigens leads to the development of antimitochondrial antibodies (AMA) and immunologic destruction of the biliary epithelial cells of small size bile ducts.

PBC is typically suspected when liver tests are abnormal and the diagnosis can be made when at least 2 of 3 criteria are met,[2,3] including persistent elevation of alkaline phosphatase (ALP) for more than 6 months with normal imaging of the biliary tract;

a Drexel University College of Medicine, 2900 W Queen Ln, Philadelphia, PA 19129 USA;
b Division of Gastroenterology and Hepatology, University of California Davis School of Medicine, 4150 V Street, PSSB 3500, Sacramento, CA 95817, USA
* Corresponding author:
E-mail address: clbowlus@ucdavis.edu

Clin Liver Dis 26 (2022) 705–726
https://doi.org/10.1016/j.cld.2022.06.012
1089-3261/22/© 2022 Elsevier Inc. All rights reserved.

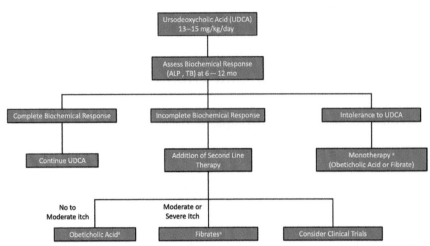

Fig. 1. Treatment algorithm for primary biliary cholangitis. Following the diagnosis of PBC, staging of fibrosis should be achieved by vibration controlled transient elastography to help guide treatment. First-line treatment with ursodeoxycholic acid (UDCA) should be given to all patients with PBC. After 6 to 12 months, biochemical response should be assessed by the GLOBE score or other criteria, with the optimal goal being normalization of ALP and total bilirubin. Second-line therapy should be considered according to the biochemical response and the stage of fibrosis. OCA should be considered unless there is pruritus or other contraindication to its use. A fibrate may be an acceptable alternative second-line agent but it is not approved for this indication by regulatory authorities. Both OCA and fibrates should be avoided in patients with decompensated cirrhosis or portal hypertension. [a]Contraindicated in PBC patients with decompensated cirrhosis or portal hypertension.

serologic reactivity to AMA or PBC-specific antinuclear antibodies, such as anti-Sp100 or anti-Gp 210; and/or histologic features of nonsuppurative obstructive cholangitis, also known as florid duct lesions, involving the interlobular bile ducts. Approximately 5% to 10% of patients with PBC have AMA-negative PBC, characterized by the lack of reactivity to AMA, and require liver biopsy for diagnosis; however, compared with individuals with AMA reactivity, clinical features and disease progression are similar.[4,5] Another 8% to 10% of patients with PBC may have features of autoimmune hepatitis as well, known as PBC/autoimmune hepatitis (AIH) overlap syndrome.[6,7] The diagnosis of PBC/AIH overlap is controversial but the Paris criteria are the most widely accepted and require a diagnosis of PBC and at least 2 of the following to be met: alanine aminotransferase (ALT) greater than 5 times the upper limit of normal (ULN), immunoglobulin G greater than 2 times the ULN or antismooth muscle antibodies greater than 1:80, and histologic evidence of periportal or periseptal lymphocytic piecemeal necrosis.[6] Presentation with fibrosis seems to be more common among patients with PBC/AIH overlap and rates of progression to liver failure, complications of portal hypertension, and death have been reported to be higher in PBC/AIH overlap compared with PBC without AIH.[8]

In the absence of treatment, PBC is a progressive disease with most patients advancing one histologic stage every 2 years and having an average survival of approximately 12 years.[9,10] Although autoimmune in nature, immune-based therapies have not been shown to be effective in PBC and current treatments are based on improving the deleterious effects of cholestasis. However, more than 3 decades since the approval of ursodeoxycholic acid (UDCA), only 1 additional drug, obeticholic acid

(OCA), has achieved regulatory approval for use in PBC reflecting the many challenges to drug development in PBC. Notably, PBC is a rare condition that, to adequately recruit for trials, requires nearly equal numbers of study sites as patients. In addition, to demonstrate definitive benefit in a randomized, controlled fashion for hard clinical outcomes such as liver transplant, a trial would require a study population of size and longevity that would not be feasible. With these limitations in mind, the efficacy of PBC treatments has largely been based on surrogate clinical endpoints, such as liver biochemistries, which have been established as robust and accurate predictors of transplant-free survival. In addition, although current treatments have efficacy to reduce the risk of transplant or death, approximately 50% of patients with PBC suffer from symptoms of fatigue and pruritus that are not affected by currently approved treatments. Thus, the optimal management of PBC should address not only the progression of liver disease but also its symptoms. However, for the purposes of this review, we will focus on those treatment options that target the liver disease.

FIRST-LINE THERAPIES
Ursodeoxycholic Acid

UDCA was the first drug approved by the US Food and Drug Administration (FDA) for use in PBC and remains the first-line therapy for all patients with PBC. UDCA protects cholangiocytes against the cytotoxicity of hydrophobic bile acids, stimulates the hepatobiliary secretion of bile acids, increases the hydrophilicity index of the circulating bile pool, and may have immunomodulatory and anti-inflammatory effects.[11] Despite several Cochrane reviews[12] in conflict with the overwhelming evidence, UDCA at a dose of 13 to 15 mg/kg/d improves biochemical indices, delays histologic progression, and most probably improves survival without transplantation. An early prospective study of 15 patients found UDCA to improve liver tests and pruritus.[13] Since that report, there have been 16 randomized controlled trials of UDCA involving more than 1400 patients with PBC.[12] Notably, these studies varied by UDCA dose, treatment length, disease stage, and outcomes measured. The results of studies of adequate duration (2 years or more) and with adequate doses of UDCA (13–15 mg/kg/d) have consistently shown biochemical and histologic benefits of UDCA (**Tables 1–3**). The notable UDCA studies include a randomized, placebo-controlled trial of 146 patients treated for 2 years in which UDCA was effective in reducing treatment failure defined as a doubling in bilirubin or development of severe complications as well as improving bilirubin, Mayo risk score, and mean histologic score.[14] In addition, during a 2-year open-label phase following the placebo-controlled trial, the previously placebo-treated patients had significantly worse transplant-free survival compared with the UDCA-treated patients with PBC.[15] These results were further corroborated by randomized, placebo-controlled trials of 222 patients and 192 patients treated for 2 years, both of which demonstrated that patients treated with UDCA had positive effects on serum bilirubin and other liver biochemistries; however, the studies were not adequately powered to determine a difference in liver transplantation or death.[16,17] Similarly, Combes *and colleagues* found UDCA even at 11 mg/kg/d for 2 years delayed histologic progression of disease but only among those with an entry bilirubin less than 2 mg/dL.[18] The longest randomized, placebo-controlled trial included 180 patients treated for 4 years in which UDCA treatment was associated with a delayed time to treatment failure defined as death, liver transplantation, histologic progression by 2 stages or to cirrhosis, development of varices, ascites, or encephalopathy, doubling of bilirubin, marked worsening of fatigue or pruritus, inability to tolerate the drug, or voluntary withdrawal for any reason.[19]

Table 1
Prospective trials of ursodeoxycholic acid for primary biliary cholangitis

Author, Year	Study Design	Inclusion Criteria	Duration	Number of Patients	UDCA Dose	Main Result
Improvement in Clinical Parameters						
Poupon[13],1987	Prospective trial	Patients with PBC	2 y	15	13–15 mg/kg/d	Improvement in GGT, ALP, ALT, bilirubin, decreased pruritus
Poupon et al,[14] 1991	Double-blind, randomized, placebo-controlled trial	Biopsy-proven PBC	2 y	146	13–15 mg/kg/d	Improvement in bilirubin, ALP, ALT, AST, GGT, cholesterol, IgM, antimitochondrial-antibody titer; improvement in Mayo risk score; improvement in mean histologic score
Lindor et al,[19] 1994	Double-blind, placebo-controlled trial	Patients with PBC	2 y	180	13–15 mg/kg/d	Delayed time to treatment failure[a]
Improvement in Histology						
Poupon et al,[20] 2003	Combined data from 4 trials	Patients with PBC with liver biopsy specimens	Variable	367	Variable	Decreased periportal necroinflammation, improved ductal proliferation, delayed histologic progression when initiated at earlier stages
Corpechot et al,[22] 2000	Randomized, double-blind, placebo-controlled trial	Patients with PBC	4 y	103	13–5 mg/kg/d	5-fold lower progression rate from early stage disease

Study	Study design	Patient population	Duration	N	Dose	Outcome
Angulo et al,[26] 1999	Study of patients enrolled in prior placebo-controlled trials	Patients with PBC with liver biopsy specimens	5–9 y	67	13–15 mg/kg/d	Decreased rate of progression to cirrhosis
Combes et al,[18] 1995	Randomized, placebo-controlled trial	PBC at least 6 mo duration, liver biopsy	2 y	151	10–12 mg/kg/d	Decreased bilirubin, improved histology, decreased complications and liver transplantation or death
Heathcote et al,[16] 1994	Randomized, placebo-controlled trial	Patients with PBC confirmed by liver biopsy and antimitochondrial antibody positive	2 y	222	14 mg/kg/d	Decreased bilirubin, ALP, AST, ALT, cholesterol, IgM, improved histologic features, however no difference in liver transplantation or death
Pares et al,[17] 2000	Randomized, double-blind, placebo-controlled trial	Patients with PBC, biopsy proven	2 y	192	14–16 mg/kg/d	Improved histology, however no change in time to death or liver transplantation
Improved Transplant-Free Survival						
Poupon et al,[15] 1994	Randomized placebo-controlled trial	Biopsy-proven PBC	4 y[b]	145	13–15 mg/kg/d	Decreased disease progression and death, reduced need for transplantation
Poupon et al,[108] 1997	Combined data from 3 trials	Biopsy-proven PBC, elevated ALP, positive AMA	2–4 y	548	Variable	Improved survival free of liver transplantation in moderate-to-severe disease

Abbreviations: ALP, alkaline phosphatase; ALT, alanine aminotransferase; AMA, antimitochondrial antibodies; AST, aspartate aminotransferase; GGT, gamma-glutamyl transferase.

[a] Treatment failure: death, liver transplantation, histologic progression by 2 stages or to cirrhosis, development of varices, ascites, or encephalopathy, doubling of bilirubin, marked worsening of fatigue or pruritus, inability to tolerate the drug, voluntary withdrawal for any reason.

[b] Initially a 2-y study, however due to benefit of UDCA, all patients received UDCA in an open trial and were monitored for 2 more years.

Table 2
Clinical trials of obeticholic acid for primary biliary cholangitis

Author, Year	Study Design	Inclusion Criteria	Duration	Number of Patients	OCA Dose	Use of UDCA	Main Result
Kowdley et al,[38] 2017	Randomized, double-blind, placebo-controlled Phase 2 study	Patients with PBC with ALP 1.5–10x ULN, off UDCA >3 mo	3 mo	60	10, 50 mg/d	No	Decrease in ALP, ALT, bilirubin, IgM, dose-dependent increase in pruritus
Hirschfield et al,[39] 2015	Randomized, double-blind, placebo-controlled trial	ALP 1.5–10× ULN	3 mo	165	10,25,50 mg/d	Yes	Decrease in ALP, GGT, ALT
Hirschfield et al,[39] 2015	Open label long-term safety extension	Completion of phase 2 trial	Study stopped after all patients had at least 23 mo in LTSE	78	10–50 mg/d	Yes	Further decrease in ALP in 10, 25 mg groups; worsened pruritus following titration to 25 mg
Nevens et al,[40] 2016	Randomized, double-blind, placebo-controlled trial	ALP 1.5–10× ULN	12 mo	216	5–10 (titration) or 10 mg/d	Yes	46% and 47% reached the primary endpoint of an ALP <1.67 ULN with a reduction of at least 15% from baseline and normal total bilirubin

Table 3
Prospective studies of fibrates in a minimum of 20 patients with primary biliary cholangitis

Author	Study Design	Inclusion Criteria	Duration	Number of Patients	Fenofibrate/ Bezafibrate Dose	Main Result
Kurihara et al,[55] 2000	Randomized trial	Biopsy proven PBC	12 mo	12 bezafibrate, 12 UDCA	Bezafibrate 400 mg/d	Decrease ALP, GGT, IgM, bezafibrate more effective than UDCA
Nakai et al,[56] 2000	Randomized trial	Patients with PBC with prior UDCA treatment	12 mo	10 UDCA + bezafibrate, 13 UDCA	Bezafibrate 400 mg/d	Decrease ALP, GGT, IgM
Kanda et al,[54] 2006	Randomized trial	Patients with PBC with elevated ALP while on UDCA	6 mo	11 UDCA + bezafibrate, 11 UDCA	Bezafibrate 400 mg/d	Decrease ALP, GGT
Kita et al,[53] 2006	Prospective case series	Patients with PBC	6 mo	22	Bezafibrate 400 mg/d	Decrease ALP, GGT, IgM
Iwasaki et al,[52] 2008	Two prospective randomized-controlled trials	Noncirrhotic patients with PBC	52 wk	Study 1: 45 Study 2: 21	Bezafibrate 400 mg/d	Study 1: bezafibrate monotherapy as effective as UDCA; Study 2: bezafibrate + UDCA improved biochemical markers in patients with incomplete response to UDCA
Levy et al,[50] 2011	Open-label pilot study	Patients with PBC with ALP >2 x ULN	12 mo	20	Fenofibrate 160 mg/d	Decrease ALP, AST, and IgM
Han et al,[49] 2012	Prospective case series	Patients with PBC treated with UDCA for at least 1 y	3–6 mo	22	Fenofibrate 200 mg/d	Decrease/normalization ALP; Decrease AST, ALT, GGT, cholesterol, TG

(continued on next page)

Table 3
(continued)

Author	Study Design	Inclusion Criteria	Duration	Number of Patients	Fenofibrate/ Bezafibrate Dose	Main Result
Lens et al,[51] 2014	Prospective case series	Patients with PBC treated with UDCA and abnormal ALP	12 mo	30	Bezafibrate 400 mg/d	Decrease/normalization ALP; Decrease ALT, GGT, cholesterol, TG, pruritus, liver stiffness unchanged
Reig et al,[57] 2017[78]	Prospective study	Patients with PBC treated with UDCA with ALP > 1.5× ULN	38 mo	48	Bezafibrate 400 mg/d	54% of patients with normalized ALP, improvement in jaundice, pruritus, liver stiffness; all but one case reported improvement in pruritus
Corpechot et al,[77] 2018[57]	Randomized, placebo-controlled trial	Patients with PBC with inadequate response to UDCA by Paris-2 criteria	24 mo	100	Bezafibrate 400 mg/d	Normalization of bilirubin, ALP, AST, ALT, albumin, PT

Combined data from these clinical trials has demonstrated that patients treated with UDCA had delayed histologic progression of disease when UDCA was initiated at early stages of disease[20] and improved transplant-free survival in those treated with UDCA at late stages of disease.[20,21] Further, Corpechot *and colleagues* used a Markov model of clinical trial data to demonstrate that UDCA therapy was associated with a 5-fold lower rate of histologic progression from early stage disease to extensive fibrosis or cirrhosis.[21–24] More recently, higher doses of UDCA (18–22 mg/kg/d) were associated with improvement in liver transplant-free survival among patients without an initial biochemical response to UDCA.[23]

Overall, the safety of UDCA has been established in these trials as well as several trials investigating other indications.[12,25] No significant differences in serious adverse events have been identified in any clinical trials. Diarrhea was the most common adverse event in trials of UDCA for gallstones occurring in 2% to 9% of patients but has not been seen in trials of PBC. Abdominal pain, nausea, and vomiting have been reported but in less than 5% of patients with PBC. Initiating UDCA at lower doses and titrating up may reduce the risk of these symptoms.

In summary, data from clinical trials in which UDCA is given at adequate doses for at least 2 years have found biochemical and histologic benefits but improvements in clinical outcomes, particularly transplant-free survival, require trials of at least 4 years duration. This is not surprisingly given that while the disease progresses even to cirrhosis, the time to liver decompensation and liver-related death may be years. In addition, the timing of liver transplantation is confounded by factors that vary with era and geography. Further, patients with early disease may be more likely to respond to treatment but are unlikely to have a clinical event even if untreated over several years of observation.

SECOND-LINE THERAPIES

Following the introduction of UDCA, long-term observation of patients with PBC treated with UDCA demonstrated a lower rate of progression to cirrhosis,[26] and there was a reduction in the number and percentage of liver transplants performed for PBC despite a trend toward increasing incidence.[27,28] However, there remained a group of patients with PBC who continued to progress despite UDCA treatment, leading to the development of response criteria to identify patients with PBC at risk of worse outcomes despite UDCA treatment and to predict transplant-free survival among with PBC. These criteria based on observational cohorts of UDCA-treated patients included the Rotterdam, Barcelona, Paris I and II, and Toronto criteria and introduced the concept of *biochemical response* to UDCA. They all demonstrated that patients who met these response criteria had a better clinical outcome and in many cases, a transplant-free survival that was not significantly different from a matched control population.[2,29] Subsequently, continuous models such as the UK-PBC and GLOBE scores, demonstrated excellent specificity and sensitivity for predicting transplant-free survival up to 10 to 15 years.[30,31] These scores quantify the relative risk of clinical outcomes rather than the qualitative biochemical response criteria, and they all assess prognosis based on either changes in or absolute levels of blood tests after 1 year of UDCA treatment. Furthermore, the GLOBE score has been shown to predict prognosis in untreated patients with PBC, suggesting its broader applicability compared with other models.[24] One limitation of these models is the absence of data on liver fibrosis stage. Recent studies have demonstrated that fibrosis stage, either by histology or by noninvasive modalities, is a predictor of clinical outcomes independent of biochemical response.[32,33]

Although nearly all patients with PBC will have some improvement in the serum ALP with UDCA, 30% to 40% will have an inadequate biochemical response and remain at risk of disease progression. This risk correlates with an increasing serum ALP more than 2 times the ULN and bilirubin even when it is less than the ULN.[34] Patients with PBC who have an inadequate response to UDCA or those few who are intolerant to UDCA should be considered for second-line therapies.

Obeticholic Acid

OCA is conditionally approved by the FDA for patients with PBC and an inadequate response to UDCA or unable to tolerate UDCA. OCA is a derivative of chenodeoxycholic acid, the natural occurring ligand of the farnesoid X receptor (FXR), which mediates the synthesis and enterohepatic circulation of bile acids. OCA is 100 times more potent as an FXR ligand compared with chenodeoxycholic acid. In the liver, FXR activation reduces the conversion of cholesterol to bile acids and increases the transport of bile acids out of hepatocytes. Activation of FXR in the ileum decreases bile acid reabsorption and increases the expression of fibroblast growth factor 19 (FGF19), which acts in the liver to further decrease bile acid synthesis. OCA may also have antifibrotic properties and may improve portal hypertension.[35–37]

The initial phase 2 studies of OCA evaluated its use as monotherapy and as add-on therapy to UDCA in patients with PBC. In a double-blind, placebo-controlled trial, placebo was compared with OCA at 10 and 50 mg daily for 3 months in 53 patients with PBC and persistently elevated ALP levels after taking UDCA for at least 6 months.[38] The groups that received OCA at 10 or 50 mg had a significant reduction from baseline in ALP (-53.9%, 95% confidence interval (CI) -62.6 to -29.3 and -37.2%, 95% CI -54.8 to 24.6, respectively) compared with placebo (-0.8%, 95% CI -6.4 to 8.7). Pruritus was the most common adverse event leading to discontinuation of 15% and 38% of patients receiving 10 and 50 mg OCA, respectively.

In the second phase 2 trial of OCA in PBC, 165 patients with PBC and a serum ALP 1.5 to 10 times the ULN despite UDCA treatment were randomized to 10, 25, or 50 mg OCA or placebo while continuing UDCA.[39] All OCA-treated groups had significantly greater reductions from baseline in serum ALP compared with placebo with the mean relative decrease of 24% (95% CI -30 to -18), 25% (95% CI -30 to -20), and 21% (95% CI -30 to -12) for the 10, 25, and 50 mg OCA groups, respectively, compared with 3% (95% CI: -7 to 2) in the placebo group. The groups that received OCA also had significant improvements in γ-glutamyl transferase and ALT but only 7% of OCA-treated patients completely normalized their ALP. Pruritus was again the only adverse event more frequent in the OCA group compared with the placebo group and was seen in terms of both frequency and severity of pruritus. In addition, there was a dose–response effect with the greatest frequency and severity seen in the 50 mg OCA group. Seventy-eight patients continued in a 12-month open-label extension with 61 patients completing the study at which time the mean final daily dose was 20 mg.

The pivotal phase 3 study (POISE) evaluated the effects of 12-month treatment of OCA in patients with PBC with an inadequate response to UDCA, defined by a serum ALP of 1.67 times the ULN or a bilirubin greater than 1 times the ULN but less than 2 times the ULN, or intolerant of UDCA.[40] Patients were randomized in a double-blind fashion (1:1:1) to receive placebo daily, OCA 10 mg daily, or OCA 5 mg daily with a titration to 10 mg after 6 months based on response and tolerability. The primary endpoint after 12 months of treatment was the combination of a serum ALP less than 1.67 times ULN with a reduction of at least 15% from baseline and a normal total bilirubin. More than 90% of the 216 patients enrolled received UDCA as background therapy. The primary endpoint was met by 47% and 46% of patients in the 10 mg and

5 to 10 mg OCA groups, respectively, compared with 10% in the placebo group ($P < .001$). In addition, significant reductions in ALP and total bilirubin occurred in the OCA-treated groups compared with the placebo group. There was no significant change in noninvasive measures of fibrosis. Pruritus was more common in the OCA group and was reported by 68% and 56% of patients in the 10 mg and 5 to 10 mg OCA treatment arms compared with 38% in the placebo arm. In addition, the severity of pruritus in the 10 mg-treated patients was reported to be more severe compared with placebo with up to 6 months of treatment but then were not significantly different at 12 months. Discontinuation due to pruritus occurred in 10% of the 10 mg OCA-treated patients compared with 1% in the 5 to 10 mg OCA group and none in the placebo group. Other common adverse effects included nasopharyngitis, headache, and fatigue.[41] Following the initial 12 months of the trial, patients were given the option to continue in an open-label long-term extension starting at 5 mg OCA and increasing to 10 mg OCA as tolerated. The majority (91%) of patients entered the extension phase and results to date support ongoing efficacy of OCA through 2 years of treatment.[42] The results of these studies led to the conditional approval of OCA for patients with PBC with an inadequate response to UDCA or who are intolerant to UDCA with an initial starting dose of 5 mg and increasing to 10 mg after 3 months based on tolerability. The definition of inadequate response is left open to clinical judgment.

A randomized confirmatory trial of OCA evaluating clinical outcomes in patients with PBC at risk of clinical events Clinical Outcomes in Patients With Primary Biliary Cholangitis (COBALT) was launched in 2014. However, due to challenges to enrollment and retention, the study was terminated in 2022 for lack of feasibility. Nevertheless, post hoc analysis of trial data, a small study of histologic improvement and real-world experience have added further support for the efficacy of OCA. In a post hoc analysis, greater percentages of patients treated with OCA, independent of dosages, compared with placebo demonstrated improvements in at least one risk stage with a combination of aspartate aminotransferase (AST) to platelet ratio index and GLOBE scores.[41] Among patients with greater risk for mortality and liver transplantation (overall GLOBE > 0.3), more patients treated with OCA achieved GLOBE score of 0.3 or lesser in 12 months compared with placebo. Furthermore, histologic fibrosis improved in 12% of patients with PBC treated with OCA for 3 years. Meanwhile, fibrosis stage remained unchanged in 59% of the study patients.[43] These findings suggest the role of OCA in reducing the likelihood of long-term complications and decreasing disease progression.

Real-world data on the efficacy of OCA have been reported. Significant reductions in key biochemical tests such as ALP and ALT were noted within 12 months of OCA treatment in 2 recent real-world data from Canadian and Italian cohorts.[44,45] In the Canadian cohort, despite of significant reduction in ALP seen in patients with cirrhosis determined by liver stiffness ($\geq$16.9 kPa), the reduction was not as substantial as patients whose liver stiffness measurements less than 16.9 kPa.[44] Similarly, lower responses to OCA treatment were noted among cirrhotic patients in the Italian cohort.[45] Both real-world data reported pruritus as the most common adverse effects of OCA.

Notably, the FDA-approved prescribing guidance advised that patients with Child-Pugh B and C cirrhosis should initiate dosing of OCA at 5 mg once weekly, which can be increased to the maximum approved dose of OCA 10 mg twice weekly. This dosing was based on modeling of the pharmacokinetic of OCA and not on any experimental evidence in patients with PBC with advanced cirrhosis. Importantly, FDA issued a new contraindication of OCA for patients with PBC with decompensated cirrhosis or portal hypertension in 2021. The revision to the Boxed Warning reflects reports of drug-induced liver injury resulting in decompensation or liver failure from 25 cases. Among the 25 cases cited by the FDA, Eaton and colleagues summarized the 8 cases of liver failure among cirrhotic patients with either PBC or primary sclerosing cholangitis (PSC) while being on OCA. A pattern of cholestatic injury was noted and 50% of the cohort underwent liver transplantation.[46]

In summary, data on OCA clearly demonstrates its ability to improve liver biochemistries including total bilirubin, which are associated with improved clinical outcomes, but the feasibility of long-term, randomized trials to confirm that this translates into clinically meaningful endpoints such as transplant-free and overall survival remains unclear. Given the limited options for patients with PBC with an incomplete response to UDCA, OCA should be considered in these patients, particularly those without significant pruritus.

Fibrates

Fibrates have anticholestatic effects mediated through the peroxisome proliferator-activated receptor. Thus, fibrates have been extensively studied as therapeutic agents because of their potential ability to reduce bile acid synthesis and bile acid-related hepatic inflammation.[47,48] Initial small pilot studies and case reports showed that fibrates, including fenofibrate in the United States and bezafibrate in Europe and Japan, improved liver biochemistries, liver stiffness measurements, and pruritus in patients with PBC.[49–71] Meta-analyses have concluded that fibrates improve liver biochemistries without an increase in adverse effects,[72,73] and a recent systematic review found the combination of fibrates and UDCA to be safe.[74] However, the long-term efficacy of bezafibrate on clinical outcomes is unclear. A systematic review did not find evidence of an effect of bezafibrate (either alone or in combination with UDCA) on mortality, liver-related morbidity, or adverse events.[75] However, a subsequent retrospective study reported concurrent UDCA and bezafibrate therapies were associated with decreases in mortality and liver transplantation compared with UDCA monotherapy.[76]

The potential therapeutic benefit of bezafibrate is supported by the phase 3 randomized, placebo-controlled Bezafibrate in Combination With Ursodeoxycholic Acid in Primary Biliary Cirrhosis (BEZURSO) trial.[77] One hundred patients with PBC and an inadequate response to UDCA by Paris-2 criteria were treated with bezafibrate 400 mg daily or placebo for 2 years. The primary endpoint was normal total bilirubin, ALP, AST, ALT, albumin, and prothrombin time at 2 years. The primary endpoint was reached more frequently in the bezafibrate group than in the placebo group (31% vs 0%, respectively). Notably, significant beneficial relative changes from baseline to 2 years were observed in serum ALP, ALT, total bilirubin, and albumin. In addition, fibrates have been noted to improve cholestatic pruritus and in a randomized trial of bezafibrate for cholestatic pruritus, including from PBC, significantly more patients on bezafibrate reached the primary endpoint of reduction in intensity of itch by 50% or greater measured by visual analog scale than those on placebo (45% vs 11%).[79]

Bezafibrate and other fibrates are associated with hepatotoxicity and elevated creatinine and creatinine kinase, which have all been observed in the treatment of PBC.[39,80] In the BEZURSO study, 3 of the 50 patients receiving bezafibrate had an ALT elevation more than 5 times the ULN compared with 1 of 50 patients receiving placebo. Similarly, 20% of patients receiving bezafibrate reported myalgias compared with 10% receiving placebo. Thus, the use of fibrates should include monitoring for these adverse effects, and their use is discouraged in patients with decompensated liver disease.[81]

OBETICHOLIC ACID AND FIBRATE COMBINATION

Both the POISE and BEZURSO studies demonstrated that despite the addition of OCA or bezafibrate to UDCA, up to 50% of patients with PBC still do not achieve an optimal biochemical response. For these patients, the concept of triple therapy (UCDA, OCA, and a fibrate) has emerged and a limited number of studies reported their effects (**Table 4**). In a multicenter, retrospective study of 58 patients with PBC treated with UDCA and either OCA or fibrate who had not had a complete biochemical response, the addition of either OCA or a fibrate, regardless of sequence, was associated with a 3-fold increase in likelihood of ALP normalization, although fibrates as the third-line therapy had a greater effect on ALP reduction than OCA.[82] An international phase 2 study of OCA and bezafibrate is ongoing. Continued study of this approach in patients with PBC refractory to dual therapy is clearly needed before evidence-based guidance can be given on triple therapy.

IMMUNOSUPPRESSANT AGENTS

Despite the vast literature supporting the concept of PBC as an autoimmune disease, immunosuppressive agents have failed to find a role for them in the treatment of PBC, except in cases of PBC/AIH overlap in which AIH component is treated the same as AIH without PBC. The reason for this lack of efficacy is unclear but may be due to the predominance of bile acid-mediated injury once bile duct injury occurs or ongoing immune activation by the environmental or autoantigen that is resistant to immunosuppressants studied to date.

Corticosteroids, including budesonide and prednisone, have been trialed in patients who do not sufficiently improve on UDCA monotherapy. [83] Two prospective randomized controlled studies have shown budesonide to be associated with improvements in liver chemistries and liver histology,[84,85] whereas a third open label study found a nonstatistically significant worsening of the Mayo score in patients receiving budesonide.[86] Adverse effects including adrenal insufficiency and decreased bone mineral density[86] are of concern, and thus, budesonide is not recommended for the treatment of PBC in the absence of AIH. A single-center, open-label trial of abatacept for 6 months in 19 patients demonstrated lack of biochemical response and no significant improvements in symptoms.[87] Other immunosuppressants, including mycophenolate mofetil,[88,89] azathioprine,[90–92] and the B-cell depleting monoclonal antibody rituximab,[93,94] have failed to demonstrate efficacy in patients with PBC. Newer approaches to induce tolerance to the antimitochondrial antigen with nanoparticles similar to that being used in celiac disease are being undertaken.[95]

TREATMENT OF ASSOCIATED CONDITIONS
Hyperlipidemia

Hypercholesterolemia is found in 75% to 95% of patients with PBC, although the clinical significance of this finding is uncertain.[96] Statin therapy is recommended for patients with PBC with hyperlipidemia and known risk factors for atherosclerotic disease. Several studies have demonstrated the safety and efficacy of statin therapy in PBC.[97–101] The effects of OCA on lipids, including increases in total cholesterol and low-density lipoprotein and decreases in high-density lipoprotein, have been observed with the treatment of PBC as well as nonalcoholic fatty liver disease but the clinical significance remains unknown. Fibrates and other peroxisome proliferator-activated receptor -agonists have beneficial effects on lipid profiles.

Table 4
Studies of Triple Therapy (ursodeoxycholic acid, obeticholic acid, and fibrate) for Primary Biliary Cholangitis

Author, Year	Study Design	Inclusion Criteria	Duration	Number of Patients	Main Result
D'amato et al,[109] 2019	Proof of concept, retrospective cohort study	Patients with PBC treated with triple-therapy of UDCA, OCA, and fibrates for at least 3 mo	3–6 mo	11	Median reduction of 29% in ALP and 3% in bilirubin; one patient discontinued due to abnormal transaminases
Soret et al,[82] 2021	Retrospective, uncontrolled	Patients with PBC treated with dual-therapy UDCA and OCA or UDCA and fibrates for at least 3 mo	3 mo	58 (29 OCA-fibrate and 29 fibrate-OCA)	Greater decrease in ALP, AST, ALT, GGT compared with dual therapy

Fatigue

Fatigue is a common symptom of PBC, although its pathogenesis is not well understood. Some of the mechanisms for fatigue in PBC including abnormalities in cerebral structures, impaired autonomic nervous system, and increased interleukin 6 have been hypothesized.[102] Fatigue in PBC has been proposed to be classified into 3 subgroups: minimal or no fatigue, fatigue associated without cognitive symptoms, and fatigue associated with significant cognitive symptoms.[103] Several interventions have been investigated for fatigue in patients with PBC. An open label study of modafinil in 21 patients with PBC reported significant improvement in fatigue scores measured by Epworth Sleepiness Scale and PBC-40 fatigue domain.[104] However, a placebo-controlled trial of modafinil did not significantly improve fatigue measured by Fisk Fatigue Impact Score.[105] An ambitious randomized trial of B-cell depletion with rituximab failed to significantly reduce fatigue.[106] A pilot study of home-based exercise in 25 patients with PBC found fatigue was significantly improved by individualized exercise programs, making this an attractive and safe approach for many patients.[107]

SUMMARY

All patients with PBC should be treated with UDCA at 13 to 15 mg/kg/d and monitored for a biochemical response using any of the available criteria and considering the disease stage. If there is an incomplete response to UDCA, then second-line therapies should be considered, namely OCA. If OCA is not tolerated or otherwise contraindicated, growing evidence supports the use of bezafibrate but its safety and dosing has not been firmly established and it is not available in the United States at this time. Data supporting the use of fenofibrate is limited but likely of similar efficacy. Importantly, the use of OCA or fibrates in advanced or decompensated cirrhosis should be avoided. For the small number of patients intolerant of UDCA, these second-line agents may also be considered. For those patients still not achieving an adequate response to dual therapy, triple therapy may have a benefit but further studies are required.

CLINICS CARE POINTS

- All patients with PBC should be monitored for a complete biochemical response after 12 months of treatment with UDCA.
- Patient with PBC who do not have a complete biochemical response to UDCA or who are intolerant to UDCA should be considered for second line treatments.

DISCLOSURE

C.L. Bowlus discloses grant funding from Intercept Pharmaceuticals, Bristol Myers Squibb, Cymabay, Gilead Biosciences, GlaxoSmithKline, Shire Pharmaceuticals, Takeda Pharmaceuticals, NGM Biosciences, and TARGET Pharmasolutions and service on advisory boards for Intercept Pharmaceuticals, Bristol Myers Squibb, GlaxoSmithKline, and Conatus; and speakers' bureau for Intercept Pharmaceuticals. GlaxoSmithKline, and Conatus; and speakers' bureau for Intercept Pharmaceuticals.

REFERENCES

1. Selmi C, Bowlus CL, Gershwin ME, et al. Primary biliary cirrhosis. Lancet 2011; 377(9777):1600–9.

2. European Association for the Study of the Liver. Electronic address eee, European Association for the Study of the L. EASL Clinical Practice Guidelines: the diagnosis and management of patients with primary biliary cholangitis. J Hepatol 2017;67(1):145–72.

3. Lindor KD, Bowlus CL, Boyer J, et al. Primary biliary cholangitis: 2021 practice guidance update from the American Association for the Study of Liver Diseases. Hepatology 2022 Apr;75(4):1012–3.

4. Siddique A, Kowdley KV. Approach to a patient with elevated serum alkaline phosphatase. Clin Liver Dis 2012;16(2):199–229.

5. Carey EJ, Ali AH, Lindor KD. Primary biliary cirrhosis. Lancet 2015;386(10003): 1565–75.

6. Chazouilleres O, Wendum D, Serfaty L, et al. Primary biliary cirrhosis-autoimmune hepatitis overlap syndrome: clinical features and response to therapy. Hepatology 1998;28(2):296–301.

7. Heurgue A, Vitry F, Diebold MD, et al. Overlap syndrome of primary biliary cirrhosis and autoimmune hepatitis: a retrospective study of 115 cases of autoimmune liver disease. Gastroenterol Clin Biol 2007;31(1):17–25.

8. Silveira MG, Talwalkar JA, Angulo P, et al. Overlap of autoimmune hepatitis and primary biliary cirrhosis: long-term outcomes. Am J Gastroenterol 2007;102(6): 1244–50.

9. Locke GR 3rd, Therneau TM, Ludwig J, et al. Time course of histological progression in primary biliary cirrhosis. Hepatology 1996;23(1):52–6.

10. Roll J, Boyer JL, Barry D, et al. The prognostic importance of clinical and histologic features in asymptomatic and symptomatic primary biliary cirrhosis. N Engl J Med 1983;308(1):1–7.

11. Poupon R. Ursodeoxycholic acid and bile-acid mimetics as therapeutic agents for cholestatic liver diseases: an overview of their mechanisms of action. Clin Res Hepatol Gastroenterol 2012;36(Suppl 1):S3–12.

12. Rudic JS, Poropat G, Krstic MN, et al. Ursodeoxycholic acid for primary biliary cirrhosis. Cochrane Database Syst Rev 2012;12:CD000551.

13. Poupon R, Chretien Y, Poupon RE, et al. Is ursodeoxycholic acid an effective treatment for primary biliary cirrhosis? Lancet 1987;1(8537):834–6.

14. Poupon RE, Balkau B, Eschwege E, et al. A multicenter, controlled trial of ursodiol for the treatment of primary biliary cirrhosis. UDCA-PBC Study Group. N Engl J Med 1991;324(22):1548–54.

15. Poupon RE, Poupon R, Balkau B. Ursodiol for the long-term treatment of primary biliary cirrhosis. The UDCA-PBC Study Group. N Engl J Med 1994;330(19): 1342–7.

16. Heathcote EJ, Cauch-Dudek K, Walker V, et al. The Canadian Multicenter Double-blind Randomized Controlled Trial of ursodeoxycholic acid in primary biliary cirrhosis. Hepatology 1994;19(5):1149–56.

17. Pares A, Caballeria L, Rodes J, et al. Long-term effects of ursodeoxycholic acid in primary biliary cirrhosis: results of a double-blind controlled multicentric trial. UDCA-Cooperative Group from the Spanish Association for the Study of the Liver. J Hepatol 2000;32(4):561–6.

18. Combes B, Carithers RL Jr, Maddrey WC, et al. A randomized, double-blind, placebo-controlled trial of ursodeoxycholic acid in primary biliary cirrhosis. Hepatology 1995;22(3):759–66.

19. Lindor KD, Dickson ER, Baldus WP, et al. Ursodeoxycholic acid in the treatment of primary biliary cirrhosis. Gastroenterology 1994;106(5):1284–90.

20. Poupon RE, Lindor KD, Pares A, et al. Combined analysis of the effect of treatment with ursodeoxycholic acid on histologic progression in primary biliary cirrhosis. J Hepatol 2003;39(1):12–6.

21. Harms MH, van Buuren HR, Corpechot C, et al. Ursodeoxycholic acid therapy and liver transplant-free survival in patients with primary biliary cholangitis. J Hepatol 2019;71(2):357–65.

22. Corpechot C, Carrat F, Bonnand AM, et al. The effect of ursodeoxycholic acid therapy on liver fibrosis progression in primary biliary cirrhosis. Hepatology 2000;32(6):1196–9.

23. Xiang X, Yang X, Shen M, et al. Ursodeoxycholic acid at 18-22 mg/kg/d showed a promising capacity for treating refractory primary biliary cholangitis. Can J Gastroenterol Hepatol 2021;2021:6691425.

24. Harms MH, de Veer RC, Lammers WJ, et al. Number needed to treat with ursodeoxycholic acid therapy to prevent liver transplantation or death in primary biliary cholangitis. Gut 2020;69(8):1502–9.

25. Hempfling W, Dilger K, Beuers U. Systematic review: ursodeoxycholic acid–adverse effects and drug interactions. Aliment Pharmacol Ther 2003;18(10): 963–72.

26. Angulo P, Batts KP, Therneau TM, et al. Long-term ursodeoxycholic acid delays histological progression in primary biliary cirrhosis. Hepatology 1999;29(3): 644–7.

27. Kuiper EM, Hansen BE, Metselaar HJ, et al. Trends in liver transplantation for primary biliary cirrhosis in The Netherlands 1988-2008. BMC Gastroenterol 2010; 10:144.

28. Lee J, Belanger A, Doucette JT, et al. Transplantation trends in primary biliary cirrhosis. Clin Gastroenterol Hepatol 2007;5(11):1313–5.

29. Pares A, Caballeria L, Rodes J. Excellent long-term survival in patients with primary biliary cirrhosis and biochemical response to ursodeoxycholic Acid. Gastroenterology 2006;130(3):715–20.

30. Lammers WJ, Hirschfield GM, Corpechot C, et al. Development and validation of a scoring system to predict outcomes of patients with primary biliary cirrhosis receiving ursodeoxycholic acid therapy. Gastroenterology 2015;149(7): 1804–1812 e1804.

31. Carbone M, Sharp SJ, Flack S, et al. The UK-PBC risk scores: Derivation and validation of a scoring system for long-term prediction of end-stage liver disease in primary biliary cholangitis. Hepatology 2016;63(3):930–50.

32. Osman KT, Maselli DB, Idilman IS, et al. Liver stiffness measured by either magnetic resonance or transient elastography is associated with liver fibrosis and is an independent predictor of outcomes among patients with primary biliary cholangitis. J Clin Gastroenterol 2021;55(5):449–57.

33. Murillo Perez CF, Hirschfield GM, Corpechot C, et al. Fibrosis stage is an independent predictor of outcome in primary biliary cholangitis despite biochemical treatment response. Aliment Pharmacol Ther 2019;50(10):1127–36.

34. Lammers WJ, van Buuren HR, Hirschfield GM, et al. Levels of alkaline phosphatase and bilirubin are surrogate end points of outcomes of patients with primary biliary cirrhosis: an international follow-up study. Gastroenterology 2014;147(6): 1338–49.e1335 [quiz: e1315].

35. Fiorucci S, Antonelli E, Rizzo G, et al. The nuclear receptor SHP mediates inhibition of hepatic stellate cells by FXR and protects against liver fibrosis. Gastroenterology 2004;127(5):1497–512.

36. Fiorucci S, Rizzo G, Antonelli E, et al. Cross-talk between farnesoid-X-receptor (FXR) and peroxisome proliferator-activated receptor gamma contributes to the antifibrotic activity of FXR ligands in rodent models of liver cirrhosis. J Pharmacol Exp Ther 2005;315(1):58–68.

37. Verbeke L, Farre R, Trebicka J, et al. Obeticholic acid, a farnesoid X receptor agonist, improves portal hypertension by two distinct pathways in cirrhotic rats. Hepatology 2014;59(6):2286–98.

38. Kowdley KV, Luketic V, Chapman R, et al. A randomized trial of obeticholic acid monotherapy in patients with primary biliary cholangitis. Hepatology 2017;67(5):1890–902.

39. Hirschfield GM, Mason A, Luketic V, et al. Efficacy of obeticholic acid in patients with primary biliary cirrhosis and inadequate response to ursodeoxycholic acid. Gastroenterology 2015;148(4):751–61, e758.

40. Nevens F, Andreone P, Mazzella G, et al. A placebo-controlled trial of obeticholic acid in primary biliary cholangitis. N Engl J Med 2016;375(7):631–43.

41. Harms MH, Hirschfield GM, Floreani A, et al. Obeticholic acid is associated with improvements in AST-to-platelet ratio index and GLOBE score in patients with primary biliary cholangitis. JHEP Rep 2021;3(1):100191.

42. Trauner M, Nevens F, Shiffman ML, et al. Long-term efficacy and safety of obeticholic acid for patients with primary biliary cholangitis: 3-year results of an international open-label extension study. Lancet Gastroenterol Hepatol 2019;4(6):445–53.

43. Bowlus CL, Pockros PJ, Kremer AE, et al. Long-term obeticholic acid therapy improves histological endpoints in patients with primary biliary cholangitis. Clin Gastroenterol Hepatol 2020;18(5):1170–8, e1176.

44. Roberts SB, Ismail M, Kanagalingam G, et al. Real-world effectiveness of obeticholic acid in patients with primary biliary cholangitis. Hepatol Commun 2020;4(9):1332–45.

45. D'Amato D, De Vincentis A, Malinverno F, et al. Real-world experience with obeticholic acid in patients with primary biliary cholangitis. JHEP Rep 2021;3(2):100248.

46. Eaton JE, Vuppalanchi R, Reddy R, et al. Liver injury in patients with cholestatic liver disease treated with obeticholic acid. Hepatology (Baltimore, Md) 2020;71(4):1511–4.

47. Suraweera D, Rahal H, Jimenez M, et al. Treatment of primary biliary cholangitis ursodeoxycholic acid non-responders: a systematic review. Liver Int 2017 Dec;37(12):1877–86.

48. Hegade VS, Khanna A, Walker LJ, et al. Long-term fenofibrate treatment in primary biliary cholangitis improves biochemistry but Not the UK-PBC Risk Score. Dig Dis Sci 2016;61(10):3037–44.

49. Han XF, Wang QX, Liu Y, et al. Efficacy of fenofibrate in Chinese patients with primary biliary cirrhosis partially responding to ursodeoxycholic acid therapy. J Dig Dis 2012;13(4):219–24.

50. Levy C, Peter JA, Nelson DR, et al. Pilot study: fenofibrate for patients with primary biliary cirrhosis and an incomplete response to ursodeoxycholic acid. Aliment Pharmacol Ther 2011;33(2):235–42.

51. Lens S, Leoz M, Nazal L, et al. Bezafibrate normalizes alkaline phosphatase in primary biliary cirrhosis patients with incomplete response to ursodeoxycholic acid. Liver Int 2014;34(2):197–203.

52. Iwasaki S, Ohira H, Nishiguchi S, et al. The efficacy of ursodeoxycholic acid and bezafibrate combination therapy for primary biliary cirrhosis: a prospective, multicenter study. Hepatol Res 2008;38(6):557–64.

53. Kita R, Takamatsu S, Kimura T, et al. Bezafibrate may attenuate biliary damage associated with chronic liver diseases accompanied by high serum biliary enzyme levels. J Gastroenterol 2006;41(7):686–92.

54. Kanda T, Yokosuka O, Imazeki F, et al. Bezafibrate treatment: a new medical approach for PBC patients? J Gastroenterol 2003;38(6):573–8.

55. Kurihara T, Niimi A, Maeda A, et al. Bezafibrate in the treatment of primary biliary cirrhosis: comparison with ursodeoxycholic acid. Am J Gastroenterol 2000; 95(10):2990–2.

56. Nakai S, Masaki T, Kurokohchi K, et al. Combination therapy of bezafibrate and ursodeoxycholic acid in primary biliary cirrhosis: a preliminary study. Am J Gastroenterol 2000;95(1):326–7.

57. Reig A, Sese P, Pares A. Effects of bezafibrate on outcome and pruritus in primary biliary cholangitis with suboptimal ursodeoxycholic acid response. Am J Gastroenterol 2018 Jan;113(1):49–55.

58. Honda A, Ikegami T, Nakamuta M, et al. Anticholestatic effects of bezafibrate in patients with primary biliary cirrhosis treated with ursodeoxycholic acid. Hepatology 2013;57(5):1931–41.

59. Takeuchi Y, Ikeda F, Fujioka S, et al. Additive improvement induced by bezafibrate in patients with primary biliary cirrhosis showing refractory response to ursodeoxycholic acid. J Gastroenterol Hepatol 2011;26(9):1395–401.

60. Hazzan R, Tur-Kaspa R. Bezafibrate treatment of primary biliary cirrhosis following incomplete response to ursodeoxycholic acid. J Clin Gastroenterol 2010;44(5):371–3.

61. Liberopoulos EN, Florentin M, Elisaf MS, et al. Fenofibrate in primary biliary cirrhosis: a pilot study. Open Cardiovasc Med J 2010;4:120–6.

62. Walker LJ, Newton J, Jones DE, et al. Comment on biochemical response to ursodeoxycholic acid and long-term prognosis in primary biliary cirrhosis. Hepatology 2009;49(1):337–8 [author reply: 338].

63. Ohmoto K, Yoshioka N, Yamamoto S. Long-term effect of bezafibrate on parameters of hepatic fibrosis in primary biliary cirrhosis. J Gastroenterol 2006;41(5): 502–3.

64. Nakamuta M, Enjoji M, Kotoh K, et al. Long-term fibrate treatment for PBC. J Gastroenterol 2005;40(5):546–7.

65. Akbar SM, Furukawa S, Nakanishi S, et al. Therapeutic efficacy of decreased nitrite production by bezafibrate in patients with primary biliary cirrhosis. J Gastroenterol 2005;40(2):157–63.

66. Itakura J, Izumi N, Nishimura Y, et al. Prospective randomized crossover trial of combination therapy with bezafibrate and UDCA for primary biliary cirrhosis. Hepatol Res 2004;29(4):216–22.

67. Dohmen K, Mizuta T, Nakamuta M, et al. Fenofibrate for patients with asymptomatic primary biliary cirrhosis. World J Gastroenterol 2004;10(6):894–8.

68. Ohira H, Sato Y, Ueno T, et al. Fenofibrate treatment in patients with primary biliary cirrhosis. Am J Gastroenterol 2002;97(8):2147–9.

69. Yano K, Kato H, Morita S, et al. Is bezafibrate histologically effective for primary biliary cirrhosis? Am J Gastroenterol 2002;97(4):1075–7.

70. Kurihara T, Maeda A, Shigemoto M, et al. Investigation into the efficacy of bezafibrate against primary biliary cirrhosis, with histological references from cases receiving long term monotherapy. Am J Gastroenterol 2002;97(1):212–4.

71. Miyaguchi S, Ebinuma H, Imaeda H, et al. A novel treatment for refractory primary biliary cirrhosis? Hepatogastroenterology 2000;47(36):1518–21.

72. Zhang Y, Chen K, Dai W, et al. Combination therapy of bezafibrate and ursodeoxycholic acid for primary biliary cirrhosis: a meta-analysis. Hepatol Res 2015;45(1):48–58.

73. Zhang Y, Li S, He L, et al. Combination therapy of fenofibrate and ursodeoxycholic acid in patients with primary biliary cirrhosis who respond incompletely to UDCA monotherapy: a meta-analysis. Drug Des Devel Ther 2015;9:2757–66.

74. Carrion AF, Lindor KD, Levy C. Safety of fibrates in cholestatic liver diseases. Liver Int 2021;41(6):1335–43.

75. Rudic JS, Poropat G, Krstic MN, et al. Bezafibrate for primary biliary cirrhosis. Cochrane Database Syst Rev 2012;1:CD009145.

76. Tanaka A, Hirohara J, Nakano T, et al. Association of bezafibrate with transplant-free survival in patients with primary biliary cholangitis. J Hepatol 2021;75(3): 565–71.

77. Corpechot C, Chazouillères O, Rousseau A, et al. A placebo-controlled trial of bezafibrate in primary biliary cholangitis. New Engl J Med 2018;378(23): 2171–81.

78. Corpechot C, CO, Rousseau D, et al. A 2-year multicenter, double-blind, randomized, placebo-controlled study of bezafibrate for the treatment of primary biliary cholangitis in patients with inadequate biochemical response to ursodeoxycholic acid therapy (Bezurso). J Hepatol 2017;66(1):S89.

79. de Vries E, Bolier R, Goet J, et al. Fibrates for itch (FITCH) in fibrosing cholangiopathies: a double-blind, randomized, placebo-controlled trial. Gastroenterology 2021;160(3):734–43, e736.

80. Davidson MH, Armani A, McKenney JM, et al. Safety considerations with fibrate therapy. Am J Cardiol 2007;99(6A):3C–18C.

81. Lindor KD, Bowlus CL, Boyer J, et al. Primary biliary cholangitis: 2018 practice guidance from the American association for the study of liver diseases. Clin Liver Dis (Hoboken) 2020;15(1):1–2.

82. Soret PA, Lam L, Carrat F, et al. Combination of fibrates with obeticholic acid is able to normalise biochemical liver tests in patients with difficult-to-treat primary biliary cholangitis. Aliment Pharmacol Ther 2021;53(10):1138–46.

83. Mitchison HC, Bassendine MF, Malcolm AJ, et al. A pilot, double-blind, controlled 1-year trial of prednisolone treatment in primary biliary cirrhosis: hepatic improvement but greater bone loss. Hepatology 1989;10(4):420–9.

84. Leuschner M, Maier KP, Schlichting J, et al. Oral budesonide and ursodeoxycholic acid for treatment of primary biliary cirrhosis: results of a prospective double-blind trial. Gastroenterology 1999;117(4):918–25.

85. Rautiainen H, Karkkainen P, Karvonen AL, et al. Budesonide combined with UDCA to improve liver histology in primary biliary cirrhosis: a three-year randomized trial. Hepatology 2005;41(4):747–52.

86. Angulo P, Jorgensen RA, Keach JC, et al. Oral budesonide in the treatment of patients with primary biliary cirrhosis with a suboptimal response to ursodeoxycholic acid. Hepatology 2000;31(2):318–23.

87. Bowlus CL, Yang GX, Liu CH, et al. Therapeutic trials of biologics in primary biliary cholangitis: an open label study of abatacept and review of the literature. J Autoimmun 2019;101:26–34.

88. Talwalkar JA, Angulo P, Keach JC, et al. Mycophenolate mofetil for the treatment of primary biliary cirrhosis in patients with an incomplete response to ursodeoxycholic acid. J Clin Gastroenterol 2005;39(2):168–71.

89. Rabahi N, Chretien Y, Gaouar F, et al. Triple therapy with ursodeoxycholic acid, budesonide and mycophenolate mofetil in patients with features of severe primary biliary cirrhosis not responding to ursodeoxycholic acid alone. Gastroenterol Clin Biol 2010;34(4–5):283–7.

90. Gong Y, Christensen E, Gluud C. Azathioprine for primary biliary cirrhosis. Cochrane Database Syst Rev 2007;3:CD006000.

91. Heathcote J, Ross A, Sherlock S. A prospective controlled trial of azathioprine in primary biliary cirrhosis. Gastroenterology 1976;70(5 PT.1):656–60.

92. Christensen E, Altman DG, Neuberger J, et al. Updating prognosis in primary biliary cirrhosis using a time-dependent Cox regression model. PBC1 and PBC2 trial groups. Gastroenterology 1993;105(6):1865–76.

93. Myers RP, Swain MG, Lee SS, et al. B-cell depletion with rituximab in patients with primary biliary cirrhosis refractory to ursodeoxycholic acid. Am J Gastroenterol 2013;108(6):933–41.

94. Tsuda M, Moritoki Y, Lian ZX, et al. Biochemical and immunologic effects of rituximab in patients with primary biliary cirrhosis and an incomplete response to ursodeoxycholic acid. Hepatology 2012;55(2):512–21.

95. Kelly CP, Murray JA, Leffler DA, et al. TAK-101 Nanoparticles Induce Gluten-specific tolerance in celiac disease: a randomized, double-blind, placebo-controlled study. Gastroenterology 2021;161(1):66–80 e68.

96. Longo M, Crosignani A, Battezzati PM, et al. Hyperlipidaemic state and cardiovascular risk in primary biliary cirrhosis. Gut 2002;51(2):265–9.

97. Stanca CM, Bach N, Allina J, et al. Atorvastatin does not improve liver biochemistries or Mayo Risk Score in primary biliary cirrhosis. Dig Dis Sci 2008;53(7):1988–93.

98. Stojakovic T, Putz-Bankuti C, Fauler G, et al. Atorvastatin in patients with primary biliary cirrhosis and incomplete biochemical response to ursodeoxycholic acid. Hepatology 2007;46(3):776–84.

99. Ritzel U, Leonhardt U, Nather M, et al. Simvastatin in primary biliary cirrhosis: effects on serum lipids and distinct disease markers. J Hepatol 2002;36(4):454–8.

100. Abu Rajab M, Kaplan MM. Statins in primary biliary cirrhosis: are they safe? Dig Dis Sci 2010;55(7):2086–8.

101. Cash WJ, O'Neill S, O'Donnell ME, et al. Randomized controlled trial assessing the effect of simvastatin in primary biliary cirrhosis. Liver Int 2013;33(8):1166–74.

102. Abbas G, Jorgensen RA, Lindor KD. Fatigue in primary biliary cirrhosis. Nat Rev Gastroenterol Hepatol 2010;7(6):313–9.

103. Phaw NA, Dyson JK, Mells G, et al. Understanding fatigue in primary biliary cholangitis. Dig Dis Sci 2021;66(7):2380–6.

104. Jones DEJ, Newton JL. An open study of modafinil for the treatment of daytime somnolence and fatigue in primary biliary cirrhosis. Aliment Pharmacol Ther 2007;25(4):471–6.

105. Silveira MG, Gossard AA, Stahler AC, et al. A randomized, placebo-controlled clinical trial of efficacy and safety: modafinil in the treatment of fatigue in patients with primary biliary cirrhosis. Am J Ther 2017;24(2):e167–76.

106. Khanna A, Jopson L, Howel D, et al. Rituximab for the treatment of fatigue in primary biliary cholangitis (formerly primary biliary cirrhosis): a randomised controlled trial. Efficacy mechanism Eval 2018;5(2):1–78.

107. Freer A, Williams F, Durman S, et al. Home-based exercise in patients with refractory fatigue associated with primary biliary cholangitis: a protocol for the

EXerCise Intervention in cholesTatic LivEr Disease (EXCITED) feasibility trial. BMJ Open Gastroenterol 2021;8(1).

108. Poupon RE, Lindor KD, Cauch-Dudek K, et al. Combined analysis of randomized controlled trials of ursodeoxycholic acid in primary biliary cirrhosis. Gastroenterology 1997;113(3):884–90.

109. D'Amato D, O'Donnell SE, Cazzagon N, et al. Additive beneficial effects of Fibrates combined with Obeticholic acid in the treatment of patients with Primary Biliary Cholangitis and inadequate response to second-line therapy: data from the Italian PBC Study Group. Dig Liver Dis 2020;52:e32.

Evaluation and Management of Pruritus in Primary Biliary Cholangitis

Miriam M. Düll, MD[a], Andreas E. Kremer, MD, PhD, MHBA[b],*

KEYWORDS

- Bezafibrate • Gabapentinoids • IBAT • Opioid receptors • Therapy • UVB

KEY POINTS

- Pruritus affects 2 out of 3 patients with PBC during their course of disease. Moderate to severe itch intensity may dramatically reduce their quality of life.
- Greater awareness of pruritus among physicians is needed to achieve the best possible treatment and symptom control.
- Other pruritic factors besides the underlying hepatobiliary disease should always be excluded.
- Treatment consists of optimal topical and—if necessary—systemic therapies such as cholestyramine, rifampicin, bezafibrate, naltrexone, sertraline, and gabapentin.
- Therapy refractory patients should be included in ongoing clinical trials or treated with ultraviolet B or invasive approaches such as albumin dialysis or biliary drainage.

INTRODUCTION

Primary biliary cholangitis (PBC) is an immune-mediated disease of the hepatobiliary system that leads to the destruction of small bile ducts, resulting in chronic intrahepatic cholestasis.[1] Laboratory chemistry is dominated by a cholestatic profile with elevated alkaline phosphatase, serum bile acids, and potentially bilirubin as a late progression marker of the disease. In PBC, intrahepatic cholestasis, which might be caused on both the hepatocellular and cholangiocellular level, is frequently associated with chronic pruritus, fatigue, sicca syndrome, arthralgia, and abdominal discomfort.[2]

[a] Department of Medicine 1, Gastroenterology, Hepatology, Pneumology, Endocrinology, University Hospital Erlangen and Friedrich-Alexander-University Erlangen-Nürnberg, Erlangen, Ulmenweg 18, 91054 Erlangen, Germany; [b] Department of Gastroenterology and Hepatology, Universitäts Spital Zürich, Rämistrasse 100, 8091 Zürich, Switzerland
* Corresponding author.
E-mail address: andreas.kremer@usz.ch

Clin Liver Dis 26 (2022) 727–745
https://doi.org/10.1016/j.cld.2022.06.009
liver.theclinics.com
1089-3261/22/© 2022 The Authors. Published by Elsevier Inc. This is an open access article under the CC BY license (http://creativecommons.org/licenses/by/4.0/).

Itch sensations lasting over 6 weeks are classified as chronic pruritus, which is often present in patients with cholestatic disorders such as PBC. Chronic pruritus may seriously reduce quality of life in these patients.[3] In particular, moderate to severe nighttime itch causes sleep deprivation, exhaustion, and significantly worsens fatigue. These factors ultimately favor the development of depression and even suicidal ideas.[4]

In addition to its unpleasant character, itching can represent a challenging symptom of PBC and is typically unresponsive to commonly applied antipruritic medication such as antihistamines.[5] Fortunately, novel therapeutic approaches for the treatment of pruritus as a symptom of PBC have been established in recent years. Nevertheless, most of these options are applied in an off-label manner or administered as part of clinical trials, of which the latter is hoped to result in more effective and approved drug treatments.[6]

This review summarizes the clinical picture, diagnostic approach, and current treatment options of pruritus in the context of PBC and provides an outlook on potential future therapeutic approaches.

CLINICAL PICTURE OF PRURITUS IN PRIMARY BILIARY CHOLANGITIS

Itching due to PBC typically affects the extremities, often involving the palms and soles.[7] However, pruritus may also be present on other body parts or is generalized in a significant number of patients. Pruritus can arise at any stage of PBC, independent of severity of cholestasis or medical interventions. Itching may present as the first symptom of PBC and sometimes precede the diagnosis for months to even years, as so-called premonitory pruritus. One study suggested that 75% of patients report pruritus preceding the diagnosis of PBC.[8] Other data reported that a substantial number of PBC patients develop pruritus after an initial asymptomatic period, with approximately 30% reporting about pruritus onset after 5 years and almost 50% after 10 years of follow-up.[9] On the other hand, in advanced stages of PBC including progression to liver cirrhosis, itching may reduce in intensity or even vanish completely despite ongoing severe cholestasis.[10] Recently, the authors' group underlined the lack of correlation between intensity of laboratory cholestasis markers, opioid metabolites, and itch intensity in patients with cholestatic liver diseases such as PBC and primary sclerosing cholangitis (PSC).[11] Although the severity of symptoms does not correlate with stage of disease in PBC, severe pruritus can point to an aggressive, ductopenic variant, which is associated with poorer prognosis.[12] Itching can become intractable, especially if resistant to currently available treatment options; therefore, it can be considered as an indication for liver transplantation, even without the presence of advanced reduction of liver function.[13] Similar to other conditions associated with chronic pruritus, itching in PBC often follows a circadian rhythm, with the highest intensity reported in the evening or late at night. A study objectively surveyed scratching activity in patients with PBC with a vibration transducer, consisting of a square piezoelectric film taped to one fingernails.[14,15] Patients scratched most intensely in the late afternoon and early evening hours; this is at least partly in accordance with other forms of chronic pruritus, which often aggravate at night, possibly due to limited sensory input and warmth in bed. Female patients particularly report about more severe intensity of pruritus during times of hormonal changes such as in the luteal phase of the menstrual cycle, in the third trimester of pregnancy, or during hormonal replacement therapy.[16] This observation points to female sex hormones as potential contributing factors in the pathophysiology of cholestatic pruritus.

EPIDEMIOLOGY OF PRURITUS IN PRIMARY BILIARY CHOLANGITIS

Data on the epidemiology of chronic pruritus in systemic diseases is still scarce. In recent years, however, more information on pruritus in patients with PBC has become available, especially through national cohort data.[17,18] Earlier research estimated a lifetime prevalence of pruritus in 70% to 80% in patients with cholestatic liver disorders, particularly in PBC.[7,19,20] The UK-PBC study group recently presented supporting data by evaluating 2194 PBC patients, of whom 73.5% experienced pruritus during their course of disease; 34.5% of patients with PBC stated persistent pruritus, with 11.7% reporting severe intensity of pruritus.[18] In an online survey of 577 patients with PBC in Germany, the authors' own group reported a point prevalence of 56% of pruritus lasting for more than 6 weeks. Around 70% of affected patients even indicated that they suffered from pruritus for many years.[21] Another study suggested that pruritus intensity might be associated with younger age at the time of the PBC diagnosis.[22] So far, no specific environmental influences including geographic or dietary factors could be associated with the presence or onset of pruritus in patients with PBC.

PATHOGENESIS OF PRURITUS IN PRIMARY BILIARY CHOLANGITIS

During the last decades, the molecular mechanisms of itch signaling have been subject to intensive research with a focus on in vitro and in vivo experiments in cellular and animal models.[23] This research discovered novel pruritogens, their receptors, and potential signaling pathways in acute and chronic itch.[24] The underlying causes of chronic pruritus in human, especially in patients with systemic diseases such as PBC, however, remain only partially understood. For hepatic pruritus, previous basic research, observations in clinical studies, and positive response of patients to certain treatments have identified several possible contributing factors (for detailed overview of potential signaling pathways see **Fig. 1**)[5,25,26]:

- Presence of cholephilic pruritogens in the enterohepatic circulation
  - Removal of bile contents improves pruritus in chronic cholestatic disorders such as PBC
    - by oral medication (anion exchange resins or inhibitors of the ileal bile acid transporter [IBAT]) or mechanically by (naso)biliary drainage.
  - Certain bile acid subspecies and potentially bilirubin activate the Mas-related G protein–coupled receptor family X4 (MRGPRX4),[27–30] which is expressed in a subset of small-diameter sensory neurons, particularly mediating itch-related signals with a major role in nonhistaminergic itch.[31]
  - The semisynthetic bile acid and selective farnesoid X receptor agonist obeticholic acid (OCA), licensed as second-line treatment in PBC, can induce and/or intensify pruritus.[32,33]
- Formation, biotransformation, and/or secretion of potential pruritogens in the liver and/or the gut
  - Effective treatment of hepatic pruritus with rifampicin, an inducer of hepatic biotransformation and pregnane X receptor (PXR) agonist,[34] and bezafibrate, a peroxisome-proliferator activated receptor (PPAR) agonist.[35]
- Influence of potential pruritogens on endogenous opioidergic and serotoninergic systems
  - Mild antipruritic effect in cholestatic pruritus of μ-opioid antagonists (eg, naltrexone), k-opioid agonists (eg, nalfurafine), and selective serotonin reuptake inhibitors (SSRIs) (eg, sertraline).

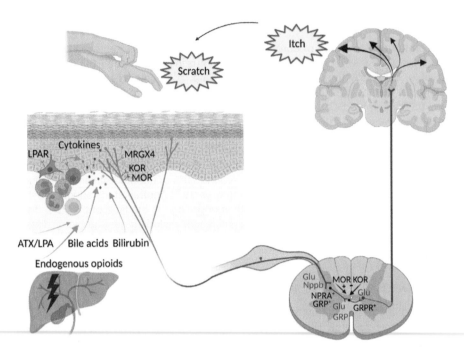

Fig. 1. Potential peripheral and central mediators and pathways of pruritus in cholestatic liver diseases such as PBC. Figure created with BioRender.com.

- o A rodent-based model with surgically induced cholestasis and a small number of patients with cholestatic PBC displayed systemically elevated opioid levels[36–39] and upregulation of opioid markers in liver tissue.[36,40,41]
- Presence of potential pruritogens in the systemic circulation
  - o Hepatic pruritus can be ameliorated by treatment with plasmapheresis, plasma separation, albumin dialysis, and anion absorption.[25]
  - o Increased concentrations of autotaxin (ATX), the enzyme hydrolyzing lyso-phosphatidic acid (LPA) from its precursor molecule lysophosphatidylcholine, were reported in sera of patients suffering from hepatic pruritus compared with nonpruritic patients with PBC and various other liver diseases. Systemic ATX activity correlated with the itch intensity in patients with PBC and other hepatobiliary diseases and decreased with successful therapeutic interventions.[42,43]

EVALUATION OF PRURITUS IN PRIMARY BILIARY CHOLANGITIS

The initial workup of a patient with PBC with pruritus should exclude other dermatologic and systemic causes such as chronic kidney disease–associated pruritus (CKDaP) and endocrine causes such as hypothyroidism, diabetes, or anemia (**Fig. 2**). Although dermatologic diseases often present with pruritic and lesional skin areas, the itchy skin of patients with PBC typically exhibits no primary efflorescences; this may change in time, as intense scratching can induce secondary skin lesions such as excoriations, lichenification, prurigo nodules, and, in case of continued skin damage, even scarring.[10,44] During the course of chronic pruritus, these secondary lesions

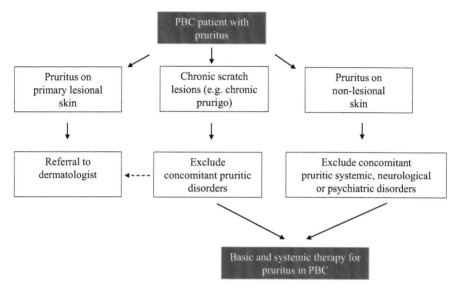

Fig. 2. Evaluation and diagnostic path of pruritus in patients with PBC.

might resemble those of primary dermatologic disorders, which can create difficulty in the differential diagnosis and treatment of pruritus (see **Fig. 2**).[25]

Because itching presents as a common and in many cases burdening symptom, the presence of pruritus should be assessed in all patients with PBC alongside other symptoms such as fatigue and arthralgia, when taking the patient's history at the time of diagnosis and throughout all follow-up visits[45] (see **Fig. 2**). Patients may not associate their itching with the underlying liver disease and will therefore not report about it without explicit enquiry by health care professionals. Consequently, patients may not receive adequate antipruritic treatment. Patients treated with OCA as a second-line drug option for PBC might also develop de-novo or intensified pruritus, which should regularly be assessed during medical follow-up visits.

If patients with PBC indicate itch sensations, it is key to collect a thorough anamnesis and clinical examination focused on properties of pruritus. The basic assessment should include intensity, time of start and time course, quality, localization, triggering, and relieving factors as well as the patient's opinion on origin and burden of pruritus.[46] Questionnaires can be helpful and timesaving tools for patients and practitioners to receive detailed self-reported information. It is also important to document other preexisting medical conditions besides PBC, as well as allergies and atopic diathesis, and to obtain a detailed list of recent drug intake including phytotherapeutics and dietary supplements. Patients with PBC, for example, often additionally suffer from hypothyroidism due to Hashimoto thyroiditis, which can add to induction of pruritus. To further evaluate the course and intensity of pruritus, patients may keep record of pruritic activity in form of a diary on paper or in a digital format, which can be assessed together with a health care professional during follow-up visits for therapeutic choices and changes.

Visual analogue scales (VAS) and numeric rating scales (NRS) are commonly used objective evaluation tools of pruritic intensity in clinical practice and studies.[47] Yet, itch sensations are intra- and interindividually very subjective, fluctuating, and remain difficult to objectify.[4] In clinical drug trials, various itch assessing tools and primary endpoints are currently applied. These different outcome variables challenge the comparability of study results, and standardized measures are warranted to increase reliability and quality of data.

The clinical examination includes inspection of the entire skin to screen for primary and secondary skin lesions including scalp and hair, nails, mucous membranes, and if indicated as itchy, the anogenital region.[46] Inspection of the patients' back is helpful to distinguish primary from secondary skin lesions. Some patients might exhibit scratch lesions with sparing of the mid-back. This so-called butterfly sign results from the inability to reach and scratch this area by hand. It is recommended to photo-document skin pathologies, to allow for comparisons throughout follow-up visits. Finally, a complete physical examination should be performed to rule out other pathologies that may be responsible for chronic pruritus.

MANAGEMENT OF PRURITUS IN PRIMARY BILIARY CHOLANGITIS
General Principles in the Management of Pruritus in Primary Biliary Cholangitis

It is important to educate patients on pruritus as a symptom of PBC and available treatment strategies depending on intensity and clinical burden. All patients should be advised on general pruritus-relieving measures for self-application[20,46]:

- Avoidance of circumstances increasing dryness and/or irritation of the skin
  - Heat (eg, sauna)
  - Very frequent washing and bathing with hot water
  - Ice packs
  - Contact of skin with possible irritants (eg, chamomile, tea-tree oil)
  - Consumption of large amounts of hot and/or spicy food, hot drinks, or alcohol
  - Tight clothing or clothes derived from animal wool
  - Use of overly scented detergents
  - Extensive rubbing of the skin after showering/bathing
  - Psychological factors, for example, stress
- Positive factors to protect the skin and decrease pruritic activity
  - Mild, nonalkaline soaps and oils for showering/bathing
  - Luke-warm water for showering or bathing, not exceeding 20 minutes
  - Mild and moisturizing topicals on the whole skin on a daily basis (eg, containing urea)
  - Topical agents with cooling and/or anesthetic effects (eg, emollients containing 1%–2% menthol or polidocanol) for pruritic skin areas
  - Soft, permeable clothes, especially cotton-based textiles
  - Shortening of fingernails to avoid severe skin damage

Psychological aspects might play a significant role, especially concerning scratching activity. Some patients could therefore benefit from relaxation techniques such as autogenic training or psychological interventions for coping with the itch-scratch circle.

Medical Treatment Options in the Management of Pruritus in Primary Biliary Cholangitis

In most cases of clinically relevant pruritus in patients with PBC, nonmedical treatment and interventions will not provide sufficient efficacy in itch reduction. Over the last decade, new treatment options for pruritus in cholestatic liver diseases have become available. Still, most currently applied therapeutic options are based on few randomized, placebo-controlled trials and cohort studies.[20] If pruritus cannot be sufficiently managed by available treatment attempts, experimental medical and interventional approaches should be taken into consideration after referral to expert centers.[48] Of note, the bile acid sequestrant cholestyramine remains the only approved drug for treating pruritus associated with cholestatic liver diseases (**Table 1**). All other drugs are applied in an "off-label" approach, on which patients have to be informed. The current EASL and AASLD guidelines include recommendations to apply a step-by-step treatment approach for pruritus in patients with PBC.[20,45,49] These recommendations can be supplemented by further therapeutic options that are presented within this review (see **Table 1**; **Table 2**). **Table 3** summarizes current clinical drug trials for pruritus in PBC.

Ursodeoxycholic acid (UDCA) remains the first-line anticholestatic treatment of PBC,[12,45] positively affecting overall and liver transplant–free survival rates. Still, UDCA does not improve pruritus, and additional medication is required.

Cholestyramine

The bile acid sequestrant and anion exchange resin cholestyramine represents the only approved and therefore guideline-recommended first-line treatment option for pruritus in hepatobiliary diseases including PBC.[45,49] In addition to bile acids, it can bind various other amphiphilic substances in the intestine, which might act as potential pruritogens.[5] Cholestyramine was effective in reducing pruritic intensity within 2 weeks in older nonplacebo-controlled trials with small patient numbers.[48] The sequestrant is most commonly applied in granular compounding with a single sachet equaling to 4 g, which is the recommended starting dosage. The intake can be increased to up to 4×4 g qd. It is important to educate patients about a 2- to 4-hour pause between the intake of cholestyramine and other medication, in particular of disease-modifying medication for PBC such as UDCA, OCA, and fibrates, to minimize risk of insufficient uptake of these drugs.[50] From clinical experience, the effect of cholestyramine on pruritic intensity is usually not sufficient to treat moderately and severely affected patients, even at higher dosages. Because of gastrointestinal adverse effects and unpalatable taste, patients are often reluctant to take cholestyramine for a longer time. In case of insufficient improvement of pruritus after 14 days of intake, we recommend to discontinue cholestyramine and to start alternative options. Interestingly, colesevelam, an anion exchange resin with a much higher adsorbing affinity to bile acids, was not superior to placebo in reducing itch intensity in a randomized, placebo-controlled study, albeit systemic bile acid concentrations dropped by almost 50%.[51] In a clinical setting, cholestyramine is often still prescribed as first-line therapy to patients with PBC and pruritus, mainly to justify a necessary change to more effective off-label treatments.

Rifampicin

Rifampicin is an agonist of the PXR as well as able to induce important liver enzymes and transporters such as cytochrome P450 3A4 or multidrug resistance–associated protein 2 involved in biotransformation and excretion of various endogenous and exogenous substances. It, therefore, holds the potential to change the hepatic metabolism and elimination of possible pruritogens.

From its original antibiotic use, rifampicin might also influence the gut and skin microbiome, possibly contributing to its antipruritic activity.[52] However, a recent study did not observe differences in stool microbiota of patients with pruritic PBC, patients with asymptomatic PBC, and a healthy control group, questioning at least the gut microbiome in the pathophysiology of pruritus in PBC.[53] Rifampicin is also able to induce downregulation of ATX expression in a PXR-dependent mechanism, which

Table 1
Systemic pharmacologic treatment options for pruritus in patients with primary biliary cholangitis.

	Cholestyramine	Rifampicin	Bezafibrate	Naltrexone	Sertraline	Gabapentin
Label	In-Label	Off-Label	Off-Label	Off-Label	Off-Label	Off-Label
Starting dose	4 g/d	150 mg/d	(200→)400 mg/d	12.5 mg/d (or low-dose naloxone)	50 mg/d	100–300 mg/d
Max. recommended dose	16 g/d	450–600 mg/d	400 mg/d	150 mg/d	100 mg/d	3600 mg/d
AE/interactions	Interference with intestinal absorption of other medication, in particular UDCA and fat-soluble vitamins (such as vitamin A, D, E, and K)	• Induction of hepatic enzymes → altered metabolism of other drugs (eg, oral anticoagulants, oral contraceptives, antiepileptic drugs) • Hepatotoxicity in up to 5% of patients • Orange-red–colored body fluids	• Dose reduction in case of impaired renal function, contraindicated in dialysis patients • Risk of myopathy as well as increased risk of rhabdomyolysis with concomitant statin use • In long-term treatment: hepatotoxicity in up to 5% of patients	AE: opioid-like withdrawal reactions (low starting dose, eg, 12.5 mg/d or naloxone), increased pain sensations, confusion	AE: hyponatremia, QT prolongation, nausea, vomiting, sleep disturbance, restlessness, change in appetite	AE: dizziness, somnolence, falls with risk of fractures, headaches • Dose reduction in case of impaired renal function, very careful use in dialysis patients (max. 100 mg/d)

Advice					
• 2- to 4-h interval to oral intake of other medication • Change to other drugs if not effectively treating pruritus after 2 wk	• Doses of 150–300 mg/d often sufficient • Monitoring of transaminases after 2, 6, and 12 wk, afterward in 12-wk intervals and in case of dose changes	• Monitoring of transaminases, creatine kinase, and retention parameters after 2, 6, and 12 wk, afterward in 12-wk intervals • Fenofibrate as less effective alternate	For in-patients or in case of severe pruritus: intravenous application of naloxone (0.002–0.2 μg/kg/min; bolus of 0.4 mg if necessary), subsequent switch to naltrexone	• Regular monitoring of sodium • ECG with QT time monitoring • Paroxetine, mirtazapine, and other SSRI may also be applied as alternates	• Regular monitoring of retention parameters • Pregabalin as alternate drug (use doses of 75–600 mg/d)

Abbreviations: AE, adverse events; ECG, electrocardiography.

Table 2
Nonpharmacological interventions for pruritus in patients with primary biliary cholangitis

UVB Phototherapy	Extracorporeal Albumin Dialysis (MARS, Prometheus, DIALIVE)	Biliary Drainage (Nasobiliary Drainage, Transcutaneous Biliary Drainage, External Biliary Diversion)

• Application 2–3 times/wk
• Broad band might be more effective than narrow band UVB light
• Precautions:
  ○ Increased risk of skin cancer in immunosuppressed patients
  ○ Avoidance of concomitant application of photo-sensitizing drugs
• Limited availability
• Application recommended in consultation with experienced dermatologists
	• 2–3 dialysis sessions on subsequent days
	• Antipruritic effect may last for weeks to months
	• Invasive method:
	  ○ Insertion of dialysis catheter needed
	  ○ Necessary hospitalization of patients
	• Additional positive effect on liver function in patients with liver transplant and graft rejection
	• Application recommended only in specialized centers with experience in the intervention
		• Invasive/surgical procedures
		• Pruritus often strongly improved during biliary drainage, with relapse after removal/discontinuation within days to weeks
		• Risk of complications from invasive procedure including infections (eg, cholangitis, pancreatitis, peritonitis), bleeding, perforation, hospitalization and mortality
		• Application recommended only in specialized centers with experience in the intervention

may decrease the amount of LPA, a suspected pruritogen in cholestatic pruritus.[42] The clinical relevance of these mechanisms in itch-reducing efficacy of rifampicin is still unclear. Rifampicin is regarded an effective and safe second-line treatment option in pruritus due to PBC with daily dosages of 150 to 600 mg.[34,54] Many patients clinically benefit from intake of 150 mg rifampicin within 2 weeks of initial application. Hepatotoxicity is a potential, but not common, serious adverse effect during treatment with rifampicin[45]; therefore, transaminases should be tested at 2, 6, and 12 weeks after begin of rifampicin and in case of dose change.[4] Other adverse effects include particularly gastrointestinal symptoms such as nausea and abdominal discomfort. Patients taking rifampicin should be advised about the possible but harmless induction of orange-red–colored body fluids such as urine, stool, or tears.

The barbiturate phenobarbital induces the enzyme CYP3A4 to a similar extent as rifampicin but reduced pruritic intensity in patients with PBC to a lower extent in an older randomized, controlled trial.[55] Phenobarbital may only be considered as an experimental off-label approach with 1 to 5 mg/kg qd in case of insufficient control of pruritus with other treatment options.

Fibrates
In recent years, bezafibrate, an unselective PPAR agonist, has been investigated for its anticholestatic and antiinflammatory as well as antipruritic activity in patients with PBC.[56] PPARs act as intracellular transcription factors and broadly affect the regulation of gene expression involved in energy metabolism, cellular differentiation, and organ growth.[57] Fibrates bind on the PPAR subtypes α, γ, and δ and have already been applied to treat dyslipidemia since the 1960s, as they lower triglyceride and low-density lipoprotein levels. Cohort studies initially in Japan and later in western countries investigated bezafibrate for its positive effects as a disease-modifying treatment option

Table 3
Recent clinical drug trials for treatment of pruritus in patients with primary biliary cholangitis

Substance Class	Drug	Dosage	Phase	Comment	Identifier
KOR agonists	Nalfurafine (TRK-820)	• 2.5–5 μg po qd • 2.5 μg po qd (12 wk)	• Licensed in Japan for uremic and hepatic pruritus • Phase IV (PBC patients)	• Not available in Europe and United States	• Kumada, Hepatol Res 2017, PMID: 27753159 • Yagi, J Gastroenterol 2018, PMID: 29663077; NCT0265996
	Difelikefalin (CR-845)	• 0.5 mg/kg iv after hemodialysis treatment • 1 mg po bid	• Intravenous application FDA approved for CKDaP • Phase II (patients with PBC)	• Currently reviewed for approval by EMA	• Fishbane, NEJM 2021, PMID: 31702883; NCT03422653; NCT03995212
IBAT inhibitors	Linerixibat (GSK2330672)	• 20 mg, 90 mg, 180 mg po qd	• II (GLIMMER)	• Primary end-point not met, 40 mg and 90 mg bid most effective doses	• NCT02966834
		• 40 mg, 90 mg po bid	• III (GLISTEN)		• NCT04950127, EudraCT: 2021-000007-21
		• n.a.	• Open-label extension		• NCT04167358, EudraCT: 2019-003158-10
	Maralixibat (SHP625, LUM001, lopixibat)	10 or 20 mg po qd	II	Not superior to placebo FDA approval to treat pruritus in Alagille syndrome[a]	Mayo MJ, Hepatol Commun 2019, PMID: 30859149
	Volixibat (SHP626, LUM002)	20 mg po bid or 80 mg po bid	II (VANTAGE)	Separate volixibat study for PSC patients	NCT05050136
MRGPRX4 inverse agonist	EP547	Single and multiple doses po	I	Healthy subjects and patients with CKDaP equally included	NCT04510090

Abbreviations: bid, twice daily; CKDaP, chronic kidney disease-associated pruritus; EMA, European Medicines Agency; FDA, US Food and Drug Administration; IBAT, ileal bile acid transporter; KOR, κ-opioid receptor; MRGPRX4, mas-related G protein-coupled receptor X4; po, per os; qd, once a day.
[a] Dose recommendation for pruritus in Alagille syndrome: day 1 to 7: 190 mg/kg po (solution) qd; from day 8 on: increase to 380 mg/kg if tolerated.

in PBC and also found an antipruritic activity in affected patients.[56,58] The randomized, placebo-controlled BEZURSO phase III study followed with application of bezafibrate 400 mg qd in 100 patients with PBC with incomplete response to UDCA according to Paris-2 criteria, of whom 66% reported about pruritus, and found a 75% reduction in itch intensity in the bezafibrate-receiving group.[59] Moreover, the Japanese PBC registry revealed a significant improved overall survival in patients with PBC on bezafibrate compared with a matched control group.[60] The recently completed placebo-controlled FITCH trial investigated bezafibrate in 70 patients with PBC or PSC/secondary sclerosing cholangitis (SSC) for treatment of moderate to severe disease-associated pruritus.[35] Bezafibrate was superior to placebo (55 vs 11%) in reducing the intensity of moderate or severe pruritus intensity by at least 50%. Bezafibrate is currently not available in all countries, for example, the United States. Fenofibrate may be used as an alternate; however, its antipruritic properties are less well established.[4] Fenofibrate exhibits different pharmacologic properties with preferential affinity to PPAR-α,[35] compared with the broader receptor binding of bezafibrate, which calls for more studies to directly compare the efficacy of both drugs. Hepatotoxicity has to be taken into consideration as a serious adverse effect of fibrates, as reported in the BEZURSO study, in which 3 (6%) patients in the Bezafibrate group had an increase in aminotransferase levels over 5 times of upper limit normal. Two of these patients had to receive steroid treatment for normalization of aminotransferase levels within 3 months, and the drug was discontinued in 2 patients.[59] Serum creatinine levels might increase mildly during intake of bezafibrate as found in the BEZURSO and FITCH trials and should be monitored throughout fibrate therapy. Fibrates commonly cause myopathy and in severe cases rhabdomyolysis. As statins may potentiate this risk, a concomitant therapy with fibrates should be prescribed with caution. Taking clinical history for muscle weakness and/or pain and laboratory assessment of creatinine kinase and myoglobin is recommended during fibrate therapy.

Modulators of the endogenous opioid system

μ-opioid receptor antagonists (naltrexone, naloxone). The μ-opioid receptor antagonist naltrexone at dosages of 25 to 50 mg qd exerted a mild effect on itch intensity of patients with cholestatic pruritus in some smaller placebo-controlled trials,[61,62] which was less pronounced compared with rifampicin in a meta-analysis.[34] Some patients may benefit from even higher dosages of up to 150 mg/d. In-patients might profit from an intravenous naloxone infusion starting at very low doses of 0.002 to 0.02 μg/kg/min with a subsequent uptitration to 0.4 mg/8 hours and later switch to oral naltrexone.[10] From clinical experience, the infusion of naloxone represents a very effective treatment option for patients with severe pruritus, especially in hospitalized patients with complications from the underlying disease, for example, decompensated cirrhosis. Of note, naltrexone dosages should be augmented slowly, as it otherwise bears the risk of opioidlike withdrawal symptoms.[63] To avoid a previously described breakthrough phenomenon of pruritus during otherwise effective treatment with naltrexone, it might be paused for 1 or 2 days a week.[64] Concurrent chronic pain symptoms due to other underlying causes might exacerbate and should be monitored during administration of μ-opioid receptor antagonists.[65] Further adverse effects can include gastrointestinal symptoms, dizziness, and headaches.

κ-opioid receptor agonists (nalfurafine, difelikefalin). Nalfurafine, a κ-opioid receptor agonist, represents another drug affecting the endogenous opioid system. In Japan, it was licensed to treat CKDaP, after positive results in some placebo-controlled trials.[66,67] Nalfurafine was later also approved for treatment of cholestatic pruritus in

Japan. An inhomogeneous patient collective of 318 patients with pruritus due to different hepatic diseases was treated with nalfurafine at dosages of 2.5 µg qd and 5 µg qd in a randomized, placebo-controlled study.[68] Pruritus intensity assessed on a VAS scale was statistically significant reduced by 8 mm compared with the placebo group at 4 and 12 weeks of administration of nalfurafine but the clinical relevance of this slight difference remains questionable. In Europe and the United States, the drug was not approved by legal authorities. In terms of adverse effects, nalfurafine can cause sleep disturbances, constipation, and nocturia.

Since 2021, the peripheral κ-opioid receptor agonist difelikefalin represents the first Food and Drug Administration–approved and licensed drug to treat moderate to severe CKDaP for adults undergoing hemodialysis treatment.[69] Difelikefalin exerts significantly less central adverse events due to its restricted peripheral mode of action. Although it is intravenously applied in this condition, a current phase II trial is investigating the effect of an oral formulation of difelikefalin on pruritus in patients with PBC. (see **Table 3**) [70]

Ileal bile acid transporter inhibitors

The IBAT mediates the reuptake of bile acids from the small intestine into the entero-hepatic circle. This receptor seems as an interesting target for the interruption of the enterohepatic circulation, as it was hypothesized and demonstrated that removal of potential pruritogens from this circulation ameliorates pruritus.[44,71,72] Inhibition of IBAT results in increased elimination of bile acids with feces.

Several IBAT inhibitors have been and are currently still investigated in various hepato-biliary disorders for their efficacy in reducing pruritus. The IBAT inhibitor linerixibat was initially applied in a phase IIa cross-over, placebo-controlled, randomized study in 21 patients with PBC at dosages of 90 mg qd for 3 days, with an increase to 180 mg qd from day 4 to 14.[73] Linerixibat reduced baseline NRS itch scores by 57% after 14 days of therapy compared with 23% in the placebo group. In a post-hoc data analysis of this study, patients with pruritic PBC exhibited higher serum bile acid and ATX levels compared with patients with PBC without pruritus and healthy controls with a significant reduction after the linerixibat treatment period.[53] The phase IIb GLIMMER trial investigated linerixibat at different dosages (20–180 mg/d) in 147 patients with PBC across 66 centers in 10 countries for dose response, safety, and tolerability. Albeit the primary endpoint was not met, preliminary positive results were presented for the 40 mg twice daily application of linerixibat in patients with moderate to severe pruritus. In 2021, the follow-up Global Linerixibat Itch Study of Efficacy and Safety (GLISTEN) in patients with PBC started as a 2-part, randomized, placebo-controlled, double-blind, multicenter, phase III trial to evaluate the efficacy and safety of linerixibat. Bile acid–induced diarrhea represents the main adverse effect of IBAT inhibitors.

In 2021, the IBAT inhibitor maralixibat was approved in the United States for the treatment of pruritus in Alagille syndrome for patients of 1 year of age or older.[74,75] In contrast, maralixibat was not superior to placebo in reducing pruritus in a phase II study in patients with PBC.[76] Odevixibat, a further IBAT inhibitor, was licensed for pruritus in Progressive familial Intrahepatic Cholestasis Europe and the United States the same year.[77,78]

Selective serotonin reuptake inhibitors

SSRIs demonstrated mild to moderate antipruritic effects in cholestatic pruritus. Sertraline reduced itch intensity in patients with various hepatobiliary disorders in a randomized, placebo-controlled cross-over trial and case series.[79,80] Paroxetine may represent an alternative drug, as it was effective in a randomized trial of patients with various systemic causes of pruritus.[81] The recommended dose for sertraline is 50 to 100 mg qd and

20 mg qd for paroxetine. Common adverse effects of SSRI may include hyponatremia, sleep disorders, reduction in appetite, and restlessness.

SUMMARY

Pruritus remains an agonizing and sometimes difficult-to-treat symptom in patients suffering from PBC. In general, greater awareness among physicians and patients is needed to achieve the best possible treatment and symptom control. After ruling out other factors that trigger chronic pruritus and applying basic care, several systemic drug therapies are available to efficiently treat pruritus in many patients with PBC (see **Table 1**).

Practical Approach to Treat Pruritus in Patients with Primary Biliary Cholangitis

Cholestyramine often still represents the first-line therapy as licensed drug to treat cholestatic pruritus, with a starting dose of 4 to 8 g qd that may be increased to 12 to 16 g qd. All other mentioned drugs represent an off-label use. In case of insufficient pruritus control within 2 to 4 weeks, the authors recommend either rifampicin at 150 mg qd or bezafibrate at (200–)400 mg qd. Rifampicin is mostly effective at 150 to 300 mg qd, and the maximum daily dose of 600 mg is rarely required. Attention should be paid in regard to augmented drug metabolism of co-administered drugs such as oral contraceptives, anticoagulants, or antiepileptic drugs. The risk for hepatotoxicity is comparable for both rifampicin and bezafibrate (see **Table 1**). Transaminases should be controlled at 2, 6, and 12 weeks after start of therapy or in case of dose change. Bezafibrate exerts additional anticholestatic properties and should therefore be considered especially in patients with an incomplete response to UDCA and moderate to severe pruritus. In OCA-treated patients with PBC suffering from pruritus both bezafibrate and rifampicin efficiently attenuate itch intensity. If symptom control is insufficient with either drug within 4 weeks or adverse effects occur, patients can be started on naltrexone. Withdrawal-like symptoms can be avoided by starting with intravenous naloxone or low doses of 12.5 mg qd and a subsequent increase in dosage every 3 days. Mostly 25 to 50 mg qd are recommended; however, some patients benefit from higher doses up to 150 mg qd. Alternative drugs are sertraline at doses of 75 to 100 mg qd or gabapentin 100 to 3600 mg qd (see **Table 1**).

In most patients with PBC, this approach will successfully attenuate chronic pruritus. Patients, unresponsive or with intolerable adverse effects to the presented drugs, should be referred to expert centers for inclusion in clinical trials or undergo experimental medical or interventional approaches, for example, ultraviolet B phototherapy, molecular adsorbent recirculating system (ie, MARS, Prometheus), external or nasobiliary drainage, plasmapheresis, plasma separation, or anion absorption (see **Table 2**). IBAT inhibitors such as linerixibat and volixibat are currently investigated in clinical trials and seem to be promising future treatment options for pruritus in PBC (see **Table 3**). Research into the molecular pathophysiological mechanisms of pruritus in cholestatic liver disorders has provided further targets for development of new therapeutics such as ATX inhibitors and MRGPRX4 antagonists, which still have to be proved beneficial in clinical trials in humans.

CLINICS CARE POINTS

- Patients with PBC shoud be actively monitored for pruritus as a potentially burdensome symptom.

- Basic measures such as applying hydrating skin care can already improve especially low-intensity pruritus.
- Cholestyramine is often not well-tolerated and effective in treating pruritus in PBC.
- Bezafibrate might also exert anti-cholestatic and anti-inflammatory effects besides its positive effect on pruritus. Still, especially transaminases levels should be closely monitored during therapy.
- IBAT inhibitors represent promising new drugs for treating pruritus in PBC, but the results of ongoing clinical trials have to be awaited.

DISCLOSURE

M.M. Düll states no commercial or financial conflicts of interest. A.E. Kremer states lecture and consulting fees for CymaBay, Escient, Falk, GSK, Intercept, Viofor, and Zambon.

REFERENCES

1. Hussain AB, Samuel R, Hegade VS, et al. Pruritus secondary to primary biliary cholangitis: a review of the pathophysiology and management with phototherapy. Br J Dermatol 2019;181(6):1138–45.
2. Dull MM, Kremer AE. Treatment of pruritus secondary to liver disease. Curr Gastroenterol Rep 2019;21(9):48.
3. Mells GF, Pells G, Newton JL, et al. Impact of primary biliary cirrhosis on perceived quality of life: the UK-PBC national study. Hepatology (Baltimore, Md) 2013;58(1):273–83.
4. Düll MM, Kremer AE. Newer approaches to the management of pruritus in cholestatic liver disease. Curr Hepatol Rep 2020;19(2):86–95.
5. Langedijk J, Beuers UH, Oude Elferink RPJ. Cholestasis-associated pruritus and its pruritogens. Front Med (Lausanne) 2021;8:639674.
6. Kremer AE. What are new treatment concepts in systemic itch? Exp Dermatol 2019;28(12):1485–92.
7. Bergasa NV, Mehlman JK, Jones EA. Pruritus and fatigue in primary biliary cirrhosis. Bailliere's best practice & research. Clin Gastroenterol 2000;14(4):643–55.
8. Rishe E, Azarm A, Bergasa NV. Itch in primary biliary cirrhosis: a patients' perspective. Acta Derm Venereol 2008;88(1):34–7.
9. Prince MI, Chetwynd A, Craig WL, et al. Asymptomatic primary biliary cirrhosis: clinical features, prognosis, and symptom progression in a large population based cohort. Gut 2004;53(6):865–70.
10. Kremer AE, Beuers U, Oude-Elferink RP, et al. Pathogenesis and treatment of pruritus in cholestasis. Drugs 2008;68(15):2163–82.
11. Dull MM, Wolf K, Vetter M, et al. Endogenous opioid levels do not correlate with itch intensity and therapeutic interventions in hepatic pruritus. Front Med (Lausanne) 2021;8:641163.
12. Hirschfield GM, Chazouillères O, Cortez-Pinto H, et al. A consensus integrated care pathway for patients with primary biliary cholangitis: a guideline-based approach to clinical care of patients. Expert Rev Gastroenterol Hepatol 2021;15(8):929–39.

13. Neuberger J, Jones EA. Liver transplantation for intractable pruritus is contraindicated before an adequate trial of opiate antagonist therapy. Eur J Gastroenterol Hepatol 2001;13(11):1393–4.
14. Bergasa NV. The itch of liver disease. Semin Cutan Med Surg 2011;30(2):93–8.
15. Bergasa NV, Jones EA. Assessment of the visual analogue score in the evaluation of the pruritus of cholestasis. J Clin Transl Hepatol 2017;5(3):203–7.
16. Bergasa NV. The pruritus of cholestasis. J Hepatol 2005;43(6):1078–88.
17. Cordell HJ, Fryett JJ, Ueno K, et al. An international genome-wide meta-analysis of primary biliary cholangitis: novel risk loci and candidate drugs. J Hepatol 2021; 75(3):572–81.
18. Hegade VS, Mells GF, Fisher H, et al. Pruritus is common and undertreated in patients with primary biliary cholangitis in the United Kingdom. Clin Gastroenterol Hepatol 2019;17(7):1379–87.e3.
19. Koulentaki M, Ioannidou D, Stefanidou M, et al. Dermatological manifestations in primary biliary cirrhosis patients: a case control study. Am J Gastroenterol 2006; 101(3):541–6.
20. European Association for the Study of the L. EASL Clinical Practice Guidelines: management of cholestatic liver diseases. J Hepatol 2009;51(2):237–67.
21. Honig S, Herder B, Kautz A, et al. Pruritus strongly reduces quality of life in PBC patients - real life data from a large national survey. J Hepatol 2018;68:S216.
22. Carbone M, Mells GF, Pells G, et al. Sex and age are determinants of the clinical phenotype of primary biliary cirrhosis and response to ursodeoxycholic acid. Gastroenterology 2013;144(3):560–9.e7 [quiz: e513–4].
23. Cevikbas F, Lerner EA. Physiology and pathophysiology of itch. Physiol Rev 2019; 100(3):945–82.
24. Meixiong J, Dong X. Mas-related G protein–coupled receptors and the biology of itch sensation. Annu Rev Genet 2017;51(1):103–21.
25. Dull MM, Kremer AE. Management of chronic hepatic itch. Dermatol Clin 2018; 36(3):293–300.
26. Kremer AE, Namer B, Bolier R, et al. Pathogenesis and management of pruritus in PBC and PSC. Dig Dis (Basel, Switzerland) 2015;33(Suppl 2):164–75.
27. Meixiong J, Vasavda C, Green D, et al. Identification of a bilirubin receptor that may mediate a component of cholestatic itch. eLife 2019;8:e44116.
28. Meixiong J, Vasavda C, Snyder SH, et al. MRGPRX4 is a G protein-coupled receptor activated by bile acids that may contribute to cholestatic pruritus. Proc Natl Acad Sci U S A 2019;116(21):10525–30.
29. Wolf K, Kühn H, Leibl V, et al. Bile salt subspecies activate the G protein-coupled receptor MRGX4 expressed on sensory neurons and cause itching in humans. Hepatology (Baltimore, Md) 2019;70(S1):769A.
30. Yu H, Zhao T, Liu S, et al. MRGPRX4 is a bile acid receptor for human cholestatic itch. eLife 2019;8:e48431.
31. Han L, Ma C, Liu Q, et al. A subpopulation of nociceptors specifically linked to itch. Nat Neurosci 2013;16(2):174–82.
32. Kowdley KV, Luketic V, Chapman R, et al. A randomized trial of obeticholic acid monotherapy in patients with primary biliary cholangitis. Hepatology (Baltimore, Md) 2018;67(5):1890–902.
33. Nevens F, Andreone P, Mazzella G, et al. A placebo-controlled trial of obeticholic acid in primary biliary cholangitis. N Engl J Med 2016;375(7):631–43.
34. Tandon P, Rowe BH, Vandermeer B, et al. The efficacy and safety of bile Acid binding agents, opioid antagonists, or rifampin in the treatment of cholestasis-associated pruritus. Am J Gastroenterol 2007;102(7):1528–36.

35. de Vries E, Bolier R, Goet J, et al. Fibrates for itch (FITCH) in fibrosing cholangio-pathies: a double-blind, randomized, placebo-controlled trial. Gastroenterology 2021;160(3):734–43.e6.
36. Bergasa NV, Vergalla J, Swain MG, et al. Hepatic concentrations of proenkephalin-derived opioids are increased in a rat model of cholestasis. Liver 1996;16(5):298–302.
37. Spivey JR, Jorgensen RA, Gores GJ, et al. Methionine-enkephalin concentrations correlate with stage of disease but not pruritus in patients with primary biliary cirrhosis. Am J Gastroenterol 1994;89(11):2028–32.
38. Swain MG, Rothman RB, Xu H, et al. Endogenous opioids accumulate in plasma in a rat model of acute cholestasis. Gastroenterology 1992;103(2):630–5.
39. Thornton JR, Losowsky MS. Opioid peptides and primary biliary cirrhosis. BMJ 1988;297(6662):1501–4.
40. Bergasa NV, Liau S, Homel P, et al. Hepatic Met-enkephalin immunoreactivity is enhanced in primary biliary cirrhosis. Liver 2002;22(2):107–13.
41. Bergasa NV, Sabol SL, Young r WS, et al. Cholestasis is associated with pre-proenkephalin mRNA expression in the adult rat liver. Am J Physiol Gastrointes-tinal Liver Physiol 1995;268(2):G346–54.
42. Kremer AE, van Dijk R, Leckie P, et al. Serum autotaxin is increased in pruritus of cholestasis, but not of other origin, and responds to therapeutic interventions. Hepatology (Baltimore, Md) 2012;56(4):1391–400.
43. Kremer AE, Martens JJ, Kulik W, et al. Lysophosphatidic acid is a potential medi-ator of cholestatic pruritus. Gastroenterology 2010;139(3):1008–18, 1018.e1001.
44. Hegade VS, Bolier R, Oude Elferink RP, et al. A systematic approach to the man-agement of cholestatic pruritus in primary biliary cirrhosis. Frontline Gastroenterol 2016;7(3):158–66.
45. European Association for the Study of the Liver. Electronic address eee, Euro-pean Association for the Study of the L. EASL Clinical Practice Guidelines: the diagnosis and management of patients with primary biliary cholangitis. J Hepatol 2017;67(1):145–72.
46. Weisshaar E, Szepietowski JC, Dalgard FJ, et al. European S2k guideline on chronic pruritus. Acta Derm Venereol. 2019;99(5):469–506.
47. Verweyen E, Stander S, Kreitz K, et al. Validation of a comprehensive set of pru-ritus assessment instruments: the chronic pruritus tools questionnaire PRURI-TOOLS. Acta Derm Venereol. 2019;99(7):657–63.
48. Kremer AE, Oude Elferink RP, Beuers U. Pathophysiology and current manage-ment of pruritus in liver disease. Clin Res Hepatol Gastroenterol 2011;35(2):89–97.
49. Lindor KD, Bowlus CL, Boyer J, et al. Primary biliary cholangitis: 2018 practice guidance from the American association for the study of liver diseases. Hepatol-ogy (Baltimore, Md) 2019;69(1):394–419.
50. Rust C, Sauter GH, Oswald M, et al. Effect of cholestyramine on bile acid pattern and synthesis during administration of ursodeoxycholic acid in man. Eur J Clin Invest 2000;30(2):135–9.
51. Kuiper EM, van Erpecum KJ, Beuers U, et al. The potent bile acid sequestrant colesevelam is not effective in cholestatic pruritus: results of a double-blind, ran-domized, placebo-controlled trial. Hepatology (Baltimore, Md) 2010;52(4):1334–40.
52. Khurana S, Singh P. Rifampin is safe for treatment of pruritus due to chronic cholestasis: a meta-analysis of prospective randomized-controlled trials. Liver Int 2006;26(8):943–8.

53. Hegade VS, Pechlivanis A, McDonald JAK, et al. Autotaxin, bile acid profile and effect of ileal bile acid transporter inhibition in primary biliary cholangitis patients with pruritus. Liver Int 2019;39(5):967–75.

54. Bachs L, Pares A, Elena M, et al. Effects of long-term rifampicin administration in primary biliary cirrhosis. Gastroenterology 1992;102(6):2077–80.

55. Bachs L, Pares A, Elena M, et al. Comparison of rifampicin with phenobarbitone for treatment of pruritus in biliary cirrhosis. Lancet 1989;1(8638):574–6.

56. Corpechot C, Poupon R, Chazouillères O. New treatments/targets for primary biliary cholangitis. JHEP Rep 2019;1(3):203–13.

57. Dunning KR, Anastasi MR, Zhang VJ, et al. Regulation of fatty acid oxidation in mouse cumulus-oocyte complexes during maturation and modulation by PPAR agonists. PloS one 2014;9(2):e87327.

58. Tanaka A, Hirohara J, Nakanuma Y, et al. Biochemical responses to bezafibrate improve long-term outcome in asymptomatic patients with primary biliary cirrhosis refractory to UDCA. J Gastroenterol 2015;50(6):675–82.

59. Corpechot C, Chazouillères O, Rousseau A, et al. A placebo-controlled trial of bezafibrate in primary biliary cholangitis. N Engl J Med 2018;378(23):2171–81.

60. Tanaka A, Hirohara J, Nakano T, et al. Association of bezafibrate with transplant-free survival in patients with primary biliary cholangitis. J Hepatol 2021;75(3):565–71.

61. Terg R, Coronel E, Sorda J, et al. Efficacy and safety of oral naltrexone treatment for pruritus of cholestasis, a crossover, double blind, placebo- controlled study. J Hepatol 2002;37(6):717–22.

62. Wolfhagen FH, Sternieri E, Hop WC, et al. Oral naltrexone treatment for cholestatic pruritus: a double-blind, placebo-controlled study. Gastroenterology 1997;113(4):1264–9.

63. Mansour-Ghanaei F, Taheri A, Froutan H, et al. Effect of oral naltrexone on pruritus in cholestatic patients. World J Gastroenterol 2006;12(7):1125–8.

64. Carson KL, Tran TT, Cotton P, et al. Pilot study of the use of naltrexone to treat the severe pruritus of cholestatic liver disease. Am J Gastroenterol 1996;91(5):1022–3.

65. McRae CA, Prince MI, Hudson M, et al. Pain as a complication of use of opiate antagonists for symptom control in cholestasis. Gastroenterology 2003;125(2):591–6.

66. Kumagai H, Ebata T, Takamori K, et al. Effect of a novel kappa-receptor agonist, nalfurafine hydrochloride, on severe itch in 337 haemodialysis patients: a Phase III, randomized, double-blind, placebo-controlled study. Nephrol Dial Transplant 2010;25(4):1251–7.

67. Wikstrom B, Gellert R, Ladefoged SD, et al. Kappa-opioid system in uremic pruritus: multicenter, randomized, double-blind, placebo-controlled clinical studies. J Am Soc Nephrol 2005;16(12):3742–7.

68. Kumada H, Miyakawa H, Muramatsu T, et al. Efficacy of nalfurafine hydrochloride in patients with chronic liver disease with refractory pruritus: a randomized, double- blind trial. Hepatol Res 2017;47(10):972–82.

69. Fishbane S, Jamal A, Munera C, et al. A phase 3 trial of difelikefalin in hemodialysis patients with pruritus. N Engl J Med 2020;382(3):222–32.

70. Deeks ED. Difelikefalin: first approval. Drugs 2021;81(16):1937–44.

71. Hegade VS, Jones DE, Hirschfield GM. Apical sodium-dependent transporter inhibitors in primary biliary cholangitis and primary sclerosing cholangitis. Dig Dis (Basel, Switzerland) 2017;35(3):267–74.

72. Hegade VS, Kendrick SF, Dobbins RL, et al. BAT117213: ileal bile acid transporter (IBAT) inhibition as a treatment for pruritus in primary biliary cirrhosis: study protocol for a randomised controlled trial. BMC Gastroenterol 2016;16(1):71.

73. Hegade VS, Kendrick SF, Dobbins RL, et al. Effect of ileal bile acid transporter inhibitor GSK2330672 on pruritus in primary biliary cholangitis: a double-blind, randomised, placebo-controlled, crossover, phase 2a study. Lancet 2017; 389(10074):1114–23.

74. Shirley M. Maralixibat: first approval. Drugs 2022;82(1):71–6.

75. Gonzales E, Hardikar W, Stormon M, et al. Efficacy and safety of maralixibat treatment in patients with Alagille syndrome and cholestatic pruritus (ICONIC): a randomised phase 2 study. Lancet 2021;398(10311):1581–92.

76. Mayo MJ, Pockros PJ, Jones D, et al. A randomized, controlled, phase 2 study of maralixibat in the treatment of itching associated with primary biliary cholangitis. Hepatol Commun 2019;3(3):365–81.

77. Baumann U, Sturm E, Lacaille F, et al. Effects of odevixibat on pruritus and bile acids in children with cholestatic liver disease: phase 2 study. Clin Res Hepatol Gastroenterol 2021;45(5):101751.

78. Deeks ED. Odevixibat: first approval. Drugs 2021;81(15):1781–6.

79. Browning J, Combes B, Mayo MJ. Long-term efficacy of sertraline as a treatment for cholestatic pruritus in patients with primary biliary cirrhosis. Am J Gastroenterol 2003;98(12):2736–41.

80. Mayo MJ, Handem I, Saldana S, et al. Sertraline as a first- line treatment for cholestatic pruritus. Hepatology (Baltimore, Md) 2007;45(3):666–74.

81. Zylicz Z, Krajnik M, Sorge AA, et al. Paroxetine in the treatment of severe non-dermatological pruritus: a randomized, controlled trial. J Pain Symptom Manag 2003;26(6):1105–12.

Novel Therapies in Primary Biliary Cholangitis
What Is in the Pipeline?

Keri-Ann Buchanan-Peart, MD[a,b], Cynthia Levy, MD[c],*

KEYWORDS

- Primary biliary cholangitis • Therapy • Novel • Ursodeoxycholic acid • OCA
- Peroxisome proliferator-activated receptor agonist • Farnesoid X receptor
- Immunomodulators

KEY POINTS

- Even with the availability of obeticholic acid as second-line therapy for patients with primary biliary cholangitis, an unmet need remains to properly address patients who are at increased risk for disease progression and to manage symptoms such as pruritus and fatigue.
- Continuous monitoring for response to treatment and symptom management is of paramount importance.
- The use of triple therapy with ursodeoxycholic acid, obeticholic acid, and fibrates in the real-world setting is associated with improved odds of alkaline phosphatase normalization.
- Novel therapies including peroxisome proliferator-activated receptor agonists and nicotinamide adenine dinucleotide phosphate oxidase 1/4 inhibitors are promising and have the potential to address both disease progression and symptoms.

INTRODUCTION

Primary biliary cholangitis (PBC) is a chronic, autoimmune disease characterized by inflammation and the progressive destruction of small intrahepatic bile ducts[1]; this leads to a reduction in bile flow, hepatocyte injury and fibrosis, and ultimately cirrhosis and liver failure requiring liver transplantation.[1,2] However, the proportion of patients progressing to advanced disease has decreased with the advent of earlier diagnosis

[a] Division of Digestive Health and Liver Diseases, University of Miami Miller School of Medicine, 1500 Northwest 12th Avenue, Suite 1101-E, Miami, FL 33136, USA; [b] Department of Internal Medicine, Jackson Memorial Hospital, 1611 NW 12th Avenue, Miami, FL 33136, USA; [c] Division of Digestive Health and Liver Diseases, Schiff Center for Liver Diseases, University of Miami Miller School of Medicine, 1500 Northwest 12th Avenue, Suite 1101-E, Miami, FL 33136, USA
* Corresponding author. Division of Digestive Health and Liver Diseases, University of Miami Miller School of Medicine, 1500 Northwest 12th Avenue, Suite 1101-E, Miami, FL 33136, USA
E-mail address: clevy@med.miami.edu

Clin Liver Dis 26 (2022) 747–764
https://doi.org/10.1016/j.cld.2022.06.013
1089-3261/22/© 2022 Elsevier Inc. All rights reserved.

and treatment initiation.[3-5] The currently approved therapeutics primarily influence bile acid physiology, with the first-line therapy being ursodeoxycholic acid (UDCA) (13–15 mg/kg/d). In addition to its cytoprotective properties against bile acid–induced injury and improved transport of bile acids, UDCA exhibits immunomodulatory and antiapoptotic properties.[6] This drug is well tolerated, and patients have shown excellent biochemical response, resulting in slowed disease progression and improved survival.[7,8] However, approximately 30% to 40% of patients have an inadequate biochemical response with UDCA monotherapy, resulting in an increased risk of progression and decreased survival free of liver transplantation[7,9]; this underscores the need for alternative therapies. Obeticholic acid (OCA), a modified bile acid Farnesoid X receptor (FXR) agonist, was approved in 2016 as a second-line combination or monotherapy treatment (5–10 mg/d). Its efficacy was demonstrated in the PBC OCA International Study of Efficacy (POISE) trial with the primary endpoint of alkaline phosphatase (ALP) less than 1.67xULN, with a reduction of at least 15% from baseline and normal total bilirubin being achieved in approximately half of the study participants.[10,11] This agent, however, is known to cause dose-dependent pruritus and has been associated with an increased risk of hepatic decompensation, limiting its use in patients with advanced cirrhosis.[12,13]

These drawbacks have propelled the drive for the development of more efficacious treatment to aid in the cessation of disease progression and improved quality of life of these patients. This article seeks to highlight the many novel therapies underway (**Fig. 1**), giving a brighter outlook for the future of PBC treatment.

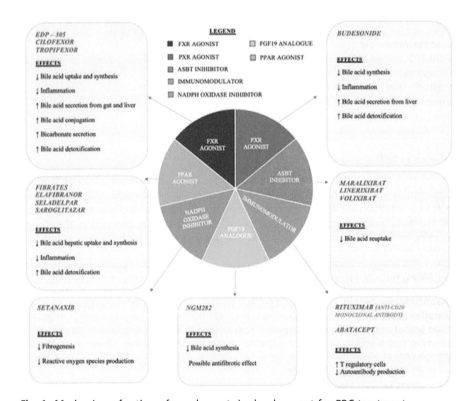

Fig. 1. Mechanism of action of novel agents in development for PBC treatment.

Therapies Aiming at Delaying Disease Progression and Improving Survival

Farnesoid X receptor agonists

FXR is a nuclear receptor expressed in the liver, kidney, intestine, and adrenal gland that plays a significant role in bile acid metabolism.[14,15] Stimulation of these receptors results in a cascade activation of multiple pathways, which reduce bile acid toxicity through decreased synthesis and uptake and increased conjugation and transport of bile acids.[15] FXR agonists demonstrate potent antiinflammatory and antifibrotic properties primarily through inhibition of the NF-kB pathway in the liver, which in turn causes downregulation of proinflammatory and profibrotic cytokines and reduces hepatic stellate cell (HSC) activation.[16,17] FXR agonists also have a direct inhibitory effect on HSC and contractility, further contributing to the antifibrotic effects. The antiinflammatory properties are further demonstrated through reduction of inducible isoform nitric oxide synthase and cyclooxygenase 2 expression and upregulation of endothelial nitric oxide synthase.[17,18] These combined effects lead to improvement in portal hypertension.[19]

Steroidal FXR agonists such as OCA, developed through the chemical modification of bile acids, have poor bioavailability and aqueous solubility due to their bile acid–like structure. Their TGR5 agonistic properties also cause the unwanted adverse effect of pruritus.[20] Hence, the development of nonsteroidal synthetic agonists such as tropifexor and cilofexor is advantageous, as it may potentially eliminate these unwanted effects while preserving their therapeutic effects. The effects of these agents are summarized in **Table 1**. The beneficial effects of OCA in PBC are described in details in Chapter 11 and will not be reviewed here. **Table 2** summarizes reports of clinical trials using non-OCA FXR agonists in PBC.

Other steroidal Farnesoid X receptor agonists

EDP-305 In mouse biliary and metabolic models of liver disease, EDP305, a potent FXR agonist, was shown to significantly reduce preexisting liver damage and hepatic fibrosis.[21] This led to a phase II randomized, double-blind, placebo-controlled study, named INTREPID. This 12-week trial looked at the safety, tolerability, pharmacokinetics, and effectiveness of EDP-305 (1 mg and 2.5 mg daily) in patients with PBC with intolerance or inadequate response to a stable dose of UDCA. At week 12, the study's primary goal was to determine the proportion of participants with a 20% decrease in ALP from pretreatment levels or ALP normalization. However, this goal was not achieved in the intention-to-treat analysis despite notable numerical response in ALP with 1 mg and 2.5 mg compared with placebo (45%, 46%, and 11%, respectively, $P = 0.06$ for placebo vs 2.5 mg/d EDP-305).[22] The most common adverse events reported were pruritus, gastrointestinal symptoms (abdominal discomfort, diarrhea, gastroesophageal reflux), headache, and sleeplessness. Treatment discontinuation owing to pruritus was 18% in the 2.5-mg EDP-305 treatment group and 3% in the 1-mg group.[22] EDP-305 will be developed further for nonalcoholic steatohepatitis (NASH) but not for PBC.

Nonsteroidal Farnesoid X receptor agonists

Tropifexor (LJN452) This highly selective non–bile acid FXR agonist exhibited potent in vivo activity in rodent models by measuring the induction of FXR target genes in numerous tissues.[23,24] In a phase II double-blind randomized controlled trial (RCT) (NCT02516605) assessing the safety, tolerability, and efficacy of tropifexor in patients with PBC and inadequate UDCA response, a reduction in gamma-glutamyl transferase (GGT) levels was chosen as the trial's endpoint to avoid confounding effects of ALP gene activation mediated by FXR. Interim analysis revealed promising results,

Table 1
Farnesoid X receptor agonist phase 2 trials and results

FXR Agonist	Steroidal/ Nonsteroidal	Number of Participants	Duration	Primary Endpoint	Result	Adverse Events	Study Design
Tropifexor 30 g, 60 g, 90 g	Nonsteroidal	61	12 wk	Reduction in GGT at 4 wk	↓ GGT (dose-dependent) ↓ AST ↓ ALP ↓ ALT	Pruritus: grade 1–2 (no discontinuations) Abdominal pain Headache Nausea	RCT
Cilofexor 30 mg and 100 mg	Nonsteroidal	71	12 wk	Reduction of ALP <1.67 ULN at week 12	↓ ALP ↓ GGT ↓ AST ↓ Bile acids	Pruritus: grade 2–3 (7% discontinuations)	RCT
EDP-305 1 mg and 2.5 mg	Steroidal	68	12 wk	20% reduction or normalization in ALP at week 12	Primary endpoint not met Secondary endpoints: ↓ ALT ↓ GGT ↓ AST	Pruritus (discontinuations in 3% in 1 mg; 18% in 2.5 mg) G.I. disturbances Headache Insomnia	RCT

Table 2
Peroxisome proliferator-activated receptor agonist notable phase 2/3 trials and results

PPAR	Isoform	Phase	Number of Participants	Duration	Primary Endpoint	Result	Adverse Event
Bezafibrate, 400 mg	α δ γ	III BEZURSO	100	2 y	Normalization of ALP, AST, ALT, bilirubin, albumin, PT	• 30% achieved endpoint goal (67% ALP normalization) • ↓liver stiffness • pruritus	• ↑Creatinine • Myalgias • Transient transaminitis
Bezafibrate, 400 mg	α δ γ	III FITCH	74	21 d	≥50% ↓pruritus	• 55% ↓pruritus in PBC • Secondary endpoints: 35% ↓ALP	• ↑ Creatinine
Seladelpar, 5 mg and 10 mg	δ	II	119	12 wk	% Change from baseline in ALP	• ↓ALP (34% and 43%)	
	δ	II	119	1 y	• ALP < 1.67 × ULN, with at least 15% reduction from baseline • Normal total bilirubin level	• ALP normalization (14% and 33%) • Composite endpoint achieved (55% and 69%) • Pruritus (58% and 93%) • ↓Bile acids	• GERD • GI disturbances • Fatigue • Nasopharyngitis
Elafibranor, 80 mg and 120 mg	α δ	II	45	12 wk	Relative change of ALP at 12 wk	• ↓ALP (67% and 79%) • ↓GGT, hsCRP, IgM	• Nausea • Diarrhea • Headache • Fatigue
Saroglitazar, 4 mg and 2 mg	α γ	II	37	16 wk	↓ALP at week 16	• ↓ALP (49% and 51%)	• ↑Aminotransferase

Abbreviations: GI, gastrointestinal; hsCRP, high-sensitivity C-reactive protein; ULN, upper limit of normal.

including a dose-dependent reduction in GGT, ALP, and hepatocellular damage (alanine aminotransferase [ALT]) after 4 weeks.[25]

Cilofexor (GS-9674) Cilofexor is a synthetic derivative of a highly selective nonsteroidal FXR agonist called GW4064.[26] A phase II double-blind RCT assessed the safety and efficacy of cilofexor in 71 patients with PBC without cirrhosis. For 12 weeks, patients were given either cilofexor, 30 mg; cilofexor, 100 mg; or a placebo once daily. Patients treated with cilofexor, particularly those who got the 100-mg dosage, exhibited substantial improvements in liver chemistries after 12 weeks when compared with placebo with a reduction of 13.8% in ALP ($P = 0.005$), 47.7% in GGT ($P < 0.001$), and 30.5% in primary bile acids ($P = 0.008$). The percentage of patients reaching the target endpoint of ALP less than 1.67 ULN was 9% and 14% in the 30-mg and 100-mg groups, respectively. Although these results are promising, 7% of patients in the 100-mg group discontinued treatment due to grade 2 to 3 pruritus, which was not reported in the 30-mg or placebo groups.[27]

Peroxisome proliferator-activated receptor agonists

These nuclear receptors have 3 isoforms, PPARα, PPARδ, and PPARγ, and are expressed in various tissues. PPARα forms are highly expressed in the liver, heart, kidney, adipose tissue, and intestines. PPARγ is found in adipose tissue and the immune system, and PPARδ expression is widespread.[28] Their effect on bile acid homeostasis and antiinflammatory properties makes them excellent candidate drugs for cholestatic diseases.

PPARα agonists decrease bile acid synthesis by suppression of 2 enzymes, the cytochrome P450 cholesterol 7α-hydroxylase (CYP7A1) and the sterol 27-hydroxylase (CYP27), and regulate bile acid transport by promoting human apical sodium–dependent bile salt transporter (ASBT) activity.[29] In addition, by inducing MDR3 expression, PPARα ligands suppress bile acid production and enhance phospholipid secretion into bile.[28] PPARγ activation inhibits inflammation and the production of proinflammatory cytokines by suppressing the transcriptional activation of inflammatory response genes in inflammatory cells and cholangiocytes.[28] PPARδ is involved in the regulation of fatty acid oxidation and mitochondrial biogenesis in several tissues. In cholangiocytes, its activation stimulates ATP-binding cassette cholesterol transporter A1 and enhances cholesterol export at the basolateral compartment affecting bile acid composition.[30]

Agonists for the different PPAR isoforms have varying affinities, including fenofibrate, which binds PPAR-α with the highest specificity, bezafibrate, which binds all 3 isoforms similarly, and seladelpar, which binds the δ isoform solely.[31] Elafibranor is a dual PPAR- α/δ agonist, and saroglitazar has a higher α/γ affinity. **Table 2** summarizes the relevant phase II/III trials conducted with PPAR agonists in PBC.

Fibrates. The 2 major fibrates studied in PBC are fenofibrate and bezafibrate. Fenofibrate is a fibric acid derivative available in the United States that is used to treat patients with hyperlipidemia.[32,33] Bezafibrate is available outside the United States.

Several modest pilot studies and nonrandomized trials were conducted evaluating fibrates in the treatment of PBC in patients with incomplete response to UDCA. In general, these studies reported reductions in liver chemistries, including ALP, ALT, GGT, as well as in bile acids and immunoglobulin M (IgM).[34–40] One such study investigated the use of fenofibrate in combination with UDCA for 20 PBC nonresponders over 12 months. This open-label study found that adding 160 mg of fenofibrate to the daily UDCA regimen helped improve serum ALP and IgM levels while also reducing proinflammatory cytokine levels.[41] Similarly, in an open-label study involving 48 patients with PBC with incomplete UDCA response, the efficacy of combination therapy with bezafibrate was studied over a 38-month period. Patients were given a daily dosage of bezafibrate (400 mg) in addition to UDCA. ALP reduction was achieved in all patients from an average of 2.4x (1.9–3.5) to 1x (0.7–1.6) UNL (P < 0.001). Older patients with mild disease were more likely to achieve ALP normalization, which was observed in 26 (54%) patients. Individuals with advanced illness, however, achieved incomplete ALP normalization. Moreover, during the course of therapy, partial (7 patients) or complete (16 patients) improvement in pruritus was observed (visual analogue scale [VAS] from 3.7 [1.2–5.6] to 0 [0–1.4]; P < 0.001). Adverse events experienced were mild, with patients only experiencing myalgia and gastrointestinal discomfort.[42]

These beneficial studies paved the way to the pivotal phase III study known as the BEZURSO trial. This trial was a 2-year double-blind RCT involving 100 patients with PBC with inadequate UDCA response.[43] Patients were randomized to receive either a combination of UDCA and bezafibrate, 400 mg/d, or UDCA and placebo. The primary endpoint was complete normalization of biochemical markers, including ALP, aspartate aminotransferase (AST), ALT, total bilirubin, albumin, and prothrombin time. This endpoint was met by 30% of patients in the bezafibrate and 0% in the placebo group. Furthermore, 67% of patients treated with bezafibrate had ALP levels normalize, compared with only 2% in the placebo group.[43] Decrease in liver stiffness and improvement in pruritus were also observed with bezafibrate, which was well tolerated. The most common adverse events were myalgias, increase in creatinine, and transient transaminase elevation.[43]

Triple therapy: ursodeoxycholic acid + obeticholic acid + fibrate. The use of combination therapy with FXR agonist, OCA, and fibrates (fenofibrate and bezafibrate) in addition to UDCA has also been explored in the real-world setting. A multicenter, uncontrolled retrospective cohort study in 58 patients with difficult-to-treat PBC aimed to investigate the efficacy of using OCA and fibrates, administered together in combination with UDCA. Half of the patients were treated with OCA as a second-line and fibrates as a third-line treatment (Group OCA-Fibrate), whereas the other half were treated in the inverse order (Group Fibrate-OCA) over a period ranging from 3 to 26 months. When compared with dual therapy, triple therapy resulted in a 22% reduction in ALP over the course of a year (95% confidence interval [CI] 12%–31%; P = 0.001). Group comparison showed a reduction in ALP level associated with triple treatment of 42% per year (95% CI 29%–53%; P = 0.001) in Group OCA-Fibrate versus 11% per year (95% CI 3% to 23%; P = 0.1) in Group Fibrate-OCA.[44]

In another larger retrospective study, conducted in 426 patients with PBC from 34 hospitals in Spain, the use of fibrates (bezafibrate or fenofibrate), OCA, or both as supplemental treatment to UDCA was evaluated. The fibrates group had a larger ALP reduction (41%) than the OCA group (19%) (P = 0.001), whereas ALT decrease was higher in individuals taking OCA. After 1 year, ALP levels were normal in 34.2% of patients (44.8% in the fibrates group and 3.5% in the OCA group, P = 0.001). Statistically significant reductions in ALP (P = 0.007) with triple therapy (UDCA + OCA + fibrates), in addition to reductions in GGT (P = 0.02), ALT (P = 0.04), and GLOBE score (P = 0.04), were also observed. Pruritus was the most common side effect reported in the OCA group (10.1%) and was not observed in the fibrate group. An important limitation was that some patients were included in more than one treatment group. As a result, the study's comparisons between OCA and fibrates therapies may be biased.[45]

Seladelpar. Seladelpar is a highly selective and potent PPAR-δ agonist with antiinflammatory and anticholestatic properties. An international open-label phase II study included 119 patients who received either 5 mg or 10 mg/d of seladelpar for 52 weeks. Subjects on the 5-mg group could be uptitrated to 10 mg after the first 12 weeks (for noncirrhotic subjects) or 26 weeks (cirrhotic subjects). At 12 weeks, ALP decreased by 34% and 43% from baseline in the 5- and 10-mg groups, respectively. These changes were sustained after 1 year of treatment, culminating at 41% and 45% reductions. The proportion of patients achieving the composite endpoint (ALP < 1.67x ULN, with at least 15% reduction from baseline and normal TB level) after 1 year of treatment was 55% and 69% in the 5-mg and 10-mg groups, respectively. ALP normalized in 14% of patients in the 5-mg group and 33% in the 10-mg group. Notably, clinically significant improvement in moderate to severe itching was also observed, especially in the 10-mg group.[46] Data on 2-year follow-up for 103 patients who entered this long-term follow-up phase indicate continued improvement with mean ALP percent change from baseline of 50% for the 10-mg group, whereas no safety signals were demonstrated.[47]

Furthermore, the effects of seladelpar treatment on pruritus and quality of life in patients with PBC were evaluated after 1 year of treatment in the open-label phase II trial. Clinically significant improvement in pruritus was observed in 58% and 93% of patients in 5-mg and 10-mg treatment groups, respectively.[48] In addition, reductions of 46% (5 mg) and 31% (10 mg) in the serum bile acid precursor C4 and up to 38% in serum bile acids were observed.[48] These combined positive results on biochemical response and pruritus indicate a dual therapeutic benefit with seladelpar.

A phase III trial (ENHANCE) was developed to investigate the safety and efficacy of seladelpar in patients with PBC with inadequate response to UDCA. Although ENHANCE was prematurely terminated due to concerns about drug-induced liver injury in the seladelpar study for NASH, this was later proved unfounded, and a new phase III trial is ongoing.[49] Safety and efficacy analyses were conducted after the termination of ENHANCE. The primary endpoint was the proportion of patients meeting the composite endpoint at week 12. A total of 78.2% of patients in the 10-mg group and 57.1% of patients in the 5-mg group achieved this response, whereas 27.3% of patients in the 10-mg group and 5.4% of patients in the 5-mg group achieved ALP normalization. The most common adverse events were pruritus and abdominal pain.[49] Patients are now being recruited for the new phase III, 52-week RESPONSE study (NCT04620733). **Table 3** lists all ongoing phase II and III clinical trials in PBC.

Elafibranor. This dual PPAR α/δ agonist was studied in a phase II, 12-week RCT aiming to assess the efficacy and safety of 2 doses (80 mg and 120 mg) of elafibranor in noncirrhotic patients with PBC who had an incomplete response to UDCA.[50] ALP reductions of 48%, 41%, and 3% were reported in the 80 mg, 120 mg, and placebo groups, respectively. The composite endpoint was achieved in 67% patients in the elafibranor 80-mg group and 79% patients in the elafibranor 120-mg group versus 6.7% patients in the placebo group. GGT, high-sensitivity C-reactive protein, and IgM, all showed considerable reductions. Patients tolerated elafibranor well with few adverse events. Pruritus was not exacerbated; in fact, it seemed to improve among subjects who were more symptomatic. On the visual analogue scale, the median change in pruritus from baseline was 7% (placebo), 24% (elafibranor, 80 mg), and 49% (elafibranor, 120 mg).[50] Limitations of the study included small sample size and short study duration. A double-blind phase III RCT (ELATIVE; NCT04526665) is now enrolling 150 patients with PBC to validate elafibranor, 80 mg, effectiveness based on changes in biochemical markers and its ability to improve pruritus and safety.

Table 3
Ongoing clinical trials in primary biliary cholangitis

Clinical Trial/ EudraCT Number	Phase	Drug	Drug Class	Primary Endpoint
NCT04950764	1	Seladelpar (includes patients with hepatic impairment)	PPAR agonist	Biochemical response
NCT04604652	2	HTD1801 (BUDCA)	Bile acid/Berberine	Biochemical response
NCT04594694	2	OCA/Bezafibrate	FXR/PPAR agonist	Biochemical response
NCT05133336	2 b/3	Saroglitazar	PPAR agonist	Biochemical response
NCT05014672	2/3	Setanaxib	NADPH oxidase inhibitor	Biochemical response
NCT04526665	3	Elafibranor	PPAR agonist	Biochemical response
NCT03301506	3	Seladelpar	PPAR agonist	Biochemical response
NCT04620733	3	Seladelpar	PPAR agonist	Biochemical response
NCT05050136	2	Volixibat	ASBT inhibitor	Pruritus
NCT03995212	2	CR845 (Difelikefalin)	Kappa opioid receptor agonist	Pruritus
NCT04950127	3	Linerixibat	ASBT inhibitor	Pruritus
NCT04167358	3	Linerixibat	ASBT inhibitor	Pruritus
NCT04893993	4	Thiamine	Vitamin B1	Fatigue

Saroglitazar. This is a novel dual PPAR (α/γ) agonist. In a recent proof-of-concept study, the safety and efficacy of saroglitazar were assessed in patients with PBC and inadequate UDCA response. For 16 weeks, 37 patients with PBC were given either saroglitazar, 4 mg (n = 13), saroglitazar, 2 mg (n = 14), or placebo (n = 10). The mean percentage reductions in ALP levels were 49% ($P < 0.001$) and 51% ($P < 0.001$) in the saroglitazar 4-mg and 2-mg groups compared with 3% in the placebo group. Because of aminotransferase elevations that quickly recovered to baseline following medication withdrawal, the study treatment was stopped in 4 patients (3 patients in the 4-mg group and 1 patient in the 2-mg group). Lower doses of 2 mg and 1 mg are currently under evaluation in the phase IIb/III study.[51]

Human pregnane X receptor agonist

Pregnane X receptor (PXR) is involved in regulating the biosynthesis, transport, and metabolism of bile acids. It affects bile acid synthesis through the downregulation of cholesterol 7α-hydroxylase (CYP7A1), the enzyme involved in the rate-limiting step of cholesterol production.[52] Its activation also results in the upregulation of certain metabolic enzymes and transporters involved in bile acid metabolism and elimination.[52] An example of a PXR agonist studied in PBC is budesonide.

Budesonide. Budesonide is a glucocorticoid that is absorbed in the small intestine. Its high first-pass effect (90%) reduces systemic bioavailability and associated adverse effects. It has dual agonist properties for both the nuclear glucocorticoid receptor and the PXR.[53,54] Budesonide and UDCA have a synergistic effect on biliary chloride/bicarbonate anion exchanger 2 expression, resulting in increased biliary bicarbonate production and stability of the biliary bicarbonate umbrella.[55]

A 2-year RCT was conducted in 39 patients who received either UDCA and budesonide combination therapy or UDCA and placebo. Patients were monitored for disease progression through liver histology before and a year after therapy. Favorable results were obtained with combination therapy as the point score of liver histology improved by 30.3%, whereas it deteriorated by 3.5% (P < 0.001) in those who received a placebo.[56] In comparison, in a phase III double-blind RCT in 62 UDCA-treated individuals with PBC with a high risk of disease progression, add-on budesonide did not provide a histologic benefit (defined as a 3-point decrease in hepatic activity index total score or no inflammatory activity according to Ishak).[57] As in other studies, improvements of surrogate biochemical markers of liver injury were noted, with 19/40 (48%) and 4/22 (18%) patients in the budesonide and placebo group, respectively, achieving ALP reduction of at least 40% from baseline. ALP normalization occurred in 35% of patients treated with budesonide and 9% with placebo (P = 0.023).[57] A total of 60/62 (97%) patients (98% and 96% in the budesonide and placebo groups, respectively) experienced adverse events, including arthralgia, osteopenia, cataract, muscle spasms, hypertension, dyspepsia, weight increase, abdominal pain, and peripheral edema. A higher discontinuation rate due to adverse events was reported in the budesonide group (9/40 patients; 23%) in comparison to the placebo group (2/22 patients; 9%). Another limitation was that the study was inadequately powered due to trial recruitment challenges attributed to the regulatory need for paired liver biopsies.[57] Budesonide use is contraindicated in patients with cirrhosis due to an increased risk of portal vein thrombosis.[54]

Antifibrotics

Setanaxib (GKT137831). This is a selective nicotinamide adenine dinucleotide phosphate oxidase (NOX) isoform 1 and 4 inhibitor. NOX is involved in tissue repair by modulating cell proliferation, angiogenesis, and fibrosis.[58] Earlier in vivo studies have demonstrated that increased production of reactive oxygen species (ROS) by NOX enzymes in response to cellular stress could induce fibrogenesis.[59] Furthermore, inhibition of NOX in multidrug-resistant mice reversed cholestatic fibrosis, suggesting that NOX inhibitors may slow or reverse disease progression in patients with cholestatic diseases.[60] Thus, the effects of setanaxib on HSC and liver fibrosis were studied in animal models, where it attenuated liver fibrosis and ROS production, reinforcing its benefit.[61]

A phase II RCT involving 111 patients with PBC with inadequate UDCA response was conducted to evaluate the safety and efficacy of setanaxib over 24 weeks. Patients were randomized to receive either 400 mg daily (OD), 400 mg bid, or placebo. After 6 weeks, GGT decreased by 7% in the placebo, 12% in the 400 mg OD, and 23% in the 400 mg BID groups (P < 0.01 for 400 mg BID vs placebo).[62]

In individuals with advanced disease (defined as liver stiffness > 9.6 kPa at baseline), setanaxib, 400 mg BID, resulted in a significant decrease (22%) in liver stiffness and substantial decreases in GGT (32.4%) and ALP (24.3%) after 24 weeks.[62,63] Smaller reductions in mean serum ALP of 5.6% in the 400 mg OD and 3.3% in the placebo groups were also observed.[63] Furthermore, reductions in mean fatigue scores were observed in comparison to baseline among patients receiving setanaxib, 400 mg bid, a finding that deserves further evaluation in upcoming trials. Setanaxib was well tolerated with no adverse events.[63] The phase III RCT, TRANSFORM, is currently enrolling.

NGM282. FGF19 is an endocrine hormone that reduces bile acid synthesis through suppression of the rate-limiting enzyme CYP7A1.[64] FGF19 may have antifibrotic effects via reduction of bile acid cytotoxicity, resolving lipotoxicity, and activation of the oxidative stress response. Notably, when unabated, oxidative stress leads to upregulation of transforming growth factor-beta, which promotes cell proliferation and fibrogenesis. However, the use of FGF-19 is limited due to an increased risk of hepatocellular carcinoma, seen in mice with overexpression of FGF19.[64]

NGM282, a nontumorigenic FGF19 analogue, was then developed. Its use as combination therapy with UDCA was studied in a phase II double-blind RCT in which 45 patients with PBC and inadequate response to UDCA were randomized to receive 0.3 mg NGM282, 3 mg NGM 282, or placebo. The primary endpoint was an absolute change in ALP from baseline to day 28. A rapid reduction in ALP levels was reported on day 7. ALP levels decreased by 15.9% in the 0.3-mg and 19.0% in the 3-mg groups compared with 1.2% in the placebo group. Secondary endpoints of GGT, AST, ALT, and IgM reductions were also achieved. The most common adverse event was diarrhea, with no worsening of pruritus reported.[65] At present, NGM282 is not undergoing further development for the treatment of PBC.

Immunomodulators

Rituximab. This anti-CD20 monoclonal antibody that selectively depletes B cells is currently used to treat lymphomas and autoimmune diseases. Smaller trials were conducted in patients with PBC and inadequate UDCA response, with marginal reductions in ALP and AMA being reported.[66,67] The drug was also well tolerated, and 60% of patients had improvement in pruritus at 12 months. However, these trials were underpowered with small sample sizes of 6 and 14 patients, respectively, with short therapeutic duration.[66,67]

Abatacept. This monoclonal antibody binds to CD80 and CD86 molecules on antigen-presenting cells and consequently downregulates T-cell activation.[68] Its use in patients with rheumatologic conditions including rheumatoid arthritis, juvenile idiopathic arthritis, and psoriatic arthritis has shown proven clinical benefit.

In an open-label study, the efficacy of abatacept in 16 patients with PBC with incomplete UDCA response was evaluated over 24 weeks. Patients received 125 mg abatacept on a weekly basis. The primary endpoint was ALP normalization or greater than 40% ALP reduction from baseline, which was achieved in only one patient (6.3%).[68] No other significant changes in ALP, total bilirubin, ALT, CRP, IgM, or liver stiffness were reported. Limitations of the study included a small sample size and the inclusion of patients with advanced liver disease (30% had cirrhosis), who may have shown more benefit at an earlier stage in the disease process.

Therapies Aiming at Improving Symptoms of Primary Biliary Cholangitis

Pruritus

The pathophysiology and overall management of pruritus are discussed in Chapter 8. Ongoing studies for the treatment of pruritus in PBC are as follows.

Bezafibrate

The FITCH trial was conducted in the Netherlands after anecdotal improvement in pruritus was observed with use of bezafibrate. Seventy-four patients with PBC, primary sclerosing cholangitis (PSC), or secondary sclerosing cholangitis were randomized to receive either once-daily bezafibrate, 400 mg, or placebo for 21 days. The primary endpoint was a clinically significant decrease ($\geq$50%) in itch severity judged on a VAS after 21 days of therapy with bezafibrate or placebo in individuals who had moderate to severe itch before starting treatment. This endpoint was attained in 45% (55% PBC, 41% PSC) of those receiving bezafibrate and only 11% for placebo ($P = 0.003$). A 35% reduction in ALP was also reported ($P = 0.03$) in the bezafibrate group versus placebo. The drug demonstrated good tolerability with only a mild increase in creatinine.[69]

Apical sodium–dependent bile acid transporter inhibitors

ASBT is predominantly expressed in the ileum in brush border membranes, where they are involved in the reuptake of bile acids and maintenance of the enterohepatic circulation. Thus, inhibition of these transporters reduces bile acid accumulation and bile toxicity.[70] The 2 ASBT inhibitors studied for the treatment of itching in PBC are maralixibat and linerixibat.

Maralixibat. Maralixibat is a selective ASBT inhibitor. In a phase II RTC, 66 patients were randomized to receive either maralixibat, 10 mg, 20 mg, or placebo. The primary outcome was a change in Adult Itch Reported Outcome from baseline to week 13 or early termination. There were no significant differences ($P = 0.48$) found in pruritus reduction between maralixibat and placebo, which was attributed to a strong placebo effect (47%). Gastrointestinal disturbances were the most common adverse events, including diarrhea, nausea, and abdominal pain.[71]

Linerixibat. Two trials investigated the effect of linerixibat on pruritus in patients with PBC. The first smaller phase IIa trial involved 22 patients, 11 treated with linerixibat and 11 who received a placebo over 14 days. In addition to a significant reduction of pruritus severity, there was also a 50% (95% CI −37 to −61, $P < 0.0001$) reduction in serum total and conjugated bile acids.[72] As seen with maralixibat, diarrhea described as mild to moderate was the most common adverse event. However, nobody discontinued treatment due to this side effect.[72]

The larger phase IIb GLIMMER trial studied 147 patients for 16 weeks, randomized into 6 groups. Patients were given linerixibat doses of 40 mg twice daily, 90 mg twice daily, 180 mg once daily, 20 mg once daily, and 90 mg once daily or placebo. The difference in worst itch score between the placebo group and those taking 40 mg twice daily, 90 mg twice daily, and 180 mg once daily was statistically significant. Only the group receiving 40 mg twice a day had statistically significant improvement in quality of life, especially in the social and emotional domains of PBC-40, indicating perhaps the ideal balance between efficacy and tolerability. As with the smaller trial, the most common adverse event was diarrhea, with 10% of patients discontinuing treatment.[73]

A 2-part phase III GLISTEN (Global linerixibat Itch study of efficacy and safety) study is currently recruiting patients. The study will include 230 participants with PBC and cholestatic pruritus and will evaluate the efficacy, safety, and impact on health-related quality of life of linerixibat compared with placebo.

Difelikefalin (CR845)

This long-acting, selective, peripheral kappa opioid receptor agonist exhibits antipruritic properties by activating kappa opioid receptors on peripheral neurons and immune cells.[74] It has been studied extensively in hemodialysis patients with pruritus.[74] The most common adverse events were diarrhea, dizziness, and vomiting. The drug is now Food and Drug Administration approved for use in patients with moderate to severe itching associated with chronic kidney disease in adults undergoing hemodialysis. Further studies are therefore needed to assess the safety and efficacy of its use as a long-term therapeutic agent in patients with liver disease. A study in patients with PBC and cholestatic itching is now underway (NCT03995212).

Fatigue

Rituximab. A phase II, double-blind RCT was conducted over 12 months to assess the efficacy of rituximab in improving moderate or severe fatigue in patients with PBC. A total of 55 patients were randomized into groups receiving either 2 infusions on days 1 and 15 or placebo. The trial's primary outcome measure was the PBC-40 fatigue domain at 3 months. Despite good tolerability, there was no statistically significant difference in fatigue score at 3 months between the rituximab and placebo arms (adjusted mean difference −0.9, 95% CI −4.6 to 3.1).[75]

Modafinil. Modafinil affects the wakefulness centers of the central nervous system; however, the exact mechanism of action is unclear. It is believed to activate noradrenergic $\alpha 1$ receptors, decrease gamma-aminobutyric acid release, and increase glutamate release.[76] Its use in patients with daytime somnolence is well known in conditions such as narcolepsy. In patients with PBC, fatigue is associated with excessive daytime somnolence.[77] A randomized, double-blind, placebo-controlled study was thus conducted to determine the safety and efficacy of modafinil for the treatment of fatigue in 40 patients with PBC. Patients were randomized to receive either modafinil, 100 mg, daily or placebo for 12 weeks. There was no difference in the proportion of patients exhibiting greater than 50% reduction in the fatigue and functional impact scale ratings after 12 weeks of therapy.[78]

Conversely, in a follow-up study including 42 patients, participants were given a 3-day trial of 100 to 200 mg modafinil. A positive response was defined as increased energy, decreased somnolence and sleep requirements, and improved daily function. Thirty-one (73%) patients achieved a complete response throughout the initial trial period and continued using the medication. Twenty-five (81%) patients continued to take 100 to 200 mg modafinil daily during a long-term follow-up (average 17.7 months).[79] Modafinil was associated with minimal adverse events, including headaches, nausea, and nervousness.

Mindfulness-based intervention. Mindfulness is the awareness of one's thoughts, feelings, body sensations, and surroundings in the present moment. In recent years, mindfulness-based interventions (MBI) have been shown to have a favorable impact on physical health and can help persons with chronic conditions manage their psychological symptoms.[80,81] Most notably, this technique has had proved clinical benefit in patients suffering from chronic fatigue in conditions such as multiple sclerosis and cancer. There is now an ongoing clinical trial assessing the efficacy of MBI in the treatment of moderate or severe fatigue in patients with PBC (NCT03684187).

SUMMARY

The management of patients with PBC has been challenging due to lack of universal response to available medical therapies and the fact that symptoms are not addressed by these drugs. As a result, the number of novel therapies being developed has multiplied over the past few years, showing encouraging results thus far. Some of these agents include the PPAR agonists that often demonstrate a dual therapeutic benefit. Their positive effect on biochemical response and pruritus makes them ideal candidates for slowing disease progression and improving quality of life. Use of an FXR agonist in combination with a fibrate is quite promising, and beneficial effects have already been suggested in real-world studies. Furthermore, FXR agonists may have an antifibrotic effect. Despite very encouraging preliminary results, we wait for confirmation of long-term safety and efficacy of these novel therapies in the many ongoing studies.

CLINICS CARE POINTS

- Early recognition of incomplete response to ursodeoxycholic acid (UDCA) is of paramount importance for risk modification in patients with PBC.

- In patients with PBC and incomplete response to UDCA, initiation of second-line therapy is indicated to prevent disease progression.
- Novel therapies aim at delaying disease progression and concurrently improving the quality of life in patients with PBC.
- Presence and severity of symptoms are unrelated to disease stage or response to UDCA. Clinicians should address and manage symptoms irrespective of response to UDCA.

DISCLOSURE

K Buchanan-Peart has nothing to disclose. C Levy advises and has received grants from Cymabay, Gilead, Genfit, Intercept, Genkyotex, GSK, Mirum, Pliant, Target RWE, and Cara; advises for Escient and Teva; and has received grants from NGM, Novartis, Zydus, Mitsubishi, and Alnylam.

REFERENCES

1. Webb GJ, Siminovitch KA, Hirschfield GM. The immunogenetics of primary biliary cirrhosis: a comprehensive review. J Autoimmun 2015;64:42–52.
2. Wong KA, Bahar R, Liu CH, et al. Current treatment options for primary biliary cholangitis. Clin Liver Dis 2018;22(3):481–500.
3. Carey EJ, Ali AH, Lindor KD. Primary biliary cirrhosis. Lancet 2015;386(10003): 1565–75 [published correction appears in Lancet. 2015;386(10003):1536].
4. Christensen E, Crowe J, Doniach D, et al. Clinical pattern and course of disease in primary biliary cirrhosis based on an analysis of 236 patients. Gastroenterology 1980;78(2):236–46.
5. Locke GR 3rd, Therneau TM, Ludwig J, et al. Time course of histological progression in primary biliary cirrhosis. Hepatology 1996;23(1):52–6.
6. Ikegami T, Matsuzaki Y. Ursodeoxycholic acid: mechanism of action and novel clinical applications. Hepatol Res 2008;38(2):123–31.
7. Patel A, Seetharam A. Primary biliary cholangitis: disease pathogenesis and implications for established and novel therapeutics. J Clin Exp Hepatol 2016;6(4): 311–8.
8. Poupon RE, Bonnand AM, Chrétien Y, et al. Ten-year survival in ursodeoxycholic acid-treated patients with primary biliary cirrhosis. The UDCA-PBC Study Group. Hepatology 1999;29(6):1668–71.
9. Cazzagon N, Floreani A. Primary biliary cholangitis: treatment. Curr Opin Gastroenterol 2021;37(2):99–104.
10. Nevens F, Andreone P, Mazzella G, et al. A placebo-controlled trial of obeticholic acid in primary biliary cholangitis. N Engl J Med 2016;375(7):631–43.
11. Hirschfield GM, Mason A, Luketic V, et al. Efficacy of obeticholic acid in patients with primary biliary cirrhosis and inadequate response to ursodeoxycholic acid. Gastroenterology 2015;148(4):751–61.e8.
12. John BV, Schwartz K, Levy C, et al. Impact of obeticholic acid exposure on decompensation and mortality in primary biliary cholangitis and cirrhosis. Hepatol Commun 2021;5(8):1426–36. Published 2021 May 6.
13. Eaton JE, Vuppalanchi R, Reddy R, et al. Liver injury in patients with cholestatic liver disease treated with obeticholic acid. Hepatology 2020;71(4):1511–4.
14. Chapman RW, Lynch KD. Obeticholic acid-a new therapy in PBC and NASH. Br Med Bull 2020;133(1):95–104.

15. Forman BM, Goode E, Chen J, et al. Identification of a nuclear receptor that is activated by farnesol metabolites. Cell 1995;81(5):687–93.

16. Calkin AC, Tontonoz P. Transcriptional integration of metabolism by the nuclear sterol-activated receptors LXR and FXR. Nat Rev Mol Cell Biol 2012;13(4):213–24. Published 2012 Mar 14.

17. Verbeke L, Mannaerts I, Schierwagen R, et al. FXR agonist obeticholic acid reduces hepatic inflammation and fibrosis in a rat model of toxic cirrhosis. Sci Rep 2016;6:33453 . Published 2016 Sep 16.

18. Verbeke L, Nevens F, Laleman W. Steroidal or non-steroidal FXR agonists - is that the question? J Hepatol 2017;66(4):680–1.

19. Schwabl P, Hambruch E, Seeland BA, et al. The FXR agonist PX20606 ameliorates portal hypertension by targeting vascular remodeling and sinusoidal dysfunction. J Hepatol 2017;66(4):724–33.

20. Verbeke L, Farre R, Trebicka J, et al. Obeticholic acid, a farnesoid X receptor agonist, improves portal hypertension by two distinct pathways in cirrhotic rats. Hepatology 2014;59(6):2286–98.

21. Alemi F, Kwon E, Poole DP, et al. The TGR5 receptor mediates bile acid-induced itch and analgesia. J Clin Invest 2013;123(4):1513–30. https://doi.org/10.1172/JCI64551.

22. An P, Wei G, Huang P, et al. A novel non-bile acid FXR agonist EDP-305 potently suppresses liver injury and fibrosis without worsening of ductular reaction. Liver Int 2020;40(7):1655–69.

23. Knowdley KV, Bonder A, Heneghan MA, et al. Final data of the phase 2a INTREPID study with EDP-305, a non-bile acid farnesoid X receptor (FXR) agonist. Hepatology 2020;72(1):746A.

24. Tully DC, Rucker PV, Chianelli D, et al. Discovery of tropifexor (LJN452), a highly potent non-bile acid FXR agonist for the treatment of cholestatic liver diseases and nonalcoholic steatohepatitis (NASH). J Med Chem 2017;60(24):9960–73. https://doi.org/10.1021/acs.jmedchem.7b00907.

25. Badman MK, Chen J, Desai S, et al. Safety, tolerability, pharmacokinetics, and pharmacodynamics of the novel non-bile acid FXR agonist tropifexor (LJN452) in healthy volunteers. Clin Pharmacol Drug Dev 2020;9(3):395–410.

26. Schramm C, Hirschfield G, Mason A, et al. Early assessment of safety and efficacy of tropifexor, a potent non-bile acid FXR agonist, in patients with primary biliary cholangitis: an interim analysis of an ongoing phase 2 study. J Hepatol 2018;68:S103.

27. Jiang L, Zhang H, Xiao D, et al. Farnesoid X receptor (FXR): structures and ligands. Comput Struct Biotechnol J 2021;19:2148–59.

28. Kowdley KV, Minuk GY, Pagadala MR, et al. The Nonsteroidal farnesoid X receptor (FXR) agonist cilofexor improves liver biochemistry in patients with primary biliary cholangitis (PBC): a phase 2, randomized, placebo-controlled trial. Hepatology 2019;70(1):31A–2A.

29. Halilbasic E, Baghdasaryan A, Trauner M. Nuclear receptors as drug targets in cholestatic liver diseases. Clin Liver Dis 2013;17(2):161–89. https://doi.org/10.1016/j.cld.2012.12.001.

30. Barbier O, Duran-Sandoval D, Pineda-Torra I, et al. Peroxisome proliferator-activated receptor alpha induces hepatic expression of the human bile acid glucuronidating UDP-glucuronosyltransferase 2B4 enzyme. J Biol Chem 2003;278(35):32852–60.

31. Xia X, Jung D, Webb P, et al. Liver X receptor β and peroxisome proliferator-activated receptor δ regulate cholesterol transport in murine cholangiocytes. Hepatology 2012;56(6):2288–96.

32. Goldstein J, Levy C. Novel and emerging therapies for cholestatic liver diseases. Liver Int 2018;38(9):1520–35. https://doi.org/10.1111/liv.13880.

33. Jones PH. Chapter 26 – fibrates. Ballantyne CM. In: Clinical lipidology. W.B. Saunders; 2009. p. 315–25.

34. Fenofibrate SE, Enna SJ, Bylund DB, editors. xPharm: the comprehensive pharmacology reference. Elsevier; 2009. p. 1–6.

35. Han XF, Wang QX, Liu Y, et al. Efficacy of fenofibrate in Chinese patients with primary biliary cirrhosis partially responding to ursodeoxycholic acid therapy. J Dig Dis 2012;13(4):219–24. https://doi.org/10.1111/j.1751-2980.2012.00574.x.

36. Ohira H, Sato Y, Ueno T, et al. Fenofibrate treatment in patients with primary biliary cirrhosis. Am J Gastroenterol 2002;97(8):2147–9. https://doi.org/10.1111/j.1572-0241.2002.05944.x.

37. Liberopoulos EN, Florentin M, Elisaf MS, et al. Fenofibrate in primary biliary cirrhosis: a pilot study. Open Cardiovasc Med J 2010;4:120–6. https://doi.org/10.2174/1874192401004010120. Published 2010 Apr 28.

38. Dohmen K, Mizuta T, Nakamuta M, et al. Fenofibrate for patients with asymptomatic primary biliary cirrhosis. World J Gastroenterol 2004;10(6):894–8. https://doi.org/10.3748/wjg.v10.i6.894.

39. Lens S, Leoz M, Nazal L, et al. Bezafibrate normalizes alkaline phosphatase in primary biliary cirrhosis patients with incomplete response to ursodeoxycholic acid. Liver Int 2014;34(2):197–203. https://doi.org/10.1111/liv.12290.

40. Takeuchi Y, Ikeda F, Fujioka S, et al. Additive improvement induced by bezafibrate in patients with primary biliary cirrhosis showing refractory response to ursodeoxycholic acid. J Gastroenterol Hepatol 2011;26(9):1395–401.

41. Honda A, Tanaka A, Kaneko T, et al. Bezafibrate improves GLOBE and UK-PBC scores and long-term outcomes in patients with primary biliary cholangitis. Hepatology 2019;70(6):2035–46. https://doi.org/10.1002/hep.30552.

42. Levy C, Peter JA, Nelson DR, et al. Pilot study: fenofibrate for patients with primary biliary cirrhosis and an incomplete response to ursodeoxycholic acid. Aliment Pharmacol Ther 2011;33(2):235–42. https://doi.org/10.1111/j.1365-2036.2010.04512.x.

43. Reig A, Sesé P, Parés A. Effects of bezafibrate on outcome and pruritus in primary biliary cholangitis with suboptimal ursodeoxycholic acid response. Am J Gastroenterol 2018;113(1):49–55. https://doi.org/10.1038/ajg.2017.287.

44. Corpechot C, Chazouilleres O, Rousseau A, et al. A 2-year multicenter, double-blind, randomized, placebo-controlled study of bezafibrate for the treatment of primary biliary cholangitis in patients with inadequate biochemical response to ursodeoxycholic acid (Bezurso). J Hepatol 2017;66(1):S89.

45. Soret PA, Lam L, Carrat F, et al. Combination of fibrates with obeticholic acid is able to normalise biochemical liver tests in patients with difficult-to-treat primary biliary cholangitis. Aliment Pharmacol Ther 2021;53(10):1138–46. https://doi.org/10.1111/apt.16336.

46. Reig A, Álvarez-Navascués C, Vergara M, et al. Obeticholic acid and fibrates in primary biliary cholangitis: comparative effects in a multicentric observational study. Am J Gastroenterol 2021;116(11):2250–7.

47. Levy C, Bowlus C, Neff G, et al. Durability of treatment response after 1 year of therapy with seladelpar in patients with primary biliary cholangitis (PBC): final results of an international phase 2 study. J Hepatol 2020;73:S464–5.

48. Mayo MJ, Vierling JM, Bowlus CL, et al. Long-term safety and efficacy of seladelpar in patients with primary biliary cholangitis (PBC): 2-year results from a long-term study. Hepatology 2021;74(S1):71–73A.
49. Kremer AE, Mayo MJ, Hirschfield G, et al. Seladelpar improved measures of pruritus, sleep, and fatigue and decreased serum bile acids in patients with primary biliary cholangitis. Liver Int 2022;42(1):112–23. https://doi.org/10.1111/liv.15039.
50. ENHANCE: safety and efficacy of seladelpar in patients with primary biliary cholangitis-A phase 3, international, randomized, placebo-controlled study. Gastroenterol Hepatol (N Y) 2021;17(2 Suppl 3):5–6.
51. Schattenberg JM, Pares A, Kowdley KV, et al. A randomized placebo-controlled trial of elafibranor in patients with primary biliary cholangitis and incomplete response to UDCA. J Hepatol 2021;74(6):1344–54. https://doi.org/10.1016/j.jhep.2021.01.013.
52. Vuppalanchi R, Caldwell SH, Pyrsopoulos N, et al. Proof-of-concept study to evaluate the safety and efficacy of saroglitazar in patients with primary biliary cholangitis. J Hepatol 2022;76(1):75–85. https://doi.org/10.1016/j.jhep.2021.08.025.
53. Ma X, Idle JR, Gonzalez FJ. The pregnane X receptor: from bench to bedside. Expert Opin Drug Metab Toxicol 2008;4(7):895–908.
54. Zimmermann C, van Waterschoot RA, Harmsen S, et al. PXR-mediated induction of human CYP3A4 and mouse Cyp3a11 by the glucocorticoid budesonide. Eur J Pharm Sci 2009;36(4–5):565–71. https://doi.org/10.1016/j.ejps.2008.12.007.
55. Hempfling W, Grunhage F, Dilger K, et al. Pharmacokinetics and pharmacodynamic action of budesonide in early- and late-stage primary biliary cirrhosis. Hepatology 2003;38(1):196–202. https://doi.org/10.1053/jhep.2003.50266.
56. Arenas F, Hervias I, Uriz M, et al. Combination of ursodeoxycholic acid and glucocorticoids upregulates the AE2 alternate promoter in human liver cells. J Clin Invest 2008;118(2):695–709.
57. Leuschner M, Maier KP, Schlichting J, et al. Oral budesonide and ursodeoxycholic acid for treatment of primary biliary cirrhosis: results of a prospective double-blind trial. Gastroenterology 1999 Oct;117(4):918–25.
58. Hirschfield GM, Beuers U, Kupcinskas L, et al. A placebo-controlled randomized trial of budesonide for PBC following an insufficient response to UDCA. J Hepatol 2021;74(2):321–9.
59. Jiang F, Zhang Y, Dusting GJ. NADPH oxidase-mediated redox signaling: roles in cellular stress response, stress tolerance, and tissue repair. Pharmacol Rev 2011;63(1):218–42.
60. Zhan SS, Jiang JX, Wu J, et al. Phagocytosis of apoptotic bodies by hepatic stellate cells induces NADPH oxidase and is associated with liver fibrosis in vivo. Hepatology 2006;43(3):435–43. https://doi.org/10.1002/hep.21093.
61. Nishio T, Hu R, Koyama Y, et al. Activated hepatic stellate cells and portal fibroblasts contribute to cholestatic liver fibrosis in MDR2 knockout mice. J Hepatol 2019;71(3):573–85.
62. Aoyama T, Paik YH, Watanabe S, et al. Nicotinamide adenine dinucleotide phosphate oxidase in experimental liver fibrosis: GKT137831 as a novel potential therapeutic agent. Hepatology 2012;56(6):2316–27. https://doi.org/10.1002/hep.25938.
63. Dalekos G, Invernizzi P, Nevens F, et al. Efficacy of GKT831 in patients with primary biliary cholangitis and inadequate response to ursodeoxycholic acid: interim efficacy results of a phase 2 clinical trial. J Hepatol 2019;70:E1–2.
64. Levy C, Carbone M, Wiesel P, et al. Setanaxib reduces cholestasis and fatigue in patients with primary biliary cholangitis and liver stiffness ≥9.6 kpa: post-hoc

analyses from a randomized, controlled, phase 2 trial. Hepatology 2021;74(S1): 782A.

65. Nicholes K, Guillet S, Tomlinson E, et al. A mouse model of hepatocellular carcinoma: ectopic expression of fibroblast growth factor 19 in skeletal muscle of transgenic mice. Am J Pathol 2002;160(6):2295–307.

66. Mayo MJ, Wigg AJ, Leggett BA, et al. NGM282 for treatment of patients with primary biliary cholangitis: a multicenter, randomized, double-blind, placebo-controlled trial. Hepatol Commun 2018;2(9):1037–50. Published 2018 Aug 30.

67. Myers RP, Swain MG, Lee SS, et al. B-cell depletion with rituximab in patients with primary biliary cirrhosis refractory to ursodeoxycholic acid. Am J Gastroenterol 2013;108(6):933–41.

68. Tsuda M, Moritoki Y, Lian ZX, et al. Biochemical and immunologic effects of rituximab in patients with primary biliary cirrhosis and an incomplete response to ursodeoxycholic acid. Hepatology 2012;55(2):512–21.

69. Bowlus CL, Yang GX, Liu CH, et al. Therapeutic trials of biologics in primary biliary cholangitis: an open label study of abatacept and review of the literature. J Autoimmun 2019;101:26–34.

70. de Vries E, Bolier R, Goet J, et al. Fibrates for Itch (FITCH) in fibrosing cholangiopathies: a double-blind, randomized, placebo-controlled trial. Gastroenterology 2021;160(3):734–43.e6.

71. Dawson PA. Role of the intestinal bile acid transporters in bile acid and drug disposition. Handb Exp Pharmacol 2011;201:169–203.

72. Mayo MJ, Pockros PJ, Jones D, et al. A randomized, controlled, phase 2 study of maralixibat in the treatment of itching associated with primary biliary cholangitis. Hepatol Commun 2019;3(3):365–81. Published 2019 Feb 1.

73. Hegade VS, Kendrick SF, Dobbins RL, et al. Effect of ileal bile acid transporter inhibitor GSK2330672 on pruritus in primary biliary cholangitis: a double-blind, randomized, placebo-controlled, crossover, phase 2a study. Lancet 2017; 389(10074):1114–23.

74. GLIMMER trial-a randomized, double-blind, placebo-controlled study of linerixibat, an inhibitor of the ileal bile acid transporter, in the treatment of cholestatic pruritus in primary biliary cholangitis. Gastroenterol Hepatol (N Y) 2021;17(2 Suppl 3):11–2.

75. Fishbane S, Jamal A, Munera C, et al. KALM-1 trial investigators. a phase 3 trial of difelikefalin in hemodialysis patients with pruritus. N Engl J Med 2020;382(3): 222–32.

76. Khanna A, Jopson L, Howel D, et al. Rituximab for the treatment of fatigue in primary biliary cholangitis (formerly primary biliary cirrhosis): a randomized controlled trial. Southampton (UK): NIHR Journals Library; 2018.

77. Scammell TE, Matheson J. Modafinil: a novel stimulant for the treatment of narcolepsy. Expert Opin Investig Drugs 1998;7(1):99–112.

78. Newton JL, Gibson GJ, Tomlinson M, et al. Fatigue in primary biliary cirrhosis is associated with excessive daytime somnolence. Hepatology 2006;44(1):91–8.

79. Silveira MG, Gossard AA, Stahler AC, et al. A randomized, placebo-controlled clinical trial of efficacy and safety: modafinil in the treatment of fatigue in patients with primary biliary cirrhosis. Am J Ther 2017;24(2):e167–76.

80. Ian Gan S, de Jongh M, Kaplan MM. Modafinil in the treatment of debilitating fatigue in primary biliary cirrhosis: a clinical experience. Dig Dis Sci 2009;54(10): 2242–6.

81. Zhang D, Lee EKP, Mak ECW, et al. Mindfulness-based interventions: an overall review. Br Med Bull 2021;138(1):41–57.

Liver Transplantation for Primary Biliary Cholangitis

Eric F. Martin, MD

KEYWORDS

- Primary biliary cholangitis • Liver transplantation • Outcomes • Recurrence
- Ursodeoxycholic acid

KEY POINTS

- Although ursodeoxycholic acid (UDCA) has significantly improved the clinical course of primary biliary cholangitis (PBC), liver transplantation (LT) remains the only effective cure.
- PBC, which was once the most common indication for LT, is now the seventh most common indication for LT.
- Graft and patient survival following LT for PBC are among the highest of all indications for LT.
- Recurrent PBC (rPBC) occurs in 22%, 36%, and 50% at 3, 5, and 10 years post-LT, respectively, and is associated with decreased patient and graft survival.
- Prophylactic UDCA in post-LT PBC patients is associated with reduced risk of rPBC, graft loss, liver-related death, and all-cause mortality.

INTRODUCTION

Primary biliary cholangitis (PBC) is an autoimmune cholestatic liver disease that is characterized by the progressive destruction of small intrahepatic bile ducts resulting in hepatocellular injury, cholestasis, fibrosis, and biliary cirrhosis. With a worldwide prevalence of 19.2 to 402 per million population, PBC is the most common cholestatic autoimmune liver disease.[1] PBC is often a serologic diagnosis in the setting of persistently elevated alkaline phosphatase (ALP) in the presence of the antimitochondrial antibody (AMA) or other PBC-specific antinuclear antibodies (eg, gp210 and sp100). However, a liver biopsy is required when there is a high suspicion for PBC in the absence of AMA (AMA-negative PBC). The characteristic histologic findings of PBC include chronic, nonsuppurative cholangitis that affects mainly interlobular and septal bile ducts.[2] Although the use of ursodeoxycholic acid (UDCA) as first-line therapy has significantly improved biochemical indices, delays histologic progression, and improves transplant-free survival, liver transplantation (LT) remains the only effective cure for end-stage liver disease caused by PBC.

Division of Digestive Health and Liver Diseases, University of Miami Miller School of Medicine, Miami Transplant Institute, Highland Professional Building, 1801 Northwest 9th Avenue, Miami, FL 33136, USA
E-mail address: efm10@miami.edu

Clin Liver Dis 26 (2022) 765–781
https://doi.org/10.1016/j.cld.2022.06.014
1089-3261/22/© 2022 Elsevier Inc. All rights reserved.

NATURAL COURSE
Signs and Symptoms

Fatigue and pruritus are the most commonly reported symptoms by patients with PBC and have a negative impact on quality of life (QOL).[3] In a large UK registry study during the pre-UDCA era in which 770 PBC patients were followed for up to 28 years, 60% of patients with PBC were asymptomatic at time of diagnosis, but only 5% remained asymptomatic after 20 years with a median time from diagnosis to appearance of symptoms of 3 to 4 years.[4] Other signs and symptoms of PBC include decreased bone mineral density (BMD), hyperlipidemia, xanthelasma, and the presence of other autoimmune diseases, such as Sjogren's syndrome, Raynaud's syndrome, Hashimoto's thyroiditis, and/or rheumatoid arthritis.[5]

Fatigue

Fatigue is the most common symptom in PBC and is present in nearly 80% of the patients. Fatigue fluctuates independently of disease activity and severity and is not alleviated by UDCA.[6–8] Fatigue related to PBC is associated with inability to work, sleep disturbance, depression, decreased QOL, and increased mortality.[9–11] Fatigue often persists after LT and, therefore, is not a unique indication for LT in patients with PBC.

Pruritus

Pruritus, which is a common manifestation of all cholestatic liver diseases, is reported in 40% to 80% of patients with PBC. A population-based study of patients with PBC from England reported a cumulate risk for developing pruritus in previously asymptomatic patients at 1, 5, and 10 years was 13%, 31%, and 47%, respectively.[12] Although there are well-defined treatment strategies for cholestatic pruritus,[13] chronic pruritus can be severe and debilitating and is associated with prolonged wound healing, skin infections, sleep disturbance, and diminished QOL.[3,7,14] A so-called "premature ductopenic variant" has been described in which severe pruritus develops due to progressive cholestasis and profound ductopenia in the absence of advanced hepatic fibrosis or cirrhosis.[15] This variant, which is reported to affect 5% to 10% of patients with PBC, is typically unresponsive to UDCA therapy and can progress quickly to require LT.[15] Unlike fatigue, pruritus dramatically resolves after LT, often within the first 24 hours after LT.[16] Therefore, intractable pruritus is a justifiable indication for LT.

Abnormal bone mineral density

As seen in other etiologies of cholestatic liver disease, patients with PBC have a higher prevalence of metabolic bone disease before and after LT.[17,18] Specifically, osteoporosis is four times more common in patients with PBC compared with age and gender-matched controls.[17,18] There is an expected bone loss of 8% to 18% within the first 6 months after LT,[19,20] with a reported incidence of fractures within the first posttransplant year of 20% to 40%.[21,22] Osteoporotic fractures significantly impact morbidity and mortality, especially those with PBC. Therefore, reducing the burden of disease from osteoporosis before and after LT is essential in the overall management of PBC. According to current American Association for the Study of Liver Diseases (AASLD) guidelines, BMD should be evaluated every year for osteopenic patients for the first 5 years after LT and every 2 to 3 year for patients with normal BMD.[2] The screening and treatment thereafter depends on the progression of BMD.

TREATMENT
Ursodeoxycholic Acid

Before the introduction of UDCA, LT was the only therapeutic option for PBC. The clinical course of PBC has significantly improved since the introduction of UDCA, which was formally approved by the Food and Drug Administration (FDA) in 1997 as the only first-line therapy for PBC. The clinical efficacy of long-term UDCA use is well established and characterized by improvement of liver biochemistries, slowing of histologic progression, delaying the onset of symptoms, and prolonging transplant-free survival.[23–27] However, up to 40% of patients treated with UDCA have an incomplete or absent biochemical response to therapy and such patients have significantly worse transplant-free survival than UDCA-responsive patients.[28–30]

Obeticholic Acid

Obeticholic acid (OCA), which is a potent activator of the nuclear farnesoid X receptor, was approved in 2016 by the FDA as a second-line therapy for use in combination with UDCA in patients with PBC patients with incomplete UDCA treatment response or as monotherapy in treatment-intolerant patients. There are emerging outcomes data that shown significant improvement in transplant-free survival for patients treated with OCA compared with two large well-established external PBC registry data sets, namely the Global PBC Study Group and UK-PBC registries.[31] Owing to reports of serious liver adverse events by the FDA in patients with advanced liver disease (Child-Pugh B or C), cautious dosing in accordance with the drug label is imperative. In the event of hepatic decompensation, OCA should be discontinued, and the patient should be referred for LT.

RISK ASSESSMENT

Multiple prognostic models were developed to assess the responsiveness to UDCA and estimate transplant-free survival specific to patients with PBC.[29,30,32–40] Of these, the GLOBE and UK-PBC scores, demonstrate superior predictive performance of biochemical response criteria compared with earlier models.

The GLOBE score was derived from an international, multicenter, prospective study of 2488 UDCA-treated patients with PBC and validated in an independent cohort of 1631 patients throughout Europe and North America.[37] The study showed that patients with risk scores greater than 0.30 had significantly shorter transplant-free survivals than matched healthy individuals ($P < .001$). Specifically, the 10-year transplant-free survival with a GLOBE score greater than 0.30 is 60%, compared with 92% with a GLOBE score $\leq$ 0.30.[37] Similarly, the UK-PBC score (http://www.uk-pbc.com/resources/tools/riskcalculator/) was derived and validated in a multicenter study including 3165 patients with UDCA-treated patients with PBC to estimate the risk of developing liver failure requiring LT within 5, 10, or 15 years from diagnosis.[33]

LIVER TRANSPLANTATION

The indications for LT for patients with PBC are similar for those with other forms of chronic liver disease. Unique to those with PBC, bilirubin greater than 6 mg/dL, Mayo risk score greater than 7.8, and intractable pruritus are other acceptable indications for LT.[35,41–43] Although the Model for End-Stage Liver Disease (MELD) score is widely used to estimate prognosis and for organ allocation in patients with end-stage liver disease of all etiologies, it remains a subject of debate as to how accurately the MELD score reflects mortality risk without taking into account the etiology of liver disease. Despite the perceived similarities of underlying autoimmune pathophysiology, PBC is often mistakenly compared with autoimmune hepatitis (AIH) and primary sclerosing cholangitis (PSC). In AIH, for example, corticosteroids and other immunosuppressive therapies can improve hepatic decompensation, even in patients previously thought to require lifesaving LT.[44] On the other hand, patients with PSC may be listed and subsequently transplanted due to recurrent cholangitis, for which they are eligible to receive MELD exceptions points on application to the National Liver Review Board (NLRB).[45] However, no such exception points exist for PBC. MELD exception points for intractable pruritus in PBC were previously granted on an individual basis by regional review boards; however, practices related to exceptions points varied widely by region.[46] Moreover, in an effort to provide a more efficient and equitable approach for waitlisted patients whose unique need for LT may not be adequately captured by their calculated MELD score, the NLRB was implemented in 2019 and replaced the prior system of 11 separate regional review boards. However, despite the high incidence of pruritus in PBC and its negative impact on QOL, the current guidance documents established by the NLRB explicitly state "there is inadequate evidence to support granting a MELD exception for pruritus in adult candidates with the typical clinical symptoms associated with this diagnosis."[45] Although intractable pruritus is a justifiable indication for LT, it is not a standard indication for MELD exception points, and therefore, it is a subject to appeal to the NLRB.

TRENDS IN LIVER TRANSPLANT FOR PRIMARY BILIARY CHOLANGITIS
Waitlist

The number of PBC patients listed for LT has declined in the United States and United Kingdom by nearly 50% since 1995.[47] The ratio of women: men with PBC waitlisted for LT decreased by 50%.[47] Although non-white patients are usually younger and with higher severity scores at time of listing compared with white patients, black and Hispanic patients remain underrepresented on the LT waitlist. Moreover, patients with PBC on the LT waitlist have a disproportionately higher waitlist mortality compared with other etiologies of chronic liver disease despite similar MELD scores.[48,49] Specifically, waitlisted patients with PBC had a higher overall and 3-month waitlist mortality when compared with patients with PSC (21.6% vs 12.7% and 5.0% vs 2.9%, respectively), despite a similar listing MELD score[49] In another study, Hispanic patients with PBC had the highest percentage of waitlist deaths (20.8%) of any ethnicity or race evaluated.[48] Compared with white patients with PBC, Hispanic patients with PBC had the lowest overall rate of undergoing LT with a significantly higher risk of death while on the waitlist and the highest proportion of waitlist removals due to clinical deterioration.[48] In fact, only patients with alcoholic liver disease combined with hepatitis C virus had a higher waitlist mortality. Waitlisted patients with PSC have a higher rate of delisting for clinical improvement than PBC (13% vs 3%).[50] As such, patients with PBC are historically considered to be disadvantaged with respect to LT due to higher waitlist mortality and lower transplant rates compared with other liver disease etiologies.

Transplant

According to data from the United Network for Organ Sharing (UNOS), other than cryptogenic cirrhosis, which accounted for 332 LT (19.4%), PBC was the most common identified indication for LT in the United States in 1988 accounting for 209 of all LTs (12.2%) compared with PSC (8.6%) and alcoholic cirrhosis (8.3%).[51] Despite an increase in the total number of LT performed in the United States by 169% since 1993, the number of LT performed for PBC decreased by 38.7% during the same time period (**Fig. 1**).[51] As a result of these trends, PBC has become a relatively uncommon indication for LT as it is now the seventh most common identified indication for LT accounting for 2.0% of all LTs in 2021, which is the lowest since such data were first collected by UNOS in 1988 (**Fig. 2**).[51] On the other hand, living donor LT (LDLT) accounted for 29 (15.9%) of all LTs performed for PBC in 2021, which was the most ever in 1 year for PBC since the first LDLT for PBC was performed in 1994.[51]

Despite the increasing overall prevalence of PBC,[52] the number of LT for PBC has declined in both North America and Europe.[2,53,54] This trend reflects the benefits of early diagnosis and treatment with UDCA as well as the availability of emerging alternative therapies for refractory disease, such as OCA.

Survival After Liver Transplant

Similar to other cholestatic liver diseases, survival rates following LT for PBC are among the highest of all indications for LT (**Table 1**). Specifically, following a more recent review of the UNOS database, the 1-year, 3-year, 5-year, and 10-year graft survival rates were 85.0%, 80.5%, 78.1%, and 71.9%, respectively, and the 1-year, 3-year, 5-year, and 10-year patient survival rates were 90.2%, 86.7%, 84.4%, and 79.0%, respectively.[55] Independent predictors of posttransplant mortality in patients with PBC included age, insurance, history of prior LT, and longer post-LT inpatient stay.[56] In a retrospective analysis of the UNOS database from 2002 to 2006, which included 99 patients with PBC who underwent LDLT, patient and graft survival following LDLT was similar to those following deceased donor liver transplant (DDLT).[57]

Disease Recurrence

Diagnosis

Recurrence of PBC after LT was originally described in 1982 by Neuberger and colleagues.[58] The diagnosis of recurrent PBC (rPBC) is often difficult because the diagnostic criteria for PBC before LT are obscured in the post-LT setting by multiple factors. First, many clinical and biochemical features of PBC that are present before LT are frequently absent in rPBC and, therefore, cannot be used alone for diagnostic

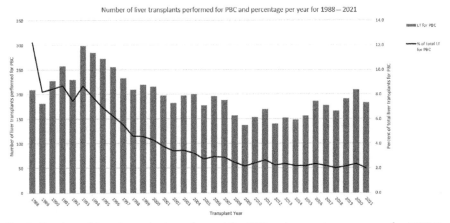

Fig. 1. Number of liver transplants performed for PBC and percentage per year for 1998 to 2021. (*Data from* https://optn.transplant.hrsa.gov/data/ (last access January 27, 2022).)

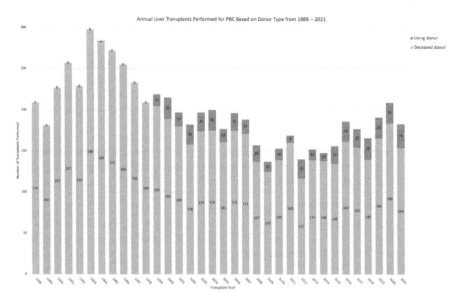

Fig. 2. Annual liver transplants performed for PBC based on donor type from 1998 to 2021. (*Data from* https://optn.transplant.hrsa.gov/data/ (last access January 27, 2022).)

purposes. In one study, only 12% of patients with rPBC reported potentially disease-related, but often nonspecific symptoms.[59] As is the case in pretransplant PBC, fatigue and pruritus were the most common symptoms, which were present in 50% of the patients with rPBC who experienced symptoms.[60] However, fatigue is nonspecific and may persist in many patients after LT unrelated to PBC.[61] Second, PBC-specific autoantibodies often persist after LT regardless of recurrence and, therefore, lose their diagnostic value for rPBC. Moreover, a cholestatic pattern of liver enzymes with an elevated ALP is also nonspecific after LT and can be found in many other clinical scenarios (**Table 2**). Owing to these limitations, histology is required to confirm the diagnosis of rPBC. In addition, the histologic features of PBC seen in the pretransplant setting, namely the immune-mediate lymphoplasmacytic injury of small bile ducts and bile duct paucity, may be mimicked in the post-LT setting by acute and chronic rejection. Therefore, the diagnosis of rPBC relies not only on the characteristic histologic features but also the exclusion of other causes of graft dysfunction (**Table 3**).[62,63]

Incidence of recurrent primary biliary cholangitis
The overall rates of rPBC are variable and range between 10% and 61% with the median time to rPBC between 3 and 5.5 years (**Table 4**).[60,64–74] The reported recurrence rates not surprisingly increase with time but vary in part due to non-standardized diagnostic criteria for rPBC with inconsistent use of protocol biopsies and variable follow-up. Using the largest PBC cohort to date, a recent study from the Global PBC Study Group reported recurrence rates of 22%, 36%, 50%, and 55% at 5, 10, 15, and 20 years, respectively.[70]

Risk factors for recurrent primary biliary cholangitis
Multiple risk factors for rPBC have been identified and are included in **Table 4**.[65,66,70,72,75,76] However, multiple previous studies reported inconsistent and contradictory results. Of all the baseline patient characteristics and immunosuppression regimens included in a recent meta-analysis included 3184 PBC patients who

Table 1
Patient and graft survival after liver transplantation for primary biliary cholangitis

Registry	Year	Cohort Size	Graft Survival (%)						Patient Survival (%)					
			1 y	3 y	5 y	10 y	15 y	20 y	1 y	3 y	5 y	10 y	15 y	20 y
UNOS[68]	1994–2009	3052	85.0	80.5	78.1	71.9	—	—	90.2	86.7	84.4	79.0	—	—
ELTR, European Liver Transplant Registry[71]	1999–2009	1929	85.0	—	78.0	—	—	—	90.0	83.0	—	—	—	—
UNOS (DDLT)[70]	2002–2006	100	85.2	82.5	80.7	—	—	—	89.6	87.0	85.1	—	—	—
UNOS (LDLT)[70]	2002–2006	100	85.6	80.9	77.4	—	—	—	92.8	90.1	86.4	—	—	—
Japanese Liver Transplant Society[72]	1994–2010	444	—	—	—	—	—	—	—	—	76.6	71.0	52.6	—
University of Tokyo Hospital[73]	1996–2010	81	—	—	—	—	—	—	90.0	88.0	80.0	—	—	—
Global PBC Group[74]	1983–2016	785	—	—	94.0	90.0	86.0	77.0	—	—	90.0	81.0	70.0	53.0

Table 2
Causes of cholestasis after liver transplantation

Early (≤6 mo)	Late (>6 mo)
Extrahepatic	Extrahepatic
Stricture: anastomotic, compressive	Stricture: anastomotic
Multiple strictures: ischemic or HAT	Multiple strictures:
Bile leak	ischemic, HAT, recurrent PSC
Cholangitis	Choledocholithiasis
Intrahepatic	Intrahepatic
Ischemia/reperfusion injury	Intrahepatic biliary strictures
ABO blood group incompatibility	Chronic rejection
HAT, hepatic artery thrombosis/stenosis	Recurrent disease
ACR	(PBC, PSC, HCV, hepatitis C virus)
Sepsis	ACR
DILI	DILI, drug-induced liver injury
Small for size CBD, common bile duct	De novo AIH
Post-LT infection	De novo viral hepatitis

underwent LT with underwent protocol or clinically driven liver biopsies, only tacrolimus and preventive UDCA were statistically and significantly associated with the risk of developing rPBC with pooled HRs of 2.62 (95% CI: 1.35–5.09; P = .004) and 0.40 (95% CI: 0.28–0.57; P<.001), respectively.[77]

Clinical impact of recurrent primary biliary cholangitis

Previous studies suggested that rPBC does not significantly affect long-term patient or graft survival.[60,67,74,78] In two previously reported cohort studies, a combined 5 out of 639 recipients required retransplantation.[60,79] rPBC after second and third LT has been described, but the proportion of graft failure due to rPBC remains low (7–14%).[67,80] However, the recently published Global PBC Study Group data challenge those conclusions. In addition to the identified risk factors for rPBC listed in **Table 4**, the study reported that rRBC was associated with graft loss and death with HR of 2.01 and 1.72, respectively.[70] For this reason, interventions to mitigate the risk of recurrent disease may play a significant role in improving posttransplant outcomes.[70]

Prevention and treatment of recurrent primary biliary cholangitis

Historically, the use of UDCA post-LT for PBC was more reactive than preventive. This approach was supported by previous data that showed the use of UDCA once rPBC was confirmed improved liver biochemistries, but did not influence patient or graft

Table 3
Proposed diagnostic criteria for recurrent primary biliary cholangitis after liver transplant

Inclusion Criteria	Exclusion Criteria
Diagnosis:	Acute and chronic rejection
Confirmed diagnosis of PBC from liver explant histology	Graft-vs-host disease
Serology"	Biliary obstruction or cholangitis
Persistence of AMA or AMA-M2	Vascular complications
Histology:	Viral hepatitis
Lymphoplasmacytic portal inflammation	DILI
Lymphoid aggregates	
Epithelioid granulomas	
Evidence of bile duct injury	

Table 4
Frequency of and risk factors for recurrent primary biliary cholangitis after liver transplantation

Reference	Registry/Study	Year	Cohort Size	Frequency	Risk Factor(s)
Liermann Garcia et al[69]	Single center (Queen Elizabeth Hospital, Birmingham, UK)	1982–1999	400	17% (3 y)	Younger age at transplant Tacrolimus
Sylvestre et al[89]	Single center (Mayo clinic)	1985–1997	100	17% (4.7 y)	Not reported
Sanchez et al[73]	Single center (Baylor University Medical Center)	1985–1999	156	10.9% (6 y)	Tacrolimus (vs cyclosporine)
Neuberger et al[72]	Single center (Queen Elizabeth Hospital, Birmingham, UK)	1982–2002	485	23%	Recipient age Tacrolimus
Jacob et al[67]	Single center (Germany)	1989–2003	100	14% (median 61 mo)	Tacrolimus
Charatcharoenwitthaya et al[60]	Single center (Mayo Clinic)	1985–2002	164	32% (3.5 y)	Older age at transplant Male sex Tacrolimus
Montano-Loza et al[71]	Single center (Alberta, Canada)	1989–2008	108	13% (5 y) 29% (10 y)	Tacrolimus Mycophenolate mofetil
Bosch et al[64]	Multicenter French and Swiss study	1988–2010	90	27% (5 y) 61% (15 y) 47% (10 y)	No significant factors
Egawa et al[66]	Japanese Liver Transplant Society Registry	1994–2010 (LDLT)	444	9.6% (5 y) 20.6% (10 y)	Younger age at transplant (48 y) IgM, immunoglobulin M > 554 mg/dL Gender mismatch Cyclosporin A as initial immunosuppression
Morioka et al[90]	Single center (Tokyo)	1994–2004 (LDLT)	50	9%	Average tacrolimus trough level within first year of LT LDLT HLA-DR, Human Leukocyte Antigen-DR locus mismatching

(continued on next page)

Table 4
(continued)

Reference	Registry/Study	Year	Cohort Size	Frequency	Risk Factor(s)
Kogiso et al[68]	Japanese Liver Transplant Society Registry	1994-2010	388 (LDLT)	14% (4.6 y)	Younger recipient age Higher serum IgM Donor sex mismatch Human leukocyte antigen B60 and DR8 Cyclosporin A as initial immunosuppression
Montano-Loza et al[70]	Global PBC Study Group	1983-2016	785	22% (5 y) 36% (10 y)	Biochemical cholestasis within first 6 mo after LT Age at diagnosis (<50 y) Age at LT (<60 y) Tacrolimus
Corpechot et al[65]	Global PBC Study Group	1983-2017	780	18% (5 y) 31% (10 y)	Tacrolimus

survival.[60] However, recently published data from the Global PBC Study showed that preventive administration of UDCA (10–15 mg/kd/d) is associated with lower risk of rPBC, graft loss, liver-related death, and all-cause mortality compared with no treatment.[65] These findings strongly support the use of UDCA after LT to not only help prevent rPBC but also improve graft and patient survival.[65] These findings were confirmed in two subsequent meta-analyses.[77,81] Further studies are needed to determine the utility of second-line therapies, such as OCA, as an alternative therapeutic option for post-LT PBC patients.

Immunosuppressive therapy

The primary maintenance immunosuppressants used after LT in the United States and Europe are calcineurin inhibitors (CNIs) of which tacrolimus is the drug of choice. However, CNI use is often limited by numerous side effects, particularly those related to renal toxicity. As such, there is a growing trend toward the use of antimetabolites such as mycophenolate mofetil (MMF) on account of its more acceptable safety profile.[41,82,83] However, there are growing data to suggest these trends may not be the most efficacious when PBC is the indication for LT. Before two recently published multicenter studies by the Global PBC Study Group, many of the previous studies reported inconsistent findings on the impact of immunosuppressants after LT in patients with PBC. The first study by Motano-Loza and colleagues, reported that tacrolimus was associated with a higher risk of rPBC (HR 2.31, 95% CI 1.72–3.10, $P < .001$) compared with MMF (HR 1.56, 95% CI: 1.19–2.04; $P = .001$) and cyclosporine (HR 0.62, 95% CI: 0.46–0.82; $P = .001$).[70] The second study published by Corphechot and colleagues supported the use of cyclosporine A in post-LT PBC patients, whereas it confirmed the previous results reporting that tacrolimus significantly increased the risk of rPBC (HR 2.06, 95% CI: 1.44–2.94; $P < .001$).[65] In addition, the Global PBC Study Group also observed an additive beneficial effect of cyclosporine compared with tacrolimus, which strongly supports the use of cyclosporine and preventive UDCA combination therapy in post-LT PBC patients.[65] Although there is no universal immunosuppression protocol for all post-LT patients, these results support a more individualized immunosuppression regimen based on the indication, one that is based on the knowledge of risk factors for disease recurrence while balancing the risk of potential medication side effects, rejection, and graft and patient mortality. Based on the growing evidence that cyclosporine A reduces PBC recurrence, it should be considered over tacrolimus as the primary immunosuppressant after LT for PBC.

Rejection

Similar to other forms of autoimmune liver disease, PBC is associated with an increased risk of rejection after LT.[84]

Rates of acute cellular rejection (ACR) after LT for PBC range from 21.7% to 83.3%.[67,85,86] ACR is associated with decreased recipient and graft survival but may also play a negative role in the development of the rPBC.[86,87] In addition, 16% of patients with PBC who underwent LT are at risk of developing late onset acute cellular rejection (LAR). In addition to previous graft failure and younger recipient age, a history of PBC was identified as an independent negative predicator of LAR with odds ratio of 2.1 and is associated with worsened graft survival.[88]

SUMMARY

The number of LT performed for PBC has declined over the years, which likely reflects the benefits of earlier diagnosis and treatment. Nonetheless, LT remains an important option and the only cure for patients with progressive PBC despite medical therapy with survival rates among the highest of all indications for LT.

As such, patients are living longer and are at risk for developing clinically relevant recurrent disease and other complications related to chronic immunosuppression. The recent landmark publications from the Global PBC Study Group provide valuable insight into the changing landscape of PBC before and after LT. Although the incidence of rPBC is improved with preventive UDCA, rPBC is associated with decreased patient and graft survival.

CLINICS CARE POINTS

- Although intractable pruritus is a justifiable indication for liver transplantation (LT) for primary biliary cholangitis (PBC), it is not a standard indication for MELD exception points, and therefore, it is a subject to appeal to the National Liver Review Board (NLRB).
- Liver biopsy is required to confirm the diagnosis of recurrent PBC (rPBC).
- The preventive administration of UDCA after LT to not only helps prevent rPBC but also improves graft and patient survival.
- Based on the growing evidence that cyclosporine A reduces PBC recurrence, it should be considered over tacrolimus as the primary immunosuppressant after LT for PBC.

REFERENCES

1. Lleo A, Colapietro F. Changes in the epidemiology of primary biliary cholangitis. Clin Liver Dis 2018;22(3):429–41.
2. Lindor KD, Bowlus CL, Boyer J, et al. Primary biliary cholangitis: 2018 practice guidance from the American association for the study of liver diseases. Hepatology 2019;69(1):394–419.
3. Mells GF, Pells G, Newton JL, et al. Impact of primary biliary cirrhosis on perceived quality of life: the UK-PBC national study. Hepatology 2013;58(1): 273–83.
4. Prince M, Chetwynd A, Newman W, et al. Survival and symptom progression in a geographically based cohort of patients with primary biliary cirrhosis: follow-up for up to 28 years. Gastroenterology 2002;123(4):1044–51.
5. Carey EJ, Ali AH, Lindor KD. Primary biliary cirrhosis. Lancet 2015;386(10003): 1565–75.
6. Goldblatt J, Taylor PJ, Lipman T, et al. The true impact of fatigue in primary biliary cirrhosis: a population study. Gastroenterology 2002;122(5):1235–41.
7. Kuo A, Kuo A, Bowlus CL. Management of symptom complexes in primary biliary cholangitis. Curr Opin Gastroenterol 2016;32(3):204–9.
8. Onofrio FQ, Hirschfield GM, Gulamhusein AF. A practical review of primary biliary cholangitis for the gastroenterologist. Gastroenterol Hepatol (N Y) 2019;15(3): 145–54.
9. Bjornsson E, Kalaitzakis E, Neuhauser M, et al. Fatigue measurements in patients with primary biliary cirrhosis and the risk of mortality during follow-up. Liver Int 2010;30(2):251–8.
10. Newton JL, Gibson GJ, Tomlinson M, et al. Fatigue in primary biliary cirrhosis is associated with excessive daytime somnolence. Hepatology 2006;44(1):91–8.
11. Stanca CM, Bach N, Krause C, et al. Evaluation of fatigue in U.S. patients with primary biliary cirrhosis. Am J Gastroenterol 2005;100(5):1104–9.

12. Mayo MJ. Natural history of primary biliary cirrhosis. Clin Liver Dis 2008;12(2): 277–88, viii.

13. Carrion AF, Rosen JD, Levy C. Understanding and treating pruritus in primary biliary cholangitis. Clin Liver Dis 2018;22(3):517–32.

14. Bunchorntavakul C, Reddy KR. Pruritus in chronic cholestatic liver disease. Clin Liver Dis 2012;16(2):331–46.

15. Vleggaar FP, van Buuren HR, Zondervan PE, et al. Jaundice in non-cirrhotic primary biliary cirrhosis: the premature ductopenic variant. Gut 2001;49(2):276–81.

16. Gross CR, Malinchoc M, Kim WR, et al. Quality of life before and after liver transplantation for cholestatic liver disease. Hepatology 1999;29(2):356–64.

17. Guanabens N, Cerda D, Monegal A, et al. Low bone mass and severity of cholestasis affect fracture risk in patients with primary biliary cirrhosis. Gastroenterology 2010;138(7):2348–56.

18. Trautwein C, Possienke M, Schlitt HJ, et al. Bone density and metabolism in patients with viral hepatitis and cholestatic liver diseases before and after liver transplantation. Am J Gastroenterol 2000;95(9):2343–51.

19. Bjoro K, Brandsaeter B, Wiencke K, et al. Secondary osteoporosis in liver transplant recipients: a longitudinal study in patients with and without cholestatic liver disease. Scand J Gastroenterol 2003;38(3):320–7.

20. Guichelaar MM, Malinchoc M, Sibonga JD, et al. Bone histomorphometric changes after liver transplantation for chronic cholestatic liver disease. J Bone Miner Res 2003;18(12):2190–9.

21. Butin S, Griffoul I, Espitalier F, et al. High incidence of vertebral osteoporotic fracture within the first year after liver transplantation. Clin Exp Rheumatol 2017;35(6): 913–8.

22. Meys E, Fontanges E, Fourcade N, et al. Bone loss after orthotopic liver transplantation. Am J Med 1994;97(5):445–50.

23. Angulo P, Batts KP, Therneau TM, et al. Long-term ursodeoxycholic acid delays histological progression in primary biliary cirrhosis. Hepatology 1999;29(3): 644–7.

24. Harms MH, van Buuren HR, Corpechot C, et al. Ursodeoxycholic acid therapy and liver transplant-free survival in patients with primary biliary cholangitis. J Hepatol 2019;71(2):357–65.

25. Lammers WJ, van Buuren HR, Hirschfield GM, et al. Levels of alkaline phosphatase and bilirubin are surrogate end points of outcomes of patients with primary biliary cirrhosis: an international follow-up study. Gastroenterology 2014;147(6): 1338–49.e5 [quiz: e15].

26. Poupon RE, Lindor KD, Pares A, et al. Combined analysis of the effect of treatment with ursodeoxycholic acid on histologic progression in primary biliary cirrhosis. J Hepatol 2003;39(1):12–6.

27. Prince MI, Chetwynd A, Craig WL, et al. Asymptomatic primary biliary cirrhosis: clinical features, prognosis, and symptom progression in a large population based cohort. Gut 2004;53(6):865–70.

28. Cheung AC, Lammers WJ, Murillo Perez CF, et al. Effects of age and Sex of response to ursodeoxycholic acid and transplant-free survival in patients with primary biliary cholangitis. Clin Gastroenterol Hepatol 2019;17(10):2076–2084 e2.

29. Corpechot C, Chazouilleres O, Poupon R. Early primary biliary cirrhosis: biochemical response to treatment and prediction of long-term outcome. J Hepatol 2011;55(6):1361–7.

30. Kuiper EM, Hansen BE, de Vries RA, et al. Improved prognosis of patients with primary biliary cirrhosis that have a biochemical response to ursodeoxycholic acid. Gastroenterology 2009;136(4):1281–7.

31. Perez C, Fisher H, Hiu S, et al. Patients with Primary Biliary Cholangitis Treated with Long-term Obeticholic Acid in a Trial-setting Demonstrate Better Transplant-free Survival than External Controls from the GLOBAL PBC and UK-PBC Study Groups. Oral Presentation at AASLD: The Liver Meeting 2021, Anaheim, California; November 12-15, 2021. 2021.

32. Angulo P, Lindor KD, Therneau TM, et al. Utilization of the Mayo risk score in patients with primary biliary cirrhosis receiving ursodeoxycholic acid. Liver 1999; 19(2):115–21.

33. Carbone M, Sharp SJ, Flack S, et al. The UK-PBC risk scores: derivation and validation of a scoring system for long-term prediction of end-stage liver disease in primary biliary cholangitis. Hepatology 2016;63(3):930–50.

34. Corpechot C, Abenavoli L, Rabahi N, et al. Biochemical response to ursodeoxycholic acid and long-term prognosis in primary biliary cirrhosis. Hepatology 2008; 48(3):871–7.

35. Dickson ER, Grambsch PM, Fleming TR, et al. Prognosis in primary biliary cirrhosis: model for decision making. Hepatology 1989;10(1):1–7.

36. Kumagi T, Guindi M, Fischer SE, et al. Baseline ductopenia and treatment response predict long-term histological progression in primary biliary cirrhosis. Am J Gastroenterol 2010;105(10):2186–94.

37. Lammers WJ, Hirschfield GM, Corpechot C, et al. Development and validation of a scoring system to predict outcomes of patients with primary biliary cirrhosis receiving ursodeoxycholic acid therapy. Gastroenterology 2015;149(7): 1804–12.e4.

38. Momah N, Silveira MG, Jorgensen R, et al. Optimizing biochemical markers as endpoints for clinical trials in primary biliary cirrhosis. Liver Int 2012;32(5):790–5.

39. Pares A, Caballeria L, Rodes J. Excellent long-term survival in patients with primary biliary cirrhosis and biochemical response to ursodeoxycholic Acid. Gastroenterology 2006;130(3):715–20.

40. Trivedi PJ, Bruns T, Cheung A, et al. Optimising risk stratification in primary biliary cirrhosis: AST/platelet ratio index predicts outcome independent of ursodeoxycholic acid response. J Hepatol 2014;60(6):1249–58.

41. European Association for the Study of the Liver. Electronic address eee. EASL clinical practice guidelines: liver transplantation. J Hepatol 2016;64(2):433–85.

42. Martin P, DiMartini A, Feng S, et al. Evaluation for liver transplantation in adults: 2013 practice guideline by the American association for the study of liver diseases and the American Society of transplantation. Hepatology 2014;59(3): 1144–65.

43. Neuberger J, Jones EA. Liver transplantation for intractable pruritus is contraindicated before an adequate trial of opiate antagonist therapy. Eur J Gastroenterol Hepatol 2001;13(11):1393–4.

44. Biewenga M, Inderson A, Tushuizen ME, et al. Early predictors of Short-term prognosis in acute and acute severe autoimmune hepatitis. Liver Transplant 2020;26(12):1573–81.

45. Guidance to liver transplant programs and the national liver review board for: adult MELD exception review. Available at: https://optn.transplant.hrsa.gov/media/2847/liver_guidance_adult_meld_201706.pdf. Accessed January 27, 2022.

46. Argo CK, Stukenborg GJ, Schmitt TM, et al. Regional variability in symptom-based MELD exceptions: a response to organ shortage? Am J Transplant 2011;11(11):2353–61.

47. Webb GJ, Rana A, Hodson J, et al. Twenty-year comparative analysis of patients with autoimmune liver diseases on transplant waitlists. Clin Gastroenterol Hepatol 2018;16(2):278–287 e7.

48. Cholankeril G, Gonzalez HC, Satapathy SK, et al. Increased waitlist mortality and lower rate for liver transplantation in hispanic patients with primary biliary cholangitis. Clin Gastroenterol Hepatol 2018;16(6):965–973 e2.

49. Singal AK, Fang X, Kaif M, et al. Primary biliary cirrhosis has high wait-list mortality among patients listed for liver transplantation. Transplant Int 2017;30(5):454–62.

50. Staufer K, Kivaranovic D, Rasoul-Rockenschaub S, et al. Waitlist mortality and post-transplant survival in patients with cholestatic liver disease - impact of changes in allocation policy. HPB (Oxford) 2018;20(10):916–24.

51. Available at: https://optn.transplant.hrsa.gov/data/. Accessed January 27, 2022.

52. Boonstra K, Beuers U, Ponsioen CY. Epidemiology of primary sclerosing cholangitis and primary biliary cirrhosis: a systematic review. J Hepatol 2012;56(5):1181–8.

53. Corpechot C, Poupon R. Geotherapeutics of primary biliary cirrhosis: bright and sunny around the Mediterranean but still cloudy and foggy in the United Kingdom. Hepatology 2007;46(4):963–5.

54. Jones DE, Watt FE, Metcalf JV, et al. Familial primary biliary cirrhosis reassessed: a geographically-based population study. J Hepatol 1999;30(3):402–7.

55. Singal AK, Guturu P, Hmoud B, et al. Evolving frequency and outcomes of liver transplantation based on etiology of liver disease. Transplantation 2013;95(5):755–60.

56. Sayiner M, Stepanova M, De Avila L, et al. Outcomes of liver transplant candidates with primary biliary cholangitis: the data from the Scientific registry of transplant recipients. Dig Dis Sci 2020;65(2):416–22.

57. Kashyap R, Safadjou S, Chen R, et al. Living donor and deceased donor liver transplantation for autoimmune and cholestatic liver diseases–an analysis of the UNOS database. J Gastrointest Surg 2010;14(9):1362–9.

58. Neuberger J, Portmann B, Macdougall BR, et al. Recurrence of primary biliary cirrhosis after liver transplantation. N Engl J Med 1982;306(1):1–4.

59. Silveira MG, Talwalkar JA, Lindor KD, et al. Recurrent primary biliary cirrhosis after liver transplantation. Am J Transplant 2010;10(4):720–6.

60. Charatcharoenwitthaya P, Pimentel S, Talwalkar JA, et al. Long-term survival and impact of ursodeoxycholic acid treatment for recurrent primary biliary cirrhosis after liver transplantation. Liver Transplant 2007;13(9):1236–45.

61. Carbone M, Bufton S, Monaco A, et al. The effect of liver transplantation on fatigue in patients with primary biliary cirrhosis: a prospective study. J Hepatol 2013;59(3):490–4.

62. Hubscher SG, Elias E, Buckels JA, et al. Primary biliary cirrhosis. Histological evidence of disease recurrence after liver transplantation. J Hepatol 1993;18(2):173–84.

63. Neuberger J. Recurrent primary biliary cirrhosis. Liver Transplant 2003;9(6):539–46.

64. Bosch A, Dumortier J, Maucort-Boulch D, et al. Preventive administration of UDCA after liver transplantation for primary biliary cirrhosis is associated with a lower risk of disease recurrence. J Hepatol 2015;63(6):1449–58.

65. Corpechot C, Chazouilleres O, Belnou P, et al. Long-term impact of preventive UDCA therapy after transplantation for primary biliary cholangitis. J Hepatol 2020;73(3):559–65.

66. Egawa H, Sakisaka S, Teramukai S, et al. Long-term outcomes of living-donor liver transplantation for primary biliary cirrhosis: a Japanese multicenter study. Am J Transplant 2016;16(4):1248–57.

67. Jacob DA, Neumann UP, Bahra M, et al. Long-term follow-up after recurrence of primary biliary cirrhosis after liver transplantation in 100 patients. Clin Transplant 2006;20(2):211–20.

68. Kogiso T, Egawa H, Teramukai S, et al. Risk factors for recurrence of primary biliary cholangitis after liver transplantation in female patients: a Japanese multi-center retrospective study. Hepatol Commun 2017;1(5):394–405.

69. Liermann Garcia RF, Evangelista Garcia C, McMaster P, et al. Transplantation for primary biliary cirrhosis: retrospective analysis of 400 patients in a single center. Hepatology 2001;33(1):22–7.

70. Montano-Loza AJ, Hansen BE, Corpechot C, et al. Factors associated with recurrence of primary biliary cholangitis after liver transplantation and effects on graft and patient survival. Gastroenterology 2019;156(1):96–107 e1.

71. Montano-Loza AJ, Wasilenko S, Bintner J, et al. Cyclosporine A protects against primary biliary cirrhosis recurrence after liver transplantation. Am J Transplant 2010;10(4):852–8.

72. Neuberger J, Gunson B, Hubscher S, et al. Immunosuppression affects the rate of recurrent primary biliary cirrhosis after liver transplantation. Liver Transplant 2004;10(4):488–91.

73. Sanchez EQ, Levy MF, Goldstein RM, et al. The changing clinical presentation of recurrent primary biliary cirrhosis after liver transplantation. Transplantation 2003; 76(11):1583–8.

74. Sylvestre PB, Batts KP, Burgart LJ, et al. Recurrence of primary biliary cirrhosis after liver transplantation: histologic estimate of incidence and natural history. Liver Transplant 2003;9(10):1086–93.

75. Guy JE, Qian P, Lowell JA, et al. Recurrent primary biliary cirrhosis: peritransplant factors and ursodeoxycholic acid treatment post-liver transplant. Liver Transplant 2005;11(10):1252–7.

76. Morioka D, Egawa H, Kasahara M, et al. Impact of human leukocyte antigen mismatching on outcomes of living donor liver transplantation for primary biliary cirrhosis. Liver Transplant 2007;13(1):80–90.

77. Li X, Peng J, Ouyang R, et al. Risk factors for recurrent primary biliary cirrhosis after liver transplantation: a systematic review and meta-analysis. Dig Liver Dis 2021;53(3):309–17.

78. Rowe IA, Webb K, Gunson BK, et al. The impact of disease recurrence on graft survival following liver transplantation: a single centre experience. Transplant Int 2008;21(5):459–65.

79. Jacob DA, Neumann UP, Bahra M, et al. Liver transplantation for primary biliary cirrhosis: influence of primary immunosuppression on survival. Transplant Proc 2005;37(4):1691–2.

80. Jacob DA, Bahra M, Schmidt SC, et al. Mayo risk score for primary biliary cirrhosis: a useful tool for the prediction of course after liver transplantation? Ann Transplant 2008;13(3):35–42.

81. Pedersen MR, Greenan G, Arora S, et al. Ursodeoxycholic acid decreases incidence of primary biliary cholangitis and biliary complications after liver transplantation: a meta-analysis. Liver Transplant 2021;27(6):866–75.

82. Lucey MR, Terrault N, Ojo L, et al. Long-term management of the successful adult liver transplant: 2012 practice guideline by the American Association for the Study of Liver Diseases and the American Society of Transplantation. Liver Transplant 2013;19(1):3–26.

83. Wiesner RH, Fung JJ. Present state of immunosuppressive therapy in liver transplant recipients. Liver Transplant 2011;17(Suppl 3):S1–9.

84. Berlakovich GA, Imhof M, Karner-Hanusch J, et al. The importance of the effect of underlying disease on rejection outcomes following orthotopic liver transplantation. Transplantation 1996;61(4):554–60.

85. Hayashi M, Keeffe EB, Krams SM, et al. Allograft rejection after liver transplantation for autoimmune liver diseases. Liver Transplant Surg 1998;4(3):208–14.

86. Satapathy SK, Jones OD, Vanatta JM, et al. Outcomes of liver transplant recipients with autoimmune liver disease using long-term dual immunosuppression regimen without corticosteroid. Transplant Direct 2017;3(7):e178.

87. Levitsky J, Goldberg D, Smith AR, et al. Acute rejection increases risk of graft failure and death in recent liver transplant recipients. Clin Gastroenterol Hepatol 2017;15(4):584–593 e2.

88. Thurairajah PH, Carbone M, Bridgestock H, et al. Late acute liver allograft rejection; a study of its natural history and graft survival in the current era. Transplantation 2013;95(7):955–9.

UNITED STATES POSTAL SERVICE ®

Statement of Ownership, Management, and Circulation
(All Periodicals Publications Except Requester Publications)

1. Publication Title	2. Publication Number		3. Filing Date
CLINICS IN LIVER DISEASE	016 – 754		9/18/2022

4. Issue Frequency	5. Number of Issues Published Annually	6. Annual Subscription Price
FEB, MAY, AUG, NOV	4	$329.00

7. Complete Mailing Address of Known Office of Publication (Not printer) (Street, city, county, state, and ZIP+4®)	Contact Person
ELSEVIER INC.	Malathi Samayan
230 Park Avenue, Suite 800	Telephone (include area code)
New York, NY 10169	91-44-4299-4507

8. Complete Mailing Address of Headquarters or General Business Office of Publisher (Not printer)

ELSEVIER INC.
230 Park Avenue, Suite 800
New York, NY 10169

9. Full Names and Complete Mailing Addresses of Publisher, Editor, and Managing Editor (Do not leave blank)

Publisher (Name and complete mailing address)
Dolores Meloni, ELSEVIER INC.
1600 JOHN F KENNEDY BLVD. SUITE 1800
PHILADELPHIA, PA 19103-2899

Editor (Name and complete mailing address)
KERRY HOLLAND, ELSEVIER INC.
1600 JOHN F KENNEDY BLVD. SUITE 1800
PHILADELPHIA, PA 19103-2899

Managing Editor (Name and complete mailing address)
PATRICK MANLEY, ELSEVIER INC.
1600 JOHN F KENNEDY BLVD. SUITE 1800
PHILADELPHIA, PA 19103-2899

10. Owner (Do not leave blank. If the publication is owned by a corporation, give the name and address of the corporation immediately followed by the names and addresses of all stockholders owning or holding 1 percent or more of the total amount of stock. If not owned by a corporation, give the names and addresses of the individual owners. If owned by a partnership or other unincorporated firm, give its name and address as well as those of each individual owner. If the publication is published by a nonprofit organization, give its name and address.)

Full Name	Complete Mailing Address
WHOLLY OWNED SUBSIDIARY OF REED/ELSEVIER, US HOLDINGS	1600 JOHN F KENNEDY BLVD. SUITE 1800 PHILADELPHIA, PA 19103-2899

11. Known Bondholders, Mortgagees, and Other Security Holders Owning or Holding 1 Percent or More of Total Amount of Bonds, Mortgages, or Other Securities. If none, check box ► ☐ None

Full Name	Complete Mailing Address
N/A	

12. Tax Status (For completion by nonprofit organizations authorized to mail at nonprofit rates) (Check one)
The purpose, function, and nonprofit status of this organization and the exempt status for federal income tax purposes:
☒ Has Not Changed During Preceding 12 Months
☐ Has Changed During Preceding 12 Months (Publisher must submit explanation of change with this statement)

PS Form **3526**, July 2014 [Page 1 of 4 (see instructions page 4)] PSN: 7530-01-000-9931 PRIVACY NOTICE: See our privacy policy on www.usps.com.

---

13. Publication Title		14. Issue Date for Circulation Data Below
CLINICS IN LIVER DISEASE		MAY 2022

15. Extent and Nature of Circulation			Average No. Copies Each Issue During Preceding 12 Months	No. Copies of Single Issue Published Nearest to Filing Date
a. Total Number of Copies (Net press run)			108	101
b. Paid Circulation (By Mail and Outside the Mail)	(1)	Mailed Outside-County Paid Subscriptions Stated on PS Form 3541 (include paid distribution above nominal rate, advertiser's proof copies, and exchange copies)	41	37
	(2)	Mailed In-County Paid Subscriptions Stated on PS Form 3541 (include paid distribution above nominal rate, advertiser's proof copies, and exchange copies)	0	0
	(3)	Paid Distribution Outside the Mails Including Sales Through Dealers and Carriers, Street Vendors, Counter Sales, and Other Paid Distribution Outside USPS®	37	35
	(4)	Paid Distribution by Other Classes of Mail Through the USPS (e.g., First-Class Mail®)	0	0
c. Total Paid Distribution (Sum of 15b (1), (2), (3), and (4))			78	72
d. Free or Nominal Rate Distribution (By Mail and Outside the Mail)	(1)	Free or Nominal Rate Outside-County Copies Included on PS Form 3541	15	14
	(2)	Free or Nominal Rate In-County Copies Included on PS Form 3541	0	0
	(3)	Free or Nominal Rate Copies Mailed at Other Classes Through the USPS (e.g., First-Class Mail)	0	0
	(4)	Free or Nominal Rate Distribution Outside the Mail (Carriers or other means)	0	0
e. Total Free or Nominal Rate Distribution (Sum of 15d (1), (2), (3) and (4))			15	14
f. Total Distribution (Sum of 15c and 15e)			93	86
g. Copies not Distributed (See Instructions to Publishers #4 (page #3))			15	15
h. Total (Sum of 15f and g)			108	101
i. Percent Paid (15c divided by 15f times 100)				

16. Electronic Copy Circulation		Average No. Copies Each Issue During Preceding 12 Months	No. Copies of Single Issue Published Nearest to Filing Date
a. Paid Electronic Copies	►		
b. Total Paid Print Copies (Line 15c) + Paid Electronic Copies (Line 16a)	►		
c. Total Print Distribution (Line 15f) + Paid Electronic Copies (Line 16a)	►		
d. Percent Paid (Both Print & Electronic Copies) (16b divided by 16c × 100)	►		

☒ I certify that 50% of all my distributed copies (electronic and print) are paid above a nominal price.

17. Publication of Statement of Ownership
☒ If the publication is a general publication, publication of this statement is required. Will be printed in the NOVEMBER 2022 issue of this publication. ☐ Publication not required.

18. Signature and Title of Editor, Publisher, Business Manager, or Owner		Date
Malathi Samayan		9/18/2022
Malathi Samayan - Distribution Controller		

I certify that all information furnished on this form is true and complete. I understand that anyone who furnishes false or misleading information on this form or who omits material or information requested on the form may be subject to criminal sanctions (including fines and imprisonment) and/or civil sanctions (including civil penalties).

PS Form **3526**, July 2014 (Page 3 of 4) PRIVACY NOTICE: See our privacy policy on www.usps.com.

Moving?

Make sure your subscription moves with you!

To notify us of your new address, find your **Clinics Account Number** (located on your mailing label above your name), and contact customer service at:

Email: journalscustomerservice-usa@elsevier.com

800-654-2452 (subscribers in the U.S. & Canada)
314-447-8871 (subscribers outside of the U.S. & Canada)

Fax number: 314-447-8029

Elsevier Health Sciences Division
Subscription Customer Service
3251 Riverport Lane
Maryland Heights, MO 63043

*To ensure uninterrupted delivery of your subscription, please notify us at least 4 weeks in advance of move.

Printed and bound by CPI Group (UK) Ltd, Croydon, CR0 4YY

03/10/2024

01040473-0005